EDITED BY ROBERT ADAMS
LENA DOMINELLI AND
MALCOLM PAYNE

CRITICAL PRACTICE IN SOCIAL WORK

SECOND EDITION

First edition 2002
Reprinted six times
Second edition 2009

Published by
PALGRAVE MACMILLAN

Palgrave Macmillan in the UK is an imprint of Macmillan Publishers Limited,
registered in England, company number 785998, of Houndmills, Basingstoke,
Hampshire RG21 6XS.

Palgrave Macmillan in the US is a division of St Martin's Press LLC,
175 Fifth Avenue, New York, NY 10010.

Palgrave Macmillan is the global academic imprint of the above companies
and has companies and representatives throughout the world.

Palgrave® and Macmillan® are registered trademarks in the United States,
the United Kingdom, Europe and other countries.

ISBN-13: 978–0–230–21863–5
ISBN-10: 0–230–21863–6

This book is printed on paper suitable for recycling and made from fully
managed and sustained forest sources. Logging, pulping and manufacturing
processes are expected to conform to the environmental regulations of the
country of origin.

A catalogue record for this book is available from the British Library.

A catalog record for this book is available from the Library of Congress.

10 9 8 7 6 5 4 3 2 1
18 17 16 15 14 13 12 11 10 09

Printed in China

CRITICAL PRACTICE
IN SOCIAL WORK

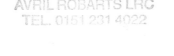

Co-edited titles by Robert Adams, Lena Dominelli and Malcolm Payne:
Social Work: Themes, Issues and Critical Debates, 3rd edn
Practising Social Work in a Complex World, 2nd edn
Reshaping Social Work Series (series editors)

Other titles by Robert Adams
Protests by Pupils; Empowerment, Schooling and the State
Prison Riots in Britain and the USA, 2nd edn*
Skilled Work with People
The Personal Social Services: Clients, Consumers or Citizens?
*Quality Social Work**
*The Abuses of Punishment**
*Social Policy for Social Work**
*Foundations of Health and Social Care**
Empowerment, Participation and Social Work, 4th edn*

Other titles by Lena Dominelli
Beyond Racial Divides: Ethnicities in Social Work (co-author)
*Feminist Social Work Theory and Practice**
Social Work: Theory and Practice for a Changing Profession
Women and Community Action
Revitalising Communities in a Globalising World
*Anti-Racist Social Work**
Introducing Social Work
*Anti-Oppressive Social Work Theory and Practice**
Revitalising Communities in a Globalising World

Other titles by Malcolm Payne
*Social Care Practice in Context**
Globalization and International Social Work: Postmodern Change and Challenge (co-author)
What is Professional Social Work?, 2nd edn
Modern Social Work Theory, 3rd edn*
*The Origins of Social Work: Continuity and Change**
Anti-bureaucratic Social Work
*Teamwork in Multiprofessional Care**
*Social Work and Community Care**
Linkages: Effective Networking in Social Care

* Also published by Palgrave Macmillan

Contents

List of figures and tables

Notes on the contributors

Robert Adams worked in the penal system for several years before running a community-based social work project for Barnardo's. He has been an external examiner on qualifying social work programmes in the UK since the mid-1980s. He has written on and researched extensively in youth and criminal justice, social work, the personal social services, protest and empowerment. He has edited more than 80 books and written more than a dozen books. He was Professor of Human Services Development at the University of Lincoln and has been Professor of Social Work at the University of Teesside for more than a decade.

Di Bailey is a Reader in Social Work at the University of Durham with 15 years' experience in interprofessional education and training. Di has a background in psychology and social work and she has worked in a variety of settings spanning the statutory and independent sector and forensic services. Her research interests include developing interdisciplinary mental health services and the involvement of service users in mental healthcare delivery.

Sarah Banks is Professor in the School of Applied Social Sciences, Durham University, and is co-editor of the journal, *Ethics and Social Welfare.* She has researched and published extensively in the field of professional ethics, particularly in relation to social, community and youth work.

Christian Beech is currently seconded from a local authority to the post of Senior Research Assistant at Swansea University. His practice experience as a qualified social worker prior to moving into policy and strategic management specialising in work with older people includes community and acute practice settings. His current research interests include critical gerontological social work with older people, partnership and interdisciplinary working, and preventive services.

Linda Briskman holds the Dr Haruhisa Handa Chair of Human Rights Education at Curtin University in Perth, Australia. She has practised, written and researched in the areas of professional ethics, Indigenous child welfare and the social work response to asylum seekers. Her most recent books are *Social Work with Indigenous Communities* and *International Perspectives on Interdiction and Deterrence of Asylum Seekers* (co-edited with A. Babacan). She convenes the People's Inquiry into Detention for the Australian Council of Heads of Schools of Social Work.

Hilary Brown is Professor of Social Care at Canterbury Christ Church University, having previously held senior posts at the Tizard Centre, University of Kent and at the School of Health and Social Welfare at the Open University. She specialises in the abuse of vulnerable adults and has conducted major research projects on the sexual abuse of people with intellectual disabilities, financial abuse of all vulnerable clients, breaches of professional boundaries and the implementation of policies to prevent and address the abuse of all vulnerable adults. She has carried out consultancy for a range of national and international bodies, including the Department of Health and the Welsh Assembly, the National Disability Authority of Ireland and the Council of Europe. She currently chairs the serious case review panel for Kent social services, conducts inquiries for other authorities, and contributes to a range of training programmes. She has taught a master class in Valencia on abuse against disabled women. She is also a qualified psychotherapist, seeing patients in the NHS and private practice, many of whom bear the scars of abuse in childhood or as adults.

Beverley Burke is Senior Lecturer at Liverpool John Moores University, UK. She has practised as a social worker in the field of childcare and has published in the areas of anti-oppressive practice, values and ethics. Beverley is co-editor of the practice section of the international peer-reviewed academic journal *Ethics and Social Welfare.*

Corinne May Chahal is Professor of Applied Social Science at Lancaster University. After 10 years as a practising social worker in local authority and voluntary agency field and residential settings, she undertook research for policy development in childcare and protection. Corinne has coordinated or partnered in several European projects that compared child welfare practices and outcomes across countries, including the Concerted Action on the Prevention of Child Abuse in Europe (CAPCAE) and the Co-ordination Action on Human Rights Violation (CAHRV). She has published widely in the childcare field and been involved in policy implementation through membership of the Home Office pilot code of practice steering group and the Family Justice Council.

Katy Cigno was, until recently, both a senior lecturer and social work practice placement organiser/supervisor, thus keeping a foot in practice and academia. She served as external examiner for the University of Reading and Queen's University Belfast, as well as regular guest lecturer for several universities in the UK and Italy. Her research is mainly in the areas of child disability and cognitive-behavioural approaches in social work.

Chris Clark is Professor of Social Work Ethics, University of Edinburgh. His research and teaching interests include professional ethics, character and decision-making.

Helen Cosis Brown is a Principal Lecturer in Social Work at Middlesex University. She also acts as an independent foster carer reviewing officer, chairs an adoption panel as well as a fostering panel. She worked as a social worker and a social work manager in inner London before moving into social work education. Her publications have included social work with lesbians and gay men as well as fostering and adoption.

Caroline Currer was, until 2007, Reader in Social Work at Anglia Ruskin University. There she led a module on loss and social work within social work programmes, for which she was also programme leader. Her background is as a psychiatric social worker in Pakistan, a sociologist with research into concepts of health and illness and a supervisor with CRUSE Bereavement Care. More recently, she has explored issues of professional suitability. She now works as an Anglican priest and on projects in the Solomon Islands as well as with Croydon council.

John Devaney is a Lecturer in Social Work at Queen's University Belfast, where he delivers teaching at undergraduate and postgraduate levels, and is involved in research in the areas of child protection, violence against the person and the impact of multiple adverse childhood experiences on later adult social exclusion. Prior to joining Queen's University in 2006, he was a Principal Social Worker and Policy Adviser to the Eastern Area Child Protection Committee in

Northern Ireland. He has advised central government on the development of strategies in relation to domestic violence and sexual violence.

Mark Doel is Research Professor of Social Work in the Centre for Health and Social Care Research at Sheffield Hallam University. He trained as a task-centred practitioner in 1981 and has used the task-centred method extensively in his practice, teaching, writing and research. He was a practitioner for almost 20 years and developed task-centred programmes with his colleague, Peter Marsh, in numerous social work agencies, including an assessed post-qualifying module with Wakefield social care department (with Catherine Sawdon). His other major publications are in practice learning and teaching, groupwork and service user narratives.

Lena Dominelli is Professor of Applied Social Sciences and Head of Social and Community and Youth Work at the University of Durham. She is an academician in the Academy of the Learned Societies for Social Sciences. From 1996 to 2004, she served as President of the International Association of Schools of Social Work. She is widely published, with a number of important sole-authored books to her name, particularly in the areas of feminism, anti-racism, globalisation and social policy.

Kevin Haines joined Swansea University in 1993 from the Institute of Criminology, University of Cambridge, where he completed an M.Phil and PhD in criminology and worked as a Research Associate. At Swansea, Kevin is Director of the Research Centre for Criminal Justice and Criminology, he is also President of the *Reseau International de Criminologie Juvenile*. Kevin has published widely on topics related to youth justice and is best known for his contribution to putting the concept 'children first' in youth justice. Current research interests include youth justice, youth crime prevention, restorative justice and risk and protective factors for juvenile offending.

Philomena Harrison is Senior Lecturer and Director of Mental Health for the Faculty of Health and Social Care at the University of Salford. Trained as a psychiatric social worker, her main practice experience has been with women, children and families. She was also involved in training social workers for 12 years at Liverpool John Moores University. Besides designing and delivering training on anti-racist and anti-oppressive practice to a range of health and social care practitioners, she has undertaken therapeutic work with children and young people on issues of 'race' and identity. She has presented work on issues of 'race' and cultural competence at national and international events.

Margaret Holloway (formerly Lloyd) is Professor of Social Work at the University of Hull. She was previously Senior Lecturer in Community Care at the University of Sheffield. Her practice experience spanned a wide range of settings including criminal justice, but as an academic, she has specialised in adult services. She undertakes research into death, dying and bereavement, with a particular interest in spirituality, and service delivery at the health and social care interface for older people and people with Parkinson's disease.

David Howe is Professor of Social Work at the University of East Anglia, Norwich. He was founding Editor of the journal, *Child and Family Social Work* (1996–2001) and is author of many books, including *Attachment Theory for Social Work Practice, Attachment Theory, Child Maltreatment and Family Support, Child Abuse and Neglect: Attachment, Development and Intervention* and *The Emotionally Intelligent Social Worker*.

Marjorie Mayo is Professor in Community Development at Goldsmiths, University of London. She has worked in the community sector and in local government as well as in higher education. Her research interests focus on strategies for participation, active citizenship and empowerment, at the local level in relation to regeneration and beyond, internationally. Her publications include *Communities and Caring: The Mixed Economy of Welfare, Imagining Tomorrow: Adult Education for Transformation, Cultures, Communities, Identities: Cultural Strategies for Participation and Empowerment* and *Global Citizens.*

Kate Morris is Head of Social Work at the University of Birmingham. She is a qualified social worker and has a longstanding interest in family involvement in professional practice. She has researched and written in the areas of family decision-making, prevention and multi-agency working. She is currently part of an international team reviewing evidence of the impact of family engagement in professional practices, and continues to evaluate and support local family-based services.

Joan Orme is Professor of Social Work at the University of Glasgow. Throughout her social work career, she has explored the impact of feminism on theory, research and practice and has written extensively in this area, including *Gender and Community Care: Social Work and Social Care Perspectives.*

Nigel Parton is NSPCC Professor of Applied Childhood Studies in the Centre of Applied Childhood Studies at the University of Huddersfield. Over the past 30 years, he has written numerous books and articles about child protection and child welfare and social work and social theory. His most recent book is *Safeguarding Childhood: Early Intervention and Surveillance in a Late Modern Society.*

Malcolm Payne is Policy and Development Adviser at St Christopher's Hospice, London, having been Director of Psychosocial and Spiritual Care there for more than five years. He is Honorary Professor, Kingston University/St George's University of London and was formerly Head of Department and Professor of Applied Community Studies at Manchester Metropolitan University. Recent publications include papers and research on aspects of palliative care, including *Creative Arts in Palliative Care* (edited with N. Hartley). He is author of *What is Professional Social Work?, Social Work Practice in Context* and *Modern Social Work Theory* (3rd edn).

Bob Pease is Chair of Social Work at Deakin University in Melbourne, Australia. His main research interests are in the fields of critical masculinity studies and critical social work practice. In the former area, his specific research focus is on men's violence against women and global perspectives on men and masculinities. In the latter area, he is interested in the application of critical theories to progressive social work practice and pro-feminist approaches to working with men in the human services. His most recent books are *International Encyclopedia of Men and Masculinities* (co-edited), *Critical Social Work Practice* (co-edited) and *Men and Gender Relations.* He is currently co-editing a book titled *Migrant Men: Critical Studies of Masculinities and the Migration Experience* and writing a book titled *Undoing Privilege: Facing the Predicament of Unearned Advantages.*

John Pinkerton is Professor of Child and Family Social Work at Queen's University Belfast. He is involved with both qualifying and post-qualification social work education. His main areas of research and publication are young people leaving care, family support and the relationship of research to practice and policy.

Mo Ray qualified as a social worker in 1990 and for many years worked with older people. She has also worked for a number of years as an independent practice teacher and tutored on a variety of social work programmes. Mo completed her PhD at Keele University. At present, Mo is a full-time Lecturer in Social Work and Director of the MA in Social Work award. Mo's research interests focus on the management of change in older age and developing gerontological social work practice. Her writing has focused on social work practice with older people.

Lena Robinson is Professor of Social Work at the University of the West of Scotland. She has published and researched widely in the field of race, culture, ethnicity and social work. Her publications include *Cross Cultural Child Development for Social Workers* and *Psychology for Social Workers: Black Perspectives* (2nd edn).

Alastair Roy is a Senior Lecturer at the International School for Communities, Rights and Inclusion, University of Central Lancashire. He has a professional background in youth and community work and spent eight years as a practitioner and manager in residential childcare. He has extensive experience as a researcher and consultant in the fields of substance misuse and juvenile justice, including commissioned work for the Home Office, the prison service and a consultancy project with UNICEF exploring international indicators for children in conflict with the law.

Bob Sapey is a Senior Lecturer in Applied Social Science at Lancaster University. His publications include *Social Work with Disabled People* (with M. Oliver, 3rd edn). Prior to his academic career, Bob was a social worker and training officer, specialising in work with disabled and older people.

Tim Stainton is Professor of Social Work at the University of British Columbia. He is author of numerous works on service and supports for people with intellectual disabilities, disability rights, individualised funding, history, ethics and theory. He is a past board member of the Canadian and the British Columbia Association for Community Living. He lives in Delta, British Columbia and has four children, one of whom lives with an intellectual disability.

Dave Ward is Professor of Social and Community Studies at De Montfort University, Leicester. The Centre for Social Action at De Montfort University promotes and undertakes practice, training and research within the principles of the anti-oppressive groupwork advocated in his chapter.

Frances Young is a Senior Lecturer at the University of Central Lancashire. She is a qualified social worker with a professional background in childcare specialising in fostering and adoption. She teaches on initial and post-qualifying social work courses focusing on childcare issues. She has undertaken a number of research projects exploring issues related to looking after children and young people. She undertook a consultancy project with UNICEF exploring international indicators for children in formal care.

Introduction

What is this book about?

This book provides material for the middle of the professional qualifying degree programme for social workers. Its theme throughout is your development as a critical practitioner, as you develop your understanding of what is involved in practising social work critically. In order to do this, you will need to study three major aspects: social work values for practice; theories and approaches to practice; and how you actually do critical practice. This is how you need to build on your understanding of the themes, issues and debates in contemporary social work, which we examined in Book 1 (Adams et al., 2009a). These three aspects of the task of developing the capacity to practise social work critically are tackled successively in the three parts of this book, through:

- looking at how values affect your personal and professional development (Part 1)
- surveying the main theoretical perspectives on, and approaches to, practice (Part 2)
- studying in more detail particular areas of social work, from the viewpoint of how you can develop your critical practice (Part 3).

How does this book fit into our trilogy of social work books?

The first book in the trilogy, *Social Work: Themes, Issues and Critical Debates* (Adams et al., 2009a), introduces the distinctive character of social work in its different settings. It tackles social work values, locates social work in its different contexts, and begins to explore some of the lasting debates that arise about practice in different practice settings. The book you are now beginning – *Critical Practice in Social Work* – is the second in the trilogy. The third book in the trilogy, *Practising Social Work in a Complex World* (Adams et al., 2009c), argues that a good understanding of the themes, issues and debates in contemporary social work and the capacity to practise social work critically need to be integrated with more complex professional skills. These include dealing with complex situations to enable practitioners to develop confidently a partnership with service users, their families, carers and communities, with other agencies and with colleagues in other professions. They also include management and leadership skills and research-based practice skills. Partnership working is essential to achieving the fundamental objective of social work: to increase the resilience of individuals, groups and communities in dealing with problems in their lives through solidarity and equality in society.

Readers of previous editions of the three books in this series will find that the topics covered in each volume have changed to reflect feedback and our own judgement about the order in which particular topics should be introduced when readers use the books in sequence.

On being critical in social work

1

In this chapter we introduce the themes that will recur through-out the book – criticality and critical practice. Our purpose is to provide the foundations of knowledge and understanding that will enable you to develop your critical thinking. We use the word 'client' throughout, rather than 'service user', because we use it as part of our argument about being critical.

Chapter overview

Embodying critical practice in social work

We began the first book in this trilogy (*Social Work: Themes, Issues and Critical Debates*, Adams et al., 2009a, referred to hereafter as *Social Work*) by providing the intellectual tools to enable you to think critically about social work. In this second book, we move on to enabling you to understand what critical practice entails, know what it feels like, and develop and practise it with skill and confidence.

In this book we provide what you need in order to embody critical practice in yourself. When a social worker sees someone in an interview room, visits a home or goes to a multiprofessional meeting, they embody 'social work' within themselves as a person. They represent (that is, present to other people) their own personality and person, which they will use in interpersonal interactions with clients, carers, families, communities and colleagues. They also embody professional social work and the social work agency they represent (that is, act on behalf of), and they bring with them the knowledge, skills and values of social work as part of the person they are. Many of these other people have only the experience of this person, here present, to understand and judge social work by. By being present, practitioners demonstrate commitment, preparedness to engage, thoughtfulness, concern, love, caring and many other things. As they experience this person, people experience social work; often it is their only experience, certainly it is their current experience. Do they think 'neat' or 'busybody' or 'another suit' or 'one of us'? It is the embodiment of social work in front of them that they judge. Does a doctor or teacher understand what social work is? It is the knowledge, skill, experience, response that they see used in responding to their concerns about a patient or student that expands their understanding of the possibilities that social work offers them.

Embodiment brings together these components of understanding, knowledge and skill in practice. They are inseparable; they cannot be separated from each other or the person and personality that represents them. Intellectually, we can separate different areas of knowledge (Pawson et al., 2003), we can identify different ways of thinking about values (Banks, 2006) and a variety of social work skills (Trevithick, 2005). However, when we meet a client or attend a multiprofessional case conference, we embody all these things together, use them simultaneously. Therefore, we have to secure them within ourselves, practising and developing constantly to do so. We do this through critical reflection and practice.

In the chapters in this book, you will have the opportunity to find yourself as a critical practitioner. We provide material that encourages you to incorporate into your practice that constellation of aspects examined in *Social Work*. You can use them as you interact with individuals in settings, organisations and communities. Thus, we go beyond *Social Work*, intellectually and in terms of understanding.

What does embodiment entail?

Let us examine the notion of 'embodiment' further. It involves your taking on the role of social worker in practice, in a particularly exciting and yet somewhat demanding way. In doing so, you become part of the 'social' in social work described in Chapter 1 of *Social Work*. We spell out now what this means in practice. It means that as a social worker, you are governed, first of all, by a code of practice. This is demanding and it does contain an ethical dimension. However, it does not require you to be a 'saint' or even a 'good person'. It does require you to be a 'good social worker' and this means a 'critical' practitioner, which is what this book is about. In order to be critical, you will have to maintain and represent to others your judgement as an independent professional. You won't always be liked by the people with whom you work. Sometimes you will need to assert your view. Colleagues may not like this either. You will need to be both understanding and yet detached and the word 'criticality' covers both these elements. Becoming part of the social and the critical in social work entails your being partly acceptable – because you embody society's values and ideals – and partly unacceptable – when you take a critical stance or act as an agent of change – in work with individuals, groups, families, communities, with colleagues in your organisation, or in work with other professionals in other organisations. There are many aspects to this. You could say it comes down to making sure social work – including social care – provides a worthwhile, high-quality service. This brings in the aspects of connectedness, receptiveness and development discussed in *Social Work* (Chapter 1) as being crucial ingredients of caring.

Sometimes, critical practice will entail taking risks. We examine risk-taking in this book. We develop the notion of calculated risks that we take in everyday life.

What do we mean by critical practice and criticality?

In this chapter we shall explore what we mean by these terms 'critical practice' and 'criticality'. Here, to begin with, are some general statements.

Critical practice means something general that we apply to all good social work practice in this book. However, we don't want to devalue the word 'critical' by saying it simply applies everywhere. It starts from being critical as a thinker as well as a practitioner. We do this by applying our judgement to situations and actions. We say whether we view them as right or wrong, a help or a hindrance. We exercise our judgement about whether people are being oppressed. We reach a view about whether the diversity in a situation is appreciated and whether the subordinate viewpoint should be upheld. Often, social work is about upholding the view of the vulnerable person, the person who is seldom heard. We encourage the development and use of critical services, based on critical – this may mean uncomfortable – understandings of the world in which we work and live.

Criticality is a stance that is prepared to consider more than one approach to a person's problems; reflecting critically entails reviewing different perspectives and options before deciding on 'best practice'. Sometimes being critical is tantamount to 'heresy'. This may entail our countenancing the view that is unorthodox, unacceptable to those around us, perhaps on behalf of a minority or excluded individual or group. We may have to advocate 'heterodoxy', that is, controversial opinions, ideas and doctrines that don't agree with the official position (orthodoxy), accepted beliefs and standards.

So, as a 'critical practitioner', we are likely to be engaged in the midst of struggle. We may be constantly struggling with our own ideas and those of others about whom we read, or whose worlds we encounter in our practice. This may continue through our work and throughout our life. We may find this a positive, although challenging, experience. It will be about reflection and rethinking, which, in the process, we turn into what is personal and everyday to us. We will be responding to each challenge to accepted orthodoxy, perhaps, by shifting our own views slightly. In a changing world, nobody's views are likely to stay the same for long. We are not talking about our values here, although we may express these differently at different times as well. We are talking about the constancy of change in our work and in the world. We shift our ideas as we come into contact with other ideas.

'Critical reflection' is part of being critical. Reflection isn't a routine action. No matter how much we reflect, it probably never becomes routine. It involves change. Considering, reconsidering and changing your mind is likely always to be a painful experience. Learning and change go hand in hand. In your social work studies, you will encounter practice teachers, tutors and people who use services. Whenever they feed back views to you, these may be painful. That is the 'downside'. There is an 'upside' to this, namely those moments of enlightenment, or moving forward – the eureka moments, perhaps, when you experience what Mezirow (1983) calls 'perspective transformation'.

Critical practice is still relevant in social work

Increasingly, social workers and other professionals are asked to follow guidelines and meet national standards. Their agencies are organised to 'deliver' through 'joined-up government'. Of course, every user of social care services wants to be dealt with consistently and gain the benefits from policy and service objectives. If they are being supervised or checked up on through social work's social policing role, they want to be treated with justice and compassion. However, meeting guidelines, standards and objectives is not simple, because nearly all of them refer to the aims we have to meet. Usually, we have to use our judgement to decide the best way of doing our job.

Furthermore, social work has greater ambitions, because it seeks growth and empowerment as human beings for the people we serve, development and social progress for the communities we work in and greater justice and equality in the societies to which we contribute. It is not that every act of social work will achieve such large goals, but these values help to guide us in using our judgement about what is best. Critical practice helps to implement these values by testing our practice against them.

Critical practice in social perspective

How can we 'be critical'? And how do we do that 'in practice'? Glaister (2008: 8) uses the term 'critical' to refer to 'open-minded, reflective approaches that take account of different perspectives, experiences and assumptions'. She sees it partly as a way of managing uncertainty. Thus, critical practice speaks to a contemporary anxiety, because, as Beck (1992) argues, the recent globalisation of economic systems brings previously separated views of the world into contact and potential conflict, raising ambiguity and controversy about what once seemed rational and ordered. Our world seems more unsafe and uncertain than it once did, and we seek mechanisms to help us to control potential risks to our equilibrium. Critical practice gives us a way of organising our thinking and action to respond to uncertainty and risk.

Critical thinking leads to critical action; the two together form critical practice. Inevitably, because critical thinking will use the experience of action and its outcomes to inform further thinking, critical practice is a cycle in which thinking is bound up with action. We see this as part of a reflexive cycle. 'Reflexivity' means being in a circular process in which social workers 'put themselves in the picture' by thinking and acting with the people they are serving, so that their understandings and actions inevitably are changed by their experiences with others. As part of the same process, they influence and change others and their social worlds.

Thinking critically: working with families

To make a start on how we might think critically in a practice setting, we consider here some ideas about working with families. So many people think that living in families is good that it is a conventional assumption in many societies. Arguments are brought up that it provides for mutual support between a couple, and allows for bringing up children while they are dependent on others. Our approach to critical thinking looks first at the language used, because this helps to test our undisclosed assumptions. The word 'good', above, immediately alerts us to the fact that this sentence makes an evaluation. It considers the value that might be attributed to families. Less obvious value words, such as 'interesting' or 'worthwhile', have a practical feel to them, causing us to miss their value-laden content. Alternatively, the tone may be positive or negative, without any specific value words being present at all. Critical practitioners remain alert to the use of language. This extends beyond values. For example, 'couple' and 'children' reveal hidden assumptions about families, potentially excluding single-parent and childless families. In the next paragraph, we indicate in square brackets some, but only some, of the language issues that you might consider critically, to remind you that this is a constant issue.

The next stage [one thing after another, rather than all entwined] of critical thinking is to explore [rather than, say, analyse] agenda-setting. In a book, the process of agenda-setting is not interactive, but in the control of one party. In this case, the people in control are us, the authors, but in social work, it is often the agency and its managers or practitioners themselves who are in control of agendas, rather than clients [tone shift from referring to 'users']. You might surmise, here, that we picked 'families' from a number of possibilities because it will allow us to make our points easily, in a topic that is universal to most human audiences. The critical reader will be thinking: 'Are there topics where it is not so easy? Do the authors' arguments work then? Is it really true that families are universal, or are there different forms?' In social work, you can imagine clients thinking similar things about why your agency is interested in them and what your aims are. Clients may accept or resist [term with historical, intellectual connections to psychoanalysis or with a different meaning to Marxism] the agendas that officials or professionals impose upon them. Whichever it is, the critical social worker will be alert to who is setting the agenda. Mostly, it is more effective [hidden value word] to make agenda-setting interactive and include [hidden value words] clients in the process [tone-setting word implying continuing participation].

Critical practice also includes considering the content of the judgements we make. Here, the content of the judgement is that living in families is good. Obviously, critical points are possible. Thinking reflexively here, we can put ourselves in notional families to interact with the idea. This allows us to see that there are families, and many of them, where there are poor relationships, leading to divorce, for example. Most murders and much violence also take place within family relationships (see Adams et al., 2009c, Ch. 3). So, in social work dealing with families, the critical social worker would want to be careful about making the assumption that the client's family is of a particular kind, which is more or less acceptable. Clients' experiences of their families may be anything but 'good'. Thinking reflexively could also mean that, rather than notional families, we put ourselves in this particular family and imagine what it might feel like to them. Social work often involves using reflexive thinking to generate empathy with the client's experience in this way. As we work critically, we often find that our professional discourse questions the assumption behind family legislation that maintaining families is a positive policy objective. We may need to question politicians' or managers' assumptions about restoring or maintaining family relationships, in general, or in a particular case. Our own experience of good or bad family life may condition how we respond to what our agency or our clients ask of us. If we are not aware of this, thinking it through and thinking reflexively how our reaction will affect the family we are working with, we are not giving clients the opportunity to participate on equal terms with us.

Critical practice also involves questioning ideology. Thinking does not emerge anew every time we come across a situation. An ideology is a system of thought, often derived from political or moral theories or principles. Ideologies are extensive or even comprehensive in the areas of personal or social action that they cover, so they offer guidance in a wide range of situations. They are logical constructions, built on evidence about the world, but they usually contain an element of belief or faith. Examples of ideologies are Marxism or feminism; religions are also ideologies. The advantage of using ideologies is that their extensive coverage means that we can take a consistent approach to a number of situations. The disadvantage is that, used everyday, an ideology seems so systematic that we forget the elements of belief and value that are integral to its system.

Oversimplifying, we could say that Marxists would see families in capitalist societies as being constituted as they are to meet the needs of the economic system – to reproduce conveniently a compliant workforce. The personal needs of the individuals involved are subordinated to these covert objectives built into society, and that is why there are conflicts and violence in families. As times change, we might identify Marxist interpretations of new situations: for example, how do we see families in newly industrialising societies such as China or India? What is the evidence of changes in the family in previous generations of industrialising societies such as Japan? What do those comparisons say about the UK, which industrialised more than two centuries ago? Feminists might say that social responses to gender differences are more important, and that society assumes patriarchy, control by men, citing the fact that most violence in families is by men against women to lend support to this view. Looking critically at another assumption underlying Marxism, it takes a 'conflict' view of society, seeing different groups in society as having opposed interests. Marxism is also 'materialist', because it proposes that economic interests, that is, material conditions, have an important impact on people's lives. An alternative 'spiritual' ideology, common in religions, emphasises shared humanity, and many people in Eastern societies would say that this is still important in understanding families there. What might the implications be if such families moved to Western societies?

Picking up on our assumptions, rather than taking them for granted, discloses that our original statement about families represents another contradictory ideology, a 'functionalist' view of society. Oversimplifying again, functionalists say that social institutions such as families perform a function in human relationships. The function knits societies together in a social 'order' or structure. Our arguments for saying that living in families is good reveal hidden functionalist assumptions. We are assuming that an ordered society is valuable, rather than, say, creative chaos, and that family life contributes to that order, rather than, say, making society inflexible and hidebound.

Although we have simplified and selected from these ideologies, trying to unpick all their implications seems complicated. Therefore, we want to re-emphasise the point that everything we act on includes assumptions that come from these complex ideological systems of thought. This is a helpful way of coping with complexity but, because many of the assumptions that underlie ideologies are taken for granted, we may not be open enough to rethinking them. Working with a client, the critical social worker would put themselves reflexively in the client's family, asking what views of the value of family life exist in this particular family, and how these views conflict or connect with wider conceptions of family life.

All this seems complicated, so we must justify working in this way. So far, we have emphasised the value of openness and how this contributes to maintaining equality, inclusion and participation between workers and clients.

Practising critically

Social work is about action, so critical thinking must lead to critical action. Practising within social work requires three aspects: thinking to inform the practice; the actions we take; and the actions and their consequences that inform continuing critical thinking. There are four aspects of critical practice that take us beyond merely thinking critically:

- Examining the evidence in detail, from different perspectives through reflexive involvement, so that we avoid risk and open up opportunities.
- Contextualising the examination of evidence by placing it explicitly within the context of theoretical and value positions and within the range of other phenomena that might have an impact on the judgements being made. Contextualising is a twin process with reflexiveness: both are about allowing ideas and actions to interact together.
- Developing an overview, so that we and others involved see the full implications of the situation.
- Presenting our judgements to an audience, such as a case conference, clients or their families, or people in the community in ways that may assist, guide or influence their own understanding and evaluation.

The idea of practice contains two partly hidden assumptions:

- The idea of 'a' practice implies that what we are doing is in some way an accepted, acknowledged method of doing something, with the authority of convention or evidence of appropriateness or the likelihood of a successful outcome to support it. We says things such as: 'It is our practice to do it this way.'
- The idea of 'practice' conveys that what we do is not, and never will be, final. We are trying it out, on the basis of its authority as an acknowledged form of action, but it is provisional. If we compare it with a musician practising, or an actor rehearsing, we are practising our activity in the way that we intend, not hope, which does not carry

the implication of a planned effort to achieve the outcome we want, but intend that it will improve the situation and improve our ways of acting in such situations.

For an actor or musical performer, practice has two elements: it intends to act on the present, but also it intends to improve similar actions for the future. Every time performers practise or rehearse, they intend to get better for the next time they practise. Eventually, performing in public, they build on the practice to present the best performance possible for them. No final complete achievement of results, therefore, exists. We sometimes sit through a wonderful performance of a piece of music or we are inspired by a striking production of a play. It may seem that nothing could be more perfect. Yet, another recording, another production next year will be a further revelation of what the work contains. This will be the result of practising in two ways. First, more people trying to make things better again and again will produce improvements in technique. Second, practice will build upon past practice but will present it in a new context.

Social work is like that. Workers have general knowledge and skills that they can apply to particular situations. That is why social work theories and training are generic. We can learn what to do in general, and then adapt the ideas and practices to dealing with, say, children's special needs or practising in groups rather than with individuals. We do this by being reflexive.

EXAMPLE

For example, when we start working with a looked-after child (Chapter 24), we apply theory about anti-oppressive practice and realise that children will often have experience of being oppressed by adults, who may forget to allow children to think things out for themselves and express their own wishes and feelings. The phrase 'wishes and feelings' is drawn from the Children Act 1989, which requires us to take young people's views into account when making decisions. In this way, we take our professional theory and legal knowledge, reflexively, into the situation with the child and use it to help us to put ourselves in the child's place, rather than being like a 'typical adult'. We are thinking critically about that way of being. By doing this, we hope that the child will react positively to our approach, and we will be able to gain a better understanding of what they are thinking and planning. This can then influence how we are going to act as a social worker and make what we do more effective, or at least more responsive to the child's wishes. These perceptions build up, so that after a while, this child comes to see us not as a 'typical adult' but a more helpful and responsive person than the general run of adults. We gain experience of how this works for us in our 'practice', which is a good basis for more 'practice' with other children in the future.

Social work is an improvisation, like jazz, built up during the moments of performance, in the style of the performer, around a theme. Jazz musicians rely on experience and develop a style of responding to the stimulus of a musical theme. They also train their skills, so that they can play in many different ways and respond to many different kinds of themes and varying contexts. All this is exactly what social workers do. One of the frightening things about being a social worker is that we cannot know what situation we will face when we knock on a front door or invite someone into the interview room. However, social workers have developed their knowledge and skills to that they can respond in the best possible way. If they are going to do social work of the best quality, they, like musicians, will take every opportunity to practise. It is not hard to find opportunities, they come with the job. Each time we do something, we have the opportunity to learn from it. Most people are accustomed to keeping information about people to contact, or about services to call on, and many teams carry out projects to build up and share information.

It is possible to do the same with skills. A skill is a capacity that has been developed and trained so that it is more clearly defined, can be used more flexibly and, in social work, can be applied to influence social situations. More widely, skills are practical, they are about how to do things in the best way. Hidden in that sentence, though, is a value statement: an assumption that we know what is best. Also hidden there is the point that using skills implies using knowledge because knowing how to do something does not tell us what to do. These points lead us to the next section, in which we discuss using theory in being critical.

Using theories in being critical

In this chapter, we have emphasised the importance of action. We said that social work is always 'action' and that being critical both is and contributes to action. Recognising this emphasis is important, because conventionally people distinguish thinking and acting, in sayings like 'look before you leap' or 'engage your brain before setting off'. Thinking and acting are bound together in social work, through the reflexive cycle. Being critical in social work means being aware of this cycle and alert to how our thinking and others' ideas affect it.

However, this approach to being critical places great emphasis on reason. That is, we are assuming that the world is an organised or ordered place. If this is so, reasoning skills allow us to think out how to act and have an impact on the world, alongside other human beings such as our clients and colleagues in our team, in the reflexive process of being critical that we have been discussing and modelling. The problem is that, as we noticed when discussing the example of views about families, this is an assumption. It is a commonplace assumption by which we organise our lives, but an assumption nevertheless.

Some social theories set out to challenge this assumption of reason and the ordered nature of the world in various ways. Because of this, they are often referred to as 'critical social theories'. There are three groups commonly referred to:

- Marxism, deriving from the work of Marx in the mid-nineteenth century
- the Frankfurt School of sociologists, such as Horkheimer (1978), Adorno (Adorno and Horkheimer, 1979) and Marcuse (1964), who were working from the 1920s and 30s
- Habermas (1984, 1987), their modern successor, writing in the late twentieth century.

When many writers discuss being critical, they mean using these theories.

Historically, much social thought depends on the assumption of a fixed social order, often based on important social beliefs, such as religion, and the authority of national leaders, such as the government. When this began to be rejected, rational thinking using the scientific method became important; this is called 'modernism'. This emphasises that understanding through gaining evidence about the world can make us more effective in dealing with the outside world. Through using such methods in physical science, human beings have achieved considerable control of natural forces. Some sociologists, such as Durkheim (1972) and Weber (Gerth and Mills, 1948), emphasise how understanding the social world enables us to operate more effectively in relation to one another. So, if we understand how social relationships work, we will be able to achieve our objectives in society. In this statement, however, there is an assumption that social relationships exist and can be clarified and understood so that we then can act upon them.

Much social work thinking is modernist in this way, and so also are many critical social theories. It assumes that we may understand what is going on in social relationships through practices such as 'assessment'. Having assessed a social situation, we can plan to do something about it through activities such as 'care management' and thus we may be able to change social relationships for the better (having made a value judgement about what is better), using interpersonal relationships between the social worker and the client.

Critical theories challenge this assumption of the existence of a social order that we may understand, and consequently they lead us to question practices that seem natural parts of it. Marx (1972) argues, for example, that we treat the current, capitalist system of economic theory as natural and given, whereas he sees capitalist societies as using a particular mode of economic organisation that has particular, and in many respects unfortunate, social consequences. Marxists would say that conventional social work practices support and extend the oppressive power of social institutions in capitalist states. For example, people with disabilities often argue that social workers' assessments of them assume a society in which they are impaired and less than human, rather than acknowledging that much of their disability stems from the way that society is organised for the able-bodied (see Chapter 30 for more discussion of this). The Frankfurt theorists argue that we treat our cultural and ideological heritage as given, whereas these elements of society are crucial elements in how we may be dominated by a capitalist, authoritarian state (for example Horkheimer, 1978). Thus, in social work, we sometimes assume, as we did earlier in this chapter, that cultural ideas such as family or community are fairly universal, whereas there are many different interpretations and uncertainties in them. Habermas (1984, 1987) distinguishes between the 'system' and the 'lifeworld', which interact and to some extent conflict with each other. By the system, he means the current mode of capitalist economic organisation, operating through such social structures as government, together with the rational mode of developing knowledge, which has had such benefits for technological and scientific progress. Recently, it also includes transnational companies that have emerged with globalisation, in which economic systems across the world are more closely interdependent, and cultures and political systems have changed to reflect this (Payne and Askeland, 2008). The lifeworld comprises such aspects of the world as education, family life and the media, which operate by a process called 'communicative reason', in which moral and social ideas are worked out in a widely shared social debate. The system and the lifeworld develop different ways of viewing and acting on the world through their different forms of reason. We might see social work as part of the lifeworld, interacting uneasily with the system of managerialism in agencies; this is among the themes of Part 3 of this book.

More recently, alternative forms of critical theory have been used as part of critical practice, particularly by Fook and her colleagues: feminism and postmodernism (Fook, 2002; Fook and Gardner, 2007). These are different from the critical social theories associated with Marxism and the Frankfurt School, because they focus on the way in which understanding of the world reflects personal experience and social and historical context. These ideas avoid focusing on social orders that change only slowly and try to explain how people behave. Instead they argue that personal experience constructs and is constructed by the societies in which we live. There are a wide variety of experiences in the world, and by listening to people's narratives carefully, we can realise that they have different experiences which see the world in different ways. The term 'narrative' has a special meaning here: it means an account of a life experience that explains the narrator's understanding of the world as part of the account. We often hear in political discourse, for example, that politicians need a 'narrative' about their policies; this means that their policy should be backed up by an explanation of how the problem arose in society that the policy is trying to solve, and the direction in which the policy is trying to move society. Narratives give direction and explanation to bald accounts of events. So feminists would say, listen to people's personal experience, have an equal dialogue with them, and you will begin to understand and be able to work with their personal views of the world. That personal view, like a politician's policy, will include their explanation about how the world came to be as they see it, and what they want to achieve in working with you. Postmodernists say there is a discourse about any social phenomenon: alternative ways of seeing it. These views compete for influence in society. For example, there are a number of ways of understanding teenage binge drinking. It might be a failure of parental socialisation of weak-willed individuals, or an example of commercial pressures to spend money in conventional entertainment, rather than encouraging participation in positive educational experiences in youth clubs, or a legitimate letting off steam in active young people. Different ways of understanding, or combinations of explanation, might lead to different ways of dealing with the problem in a town centre, and helping a young person who has become dependent on alcohol. These discourses go on all the time; by looking for alternative discourses, we can see alternative ways of acting when we are trying to help an individual or community respond to particular difficulties.

To use these theories for critical purposes in social work is beyond the scope of this book, and would require extensive study of these writers and their modern interpreters and successors. However, we take three points from their ideas.

First, they emphasise social change and the importance of developing collective action to achieve it. Much social thought assumes that there is an identifiable social structure, which we can analyse and describe. What these theories all emphasise is that society does not exist in an unchanging or slowly changing social order, but that it evolves, or may be subject to revolutions, or may be in constant flux that raises the possibility of helpful or unhelpful change. Therefore, we should be concerned with social change and what factors bring it about or act to slow it down. It is a short step from this to being concerned with how human actions can alter social structures. These theories, therefore, place importance on human agency, that is, how human beings may have an impact on the social world in which they live. Much conventional social thought assumes that general social forms have a significant impact on individuals; critical theories emphasise how human beings may act to change general social forms. This produces a very different sort of 'acting on' social relationships from the actions of assessment, care management and interpersonal change: it is a form of political agency (Batsleer and Humphries, 2000). That is, critical theory proposes that when we say social work is concerned with action, acting within interpersonal situations is always part of a wider action concerned with broader social forms. Such action is always political in the sense that interpersonal action always has an impact on the interaction of wider groups in society.

Second, critical theory focuses on intentionality. Earlier in this chapter, we stressed that thinking critically in social work leads us to act, not in a haphazard way, but with the intention of creating a planned change. Critical theories suggest that we need to scan the origins of our intent warily for exactly the same hidden value assumptions about how society is or ought to be organised. However, agency implies more than simply movement, but impulsion, towards some intention based on our values and ideologies. So, critical theories are concerned with how our everyday actions are part of continuing streams of either social change or stability. We are part of social movements that form around important ideas, such as environmentalism, feminism and social development. Some critical theorists regard it as crucial that action, intention and social movements are transformational and emancipatory in the way they work. The argument is that social movements transform the way people experience society and emancipate us from the limitations of present economic, cultural and ideological heritage.

Third, the implication for social work, and other intentional actions, of these theoretical ideas is that being critical does not only involve the use of reasoning or thinking in the technical way we have been discussing in the early part of this chapter. Being critical in practical thinking and practice takes place within social movements that are directed towards transforming societies and our intentions therefore need to be formed by our analysis of how societies are changing and might be changed towards greater freedoms for people. Thinking and acting critically therefore needs to be placed within analyses of how the limitations of social divisions such as class, gender and social assumptions about disability, sexuality and ethnic origin are created within social ideas that appear rational and that we take for granted, but are also changeable and changing. Some critical theorists argue that thinking critically in this way reveals important social movements and enables us to participate in them, pressing them forward.

The importance of language and understandings

Ideas and how they are represented in societies are, therefore, part of the process that creates our intentions. If we want to have an impact on individuals and societies, we must also be aware of ideas and their representation and how they affect the situation within which we are working. This element of critical theories reminds us of the importance of language and how we use it in expressing our understandings about the world. These came out in a pragmatic way as we were looking at thinking critically earlier. They relate to a range of ideas that are particularly in debate at the present time, arising from the work of social constructionist writers such as Shotter (1996) and Gergen (1999). What these writers propose is that our understanding of how societies, and relationships within them, operate is constructed and represented by the language that we use. We saw in the example of thinking about families that the words used revealed assumptions and ideas that we held about families. As with the critical theorists, the argument is that we express social relationships in how we behave and speak about the world. Because we come to share these social relationships through interacting with one another, we take part in a set of conventions about how the world is. Our participation means that we both mould and control and also are moulded and controlled by these ideas.

The implication of these writers for social work is that we can only become free of this control by taking apart these ideas through exploring rigorously the language and the social ideas it represents; this leads to the postmodernist idea of 'deconstruction'. By operating reflexively in social work processes, we can understand and construct or reconstruct the aspects of life that are causing people problems through developing shared social understandings and structures for action. In our professional role, by becoming reflexively part of a family with debt problems, we can see how destructive the fear of debt may be to relationships. In this way, our understanding and thinking becomes more empathic, reconstructed from a bureaucratic concern with the loss of the house. We can then help the family to explore the consequences of various possible actions. Should they run away? Should they reconstruct all their debts? Social work participation identifies options and priorities and in doing so identifies who might do what. Do we understand with the family that the credit company is oppressive in its policies? Do we confront the family with the perception that they have been unrealistic? Operating reflexively means that we have a better appreciation of what different responses may mean for the family, and what their meanings may imply for practical actions.

Practising critically in the way discussed in this chapter, therefore, moves towards greater freedom by making apparent our assumptions and representations about the world. A crucial element in this is how social work, its organisation, its language and the practices that it pursues are ideas that mould and control us and our clients as part of ideas that mould and control the social worlds in which we all move. We should not see this as a conspiracy of those in power or as an evil; this is how social worlds operate. Worlds in which people live collectively rather than as individuals inevitably generate collective understandings. It is a characteristic of social interaction that it creates these oppressions and limitations in our interactions with each other.

Conclusion

This chapter has explored some important general features of two important constituents of critical practice: critical thinking and critical action. Part 1 of this book, which concerns values, identifies an extension of critical practice beyond the interpersonal interaction between social workers and clients. Equality treats people equally, and also seeks greater social equality. Openness offers a critical dialogue between people, both clients and colleagues, and offers opportunities for creativity. Making a difference means not only pursuing betterment for clients in their world, but in the wider social worlds that we live in.

Understanding and exploring language, how it is used in interactions and how it forms our views of the world is an essential element in critical practice. Through a process of critical thinking, by interacting reflexively in relationships with others, we can examine agenda-setting, the content of judgements that we make and the ideologies that underlie them. Using these understandings, we can build a critical practice of examining evidence and perspectives in detail, contextualising information, developing an overview and then presenting our thinking effectively to our audiences. As we practise, we develop and refine skills. Part 2 builds on the value base of critical practice to identify how these processes may be applied in a multitude of practice situations. Part 3 extends this to critical management practice and the management contexts of practice.

The theoretical ideas of critical sociology, feminism and postmodernism emphasise that social work must go beyond a technical form of thinking and practice, following guidelines and standard practices to empower people, both colleagues and clients, with political agency to achieve collective and social objectives as well as personal growth. A reflexive focus on language and understanding incorporates within daily practice our wider social objectives, but grounds them in the lived experience of the people with whom we work. Critical theory and critical action thus become participation with intentionality in a critical practice within social work, extending the interpersonal towards the social. It is the value base, practice and management of these processes that the following chapters seek to capture, explore and extend.

For further discussion of critical approaches in social work, see Chapter 8, and for practising critically, see Chapter 21.

Adams, R. (2008) 'Critical social work: opportunites for change', Morag Faulds Memorial Lecture, University of the West of Scotland, 12 September, www. paisley.ac.uk/schoolsdepts/socialsciences/lecture.asp. Considers the importance of academic, management, practice and service user 'wisdoms' to a critical understanding of social work.

Payne, M. (2007) 'Performing as a "wise person" in social work practice', *Practice*, 19(2): 85–96. Explains, through detailed analysis of a case study, how different forms of social work knowledge are embodied in the practitioner, who brings them together constantly throughout a practice incident.

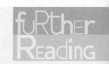

Part 1

VALUES INTO PRACTICE

Making social work values practical is so important that the first part of this book focuses on making value objectives central to practice. This book develops interpersonal practice towards enhancing collective relationships, empowerment and change; we see the aim of individual work with service users, their carers and families and with groups and communities as about achieving social solidarity and social resilience. Making a difference involves not only personal changes and gains for the better, but also seeing these as part of a movement towards empowering oppressed and disadvantaged groups in society. This means that the people we work with become stronger in dealing with their lives in the future and society is stronger because its members are more able to play their part and achieve what they are aiming for in life. This should enhance individuals and interpersonal relationships in interaction with wider social progress, so that people are not excluded from participation in it.

Chapter 2 sets the scene, and subsequent chapters tackle values from different vantage points. Chapter 3 examines the issues raised by multiple accountabilities. Chapter 4 discusses the complexities of balancing individual and social interests in a world where the rights of the individual citizen are important, as are the goals of social justice. Chapter 5 focuses on social work with asylum seekers and Indigenous people in Australia. Chapter 6 is a critical discussion of issues arising in relation to women's reproductive rights. Chapter 7 explores some of the tensions arising in relation to people's rights and choices, where questions of their mental capacity arise.

All these chapters share difficulties inherent in the lack of consensus about values in professional practice and there is clearly a reflexive element in this, in that the practitioner cannot distance personal from professional values.

Values in critical practice: contested entities with enduring qualities

2

Values guide personal and professional ethics. Professional values contain continuities arising from those posited by Father Biestek and discontinuities emanating from recent demands from service users to embed practice in notions of citizenship, human rights and social justice. These support their commitment to provisions that meet their needs and which they control.

Chapter overview

Values are concepts that provide a philosophical basis to social work practice (Compton et al., 2004). They furnish the foundation for ethics as a set of principles that guide practice and are an important part of any profession. Values underpin the norms that ensure that practitioners behave ethically and elaborate a basis for holding them accountable for their actions (Hugman, 1991). Values justify particular types of behaviour, giving validity and legitimacy to those that conform. They are used in setting parameters around what can be considered defensible behaviour in professional practice and outlining the responsibilities of different participants in a given intervention. These functions lead social workers to expect values to ensure continuity or have enduring qualities through which practice can be judged or evaluated across different settings and at distinct points in time.

Values have an aura of stability about them that enables practitioners to talk to other colleagues about their work and cross various divides, giving the impression that they are talking about similar entities, even when they hail from different countries and cultures. When discourses about values and their application in practice are explored more carefully, several problems emerge. One is that to focus on values as concepts or consider their similarities, values have to be defined at high levels of abstraction that denude them of their contexts. Another difficulty is that once values are contextualised to locate their specificity, significant differences in interpretation become more visible. Finally, different stakeholders in the social work enterprise contest values as they argue over their symbolic meanings. This can produce conflict, but it also allows growth and change to take place. The fluid movement of values through complex interactions in helping relationships suggests that the certainty and stability that surround values are illusory. Some theorists argue that social work is an exercise in ambiguity and uncertainty (Parton, 1998a).

In this chapter, I explore values in social work – their meaning and relevance for practice, their shifting nature and implications for critical practice. I conclude that values are contested entities and that, as practised, they express both continuities and discontinuities between the past, present and future of the profession. As guides to ethical behaviour, values seldom provide the clear-cut principles sought by those at the receiving end of social workers' ministrations or their employers. When trying to resolve moral and ethical dilemmas, social workers may produce new values.

Defining values

How do social workers define values? Are these defining values? The task of defining values can be an elusive one (Shardlow, 1998). There are different kinds of values: personal, professional, institutional, organisational or agency, political, religious and cultural. The list can easily be extended, but a common feature of each is that they are socially constructed and historically specific. They are usually derived from values that permeate a given society at a particular historical conjuncture. Personal values are those that an individual holds and uses in guiding individual behaviour and actions. They are important in constituting the person as a moral agent and support continuity between and across generations. Professional values are those that practitioners define as specific to their particular profession and are usually enshrined in a regulatory code of ethics that is used to control professional behaviour. Their formulation is the explicit product of discussion and agreement among professional colleagues who advise upon them and, acting as a peer group, monitor each other's activities in relation to the stipulated code. In older professions such as medicine, professional values are backed by a code of ethics that is enforced by professional peers.

In social work, professional values are promulgated through professional associations, but their enforcement is more problematic. This is particularly the case in countries where social work does not have a protected title and the professional association has no legal powers of enforcement. In Britain, social workers have a code of ethics that draws on generally held professional values that has been developed by the British Association of Social Workers (BASW). The General Council for Social Care (GCSC) has established a code of practice that it requires registered social workers to uphold. British social workers' failure to act ethically can result in their losing registration and entitlement to practice. On the international front, the International Federation of Social Workers (IFSW) and the International Association of Schools of Social Work (IASSW) have devised an international ethics document to give the profession common ethical guidance. Adherence to this document is voluntary and acts as a guide in the formulation of local, usually national codes that are devised by the relevant associations. There is considerable variability in these codes, although the dominance of Anglo-American paradigms is also evident. Some practitioners have countered Western hegemony by developing locally specific or indigenous codes, for example practitioners of First Nation (the name that the indigenous people have given themselves) descent in Canada and those with Maori origins in New Zealand. These have sought to incorporate the collectivist or community considerations and responsibilities that are missing in Western ethical models. Like Afrocentric models, these focus on continuities in values and cultural traditions that ensure the survival of ethnic groups experiencing oppression over centuries (John Baptiste, 2001). Asian writers have asked for harmony to be included in these ethical considerations (personal communication).

Organisational values can distort professional values by narrowing options while practitioners seek to broaden them. This occurs when social workers seek to increase the options available to 'clients' at the same time as organisational resources reduce them. The term client is a contested one and interchangeable with service user or consumer. Similarly, the words black and white used to refer to people should not be taken to mean homogeneity in physical, social or cultural attributes. Budgetary limitations on community care assessments exemplify this practice dilemma. The fanfare of client empowerment surrounding community care raises the question of whether organisations can be ethical if they raise false expectations about the range of choices accessible by them. Research into this issue by Khan and Dominelli (2000) demonstrates how marketisation and globalisation have skewed professional priorities and contributed to practitioner disillusionment in their ability to deliver the best quality services in their organisations (Dominelli, 2004a).

Values seem contradictory and difficult to define. Yet most social workers claim to adhere to a discrete set of values that represent their commitment to principles that guide their behaviour and help them to evaluate their performance. The most commonly recognised values in social work emanate from Biestek (1961) and consist of the following:

- Individualism
- Purposeful expression of feelings
- Controlled emotional involvement
- Non-judgemental attitude
- Self-determination
- Confidentiality.

Respect for others and the dignity of the person underpin these and are fundamental to black perspectives (Ahmad, 1990), anti-racist approaches (Dominelli, 1988) and other anti-oppressive positions. Banks (2006) argues that the underlying theme in Biestek's values is the Kantian one of 'respect for the individual person'. While this formulation of values has been criticised for its modernist bias and overreliance on scientific rationality (see Chapter 1) to back its claim to 'truth', it has been recognised by practitioners worldwide and can claim universal applicability. Healy (2001) proposes respect and dignity as essential values in international social work.

Putting to one side the question of interpretation, reducing a set of values to one statement highlights the abstract nature of these values. When boiled down to one, it reaches levels of agreement and universality, which in practice become difficult to sustain in certain circumstances. If we are asked whether respecting the person is a key social work value, the question is cast in a decontextualised form and it is hard to imagine a social worker who would not overtly endorse it. Posing the question in terms of practising values in context, the answers would be more nuanced and complex. For example, in working with a sex offender, social workers draw a distinction between the person whom they claim to respect and his (most sex offenders are men) behaviour, which they cannot condone. Although a myth, acting as if the person and behaviours are two entirely separate entities allows social workers to address the tension between not endorsing unacceptable behaviour while maintaining the validity of the principle of respect. Similar dilemmas occur with counselling people on death row to become reconciled with their demise. While their professional ethics demand respect for the person simultaneously with the sanctity of life, practitioners collude with the elimination of that person through state-sanctioned violence, the legitimacy of which has been contested. The unequal power relations that it exposes cut across the emancipatory dimensions of social work values and create oppression through practice, as the literature that challenges racism (Dominelli, 1988; Ahmad, 1990), sexism (Hanmer and Statham, 1988; Dominelli and McLeod, 1989; Dominelli, 2002a) and disablism (Oliver, 1990; Morris, 1991; Shakespeare, 1999) indicates.

Social workers have to become skilful mental acrobats who can juggle contradictory positions with ease when practising their values. A further value or principle that practitioners use to deal with ethical dilemmas is that of not treating people as a means to other ends. As demonstrated above, it is not always possible to maintain this concern. Nonetheless, it helps social workers to maintain their commitment to social justice, where they have argued that the means used to achieve a particular end must reflect the end that is being sought (Dominelli, 1996).

Biestek's (1961) principles have been criticised for being highly individualistic and culturally specific, that is, tied to Western culture. They are often used in ways that claim universal validity and applicability while disregarding other cultural traditions, especially Eastern ones that emphasise collective rather than individualistic bases to their societies. Westerners configure these concerns as irrelevant to their way of working. The issue of confidentiality becomes particularly relevant in this critique. For example, in a project that I was involved in some while ago, white community workers in a British Muslim Gujarati community in northern England expressed unease when interested members of this community accompanied a person who had a problem into the office and insisted on participating in the ensuing discussions. Several white practitioners found this behaviour incomprehensible because they defined it as one that violated their expectations about confidentiality. Their discomfort abated when it was explained to them that confidentiality was seen differently by this group of clients and that they welcomed the presence of kin and friends. At the same time, these clients were not willing to have their business discussed outside this group. Thus, they had criteria that stipulated boundaries or points at which their interpretation of confidentiality took substance, and they expected the white practitioners to honour these. These boundaries can be identified at the very beginning of an intervention by exploring the meaning of confidentiality in each specific case.

Whether Biestek's (1961) values are defining values, in the sense of being crucial to the profession or setting its parameters, is another question. Reference to them can be found in most social work texts on values. Their continued presence over the past four decades suggests that they have been influential, despite their modification to more closely reflect contemporary linguistic usage. The process of reformulation and development is indicated by empowerment, which extends self-determination in new directions. Their adaptation has also furnished them with slightly different meanings. For example, in becoming empowerment, self-determination has acquired a more active sense even though the clients' rights to make decisions about their lives remain germane to both. And, as Jane Dalrymple and Beverley Burke remind us (Adams et al., 2009a, Ch. 19), 'empowerment is overlain by contrasting and conflicting aims and expectations'.

Empowerment goes beyond the value of self-determination, in that it makes power relations an explicit part of its analytical and practice repertoire, thereby making it a more contextualised concept than self-determination as defined by Biestek (1961). The term has been developed conceptually in different directions (Humphries, 1996; Dominelli, 2000). Are the terms synonymous, as some texts suggest, or are attempts to find similarities between them exercises in futility? Dominelli (2004a) also warns that empowerment has been appropriated by the New Right to commodify and bureaucratise empowering relationships at individual and community levels. Thus, empowerment has become a trendy term conveying a sense of choice that can often be tokenistic and contrary to the idea of engaging people in power relations that place them in the driver's seat. Personalised care and direct payments or individual budgets in contemporary British social work signify a new shift for self-determination. Individual budgets empower service users by providing them with a budget that they can disburse themselves to employ personal assistants or purchase aids and services and, by shifting power away from professionals doing this on their behalf, can enhance the control that service users can exercise over their particular situations.

Some of the changes leading to innovation in social work's value system have been driven by a desire to identify values that are relevant to critical practice. Within this framework, respecting the person would remain a central one, but it would not simply focus on the individual as a decontextualised person. Instead, it would see them as a social being operating within a specific social context, which would include social institutions and a host of external factors that would have to be taken into account in translating this value into practice. Respecting the person would also be linked to dignity and the recognition that a person has socially sanctioned rights, although rights present another conceptual minefield.

In examining the relevant context, practitioners also need to look underneath the presenting problem, an important part of the holistic practice to which critical practitioners aspire (Ife, 1997). Asking probing questions to delve deeper into issues has also been part of traditional training (Compton and Galaway, 1975). So, there has been less innovation in this arena than appears at first glance.

Controlled emotional engagement is more likely to permit becoming non-judgemental. But even this value would be contextualised in today's critical practice. For, without contextualisation, it could be interpreted as meaning the acceptance of behaviour that harms others, whether this ranges from minor lying to theft or violence against the person or a cold detachment that precludes the formation of a professional helping relationship. Critical social workers would acknowledge that they are in the business of making judgements and that these are often finely balanced ones. For example, making decisions about whether a particular sex offender poses a potential risk to a given child requires practitioners to make judgements. However, as professional judgements, these are based on assessments of risk rather than arbitrary personal prejudices. Yet, risk assessments are not straightforward calculations. Their use has to be critiqued, the basis for their judgements has to be articulated and social workers have to be held accountable for the decisions they make.

What counts as acceptable or plausible remains problematic. Do these terms mean the same thing? These questions cannot be answered except in a specific context and, maybe, not even then. The complexity of implementing any set of values in practice is illustrated in Sarah Banks's example in Chapter 3 of the social worker's failure to disclose knowledge about a client with the potential to sexually abuse others.

Individualisation would now be expressed more in terms of validating the uniqueness of each individual. But, in critical practice, particularly as advocated by feminists and black people, the individual would at the same time be seen as part of a wider group. In this, identity issues would be treated as more self-determining, while a greater awareness of their diversity would be evident to simultaneously ensure that the space for the individual is safeguarded from bureaucratic encroachment.

Purposeful expression of feeling is the most awkward of Biestek's (1961) terms for use in the present day. Most contemporary social workers would subscribe to the view that professionals should not allow their personal views to impact upon their work, and would only share their feelings or experiences with clients under limited circumstances. Despite their caution in this regard, they would insist on being aware of what their personal views were to ensure that they are kept in check.

Critical practitioners would add that, in understanding themselves, practitioners would be able to handle the boundaries between the public and private domains more effectively. To some extent, their capacity to maintain the public–private divide would confirm their ability to be 'neutral' in relation to the client, in the sense of keeping a respectful objectivity or distance from them rather than being neutral, in the sense of having no views on the subject. On the other side of this boundary is the requirement that practitioners express empathy with their clients, an injunction that is at odds with the previous one.

Empathy requires the social worker to be in the clients' shoes (Egan, 1998; Chapter 1) or enter their epistemological and ontological worlds. This value is aimed at enabling practitioners to cross social divides and be with the client in a supportive way. Demonstrating empathy can be extremely difficult to achieve, as white workers tackling racist practices have found (Dominelli, 1988). Conflict between practitioners' personal and professional values can also block the realisation of empathy, especially if the former prevents them from complying with statutory duties. They may be unable to express empathy in certain cases and find that curbing their private views becomes a source of considerable personal stress. This is an issue that can easily crop up in work involving child molesters or murderers, where a practitioner may have difficulty in being empathetic. Such situations also reveal that values are experienced emotionally as well as being thought about intellectually and being implemented in practice.

On the practical level, it is crucial to ask how the values of a profession can be enforced so that ethical practice occurs as a matter of course. What are the roles of the individual practitioner, their employers and professional associations in ensuring that accepted values, standards and norms are adhered to by each of them? Who will monitor compliance? What happens when they are violated? Who will enforce them and how? None of these questions have easy, let alone automatic, answers. They constantly have to be posed and responded to in specific contexts. A practitioner's peers may overlook a colleague's reluctance to empathise with a child molester or murderer, but they would not be so forgiving of a failure to prevent harm being inflicted upon a child in their care, as social worker Lisa Arthurworrey discovered when Victoria Climbié was fatally abused by a great-aunt and her boyfriend.

These descriptions of values in action provide evidence that values are not neutral, particularly when applied in practice. Conflicts of interest between the different participants – service users, victims, practitioners, policy makers, service providers, and others, abound. Mediating conflicting interests draws on another principle – protection from harm. But in resolving conflicts, protection issues involving the self, others, workers and society can remain problematic. On what basis, that is, values, does a practitioner say that a child's right to safety overrides an adult's right to privacy and protection from the stigma caused by an investigation into an alleged abuse, especially when the case becomes 'not proven'? This scenario forms the most likely outcome in child protection investigations as most of these do not substantiate the allegations (DH, 1995a).

Social workers constantly prioritise one set of principles over another. In taking action, social workers weigh different priorities. Establishing priorities to facilitate action in particular situations is one way of creating certainty in an ambiguous and contradictory world. Without some way of finding at least a temporary or transient certainty in difficult moral and ethical terrains, social workers would be unable to act.

To make matters even more complicated, the entire basis on which professional values rest is subject to questioning. The alleged superiority of professional or expert knowledge is today challenged by clients who reject the exclusion of their voices (Wendell, 1996) and by postmodern theorists (Fook, 2002). Their demands can involve practitioners in conflict with traditional professional values that prioritise professional knowledge over client knowledge. Clients have led the way in emancipatory practice and given enormous impetus to the idea that practitioners can support their strivings for social justice. In this, service users have introduced the idea of citizenship as the basis of their relationships with caring professionals. However, citizenship in the welfare market is a limited or qualified one (Banks, 2001). The reduction of clients to users who follow an exit strategy when they cannot exercise meaningful choice in the marketplace introduces commodity relations to a non-commercial sphere (Dominelli, 2000, 2004b).

Practising values

The word 'values' is grammatically a noun, but it is derived from a verb, to value or hold in esteem. It is easy to talk about applying values or values in practice, but 'practising values' sounds odd despite portraying a dynamism crucial to (re)conceptualising values as values in action and addressing the complexities and dilemmas that realising them entails. The difficulties in defining values are replicated when applying them in practice. The problems encountered are not only differences in interpretation and meaning, but also of values in conflict or contradiction with one another. This situation is further complicated by issues of accountability.

Social workers are accountable to a range of stakeholders – service users, other practitioners, employers, policy makers, government and the general public. To begin with, these groups may or may not share the same values. So conflict can arise from these sources. But even if they do hold similar values, each has different imperatives that contextualise these. Contextual exigencies emanating from organisational priorities also have an impact on how values can be applied in practice. Practising values is not a straightforward matter. Social workers become embroiled as co-accused as a result of holding a case in situations where clients have been adversely treated and their vulnerability increased, as in the case of the death of a child on an 'at risk' register. Whether or not the practitioner was directly responsible, the social worker's practice will be subjected to intense scrutiny. The inquiry into their practice may be conducted in a manner that does not reflect the values of the profession in terms of showing respect for the person. The social worker may be scapegoated for a number of structural inadequacies, as Sarah Banks indicates in Chapter 3 when recounting the experience of an overworked, distraught social worker who is treated in a manner that ignores her own personal state. Social work practice is distinctive, in that no matter what the psychological or emotional state of the social worker is, they must not endanger the life of a client through their actions.

In this case, the abuse of one child in a home by another might have been prevented had the social worker passed on crucial information to the home manager. Banks's example also raises a number of other value-laden questions: How do social workers value or weigh the information they receive? Does knowledge that the boy had previously perpetrated sexual abuse become valued in hindsight because it is now possible to see a causal connection between knowledge and action? Would conducting a more thorough risk assessment upon the young man's admission to the home have highlighted the weightiness of this piece of information beforehand so that preventive action could have been taken? Evaluation, as Nick Frost shows (Adams et al., 2009c, Ch. 24), is not a one-way street. The social worker needs managerial support if evaluation is to become part of an ongoing process of intervention. This ingredient is in short supply in the case cited. Also, the evaluative tools at the practitioners' disposal do not always measure up to the task. Quinsey's (1995) research revealed the limited capacity of risk assessment effectively to predict dangerousness in a specific offender.

Practice at this level is hampered by our inadequate knowledge of risk. The possibility that an event may occur is not the same as its actual occurrence. We cannot readily distinguish between the two before the event. In playing safe by assuming that it will occur, individuals suspected of being potential sex offenders may find a utilitarian approach to their rights. This can mean that the presumption of innocence until proven guilty is put aside to ensure the safety of those who might become victims.

Other concerns to be addressed include issues of social justice, rights and fair play.

In Chapter 4, Chris Clark indicates that these are contentious and at times in conflict with each other. The children in a home have the right to live in an environment free of sexual abuse, and all those running the home and working within it are responsible for ensuring that it is such a place. Research by Kelly et al. (1991) reveals a high incidence of sexual abuse in society. Campbell's (1995) research shows that the majority of sex offenders have been neither identified as such nor convicted. Thus, it is possible to conclude that children who have been abused and those who are abusers are likely to be found in any general sample of the child population. In this context, it would be reasonable to assume that every home would have systems in place to take account of the possibility that they might have sexually abused children and sex offenders in their midst and thereby effectively implement its duty to protect children. This is an institutional responsibility that those working within the home discharge collectively. Practice has to be conceptualised as more than the sum of its constituent parts. This view is relevant for institutions responsible for caring for a particular child.

Formal inquiries seldom comment on institutional responsibilities except at the level of refining existing or introducing new bureaucratic procedures to hold individual practitioners more accountable in future. Institutional responsibility to ensure that employees have appropriate working conditions, including adequate support and supervision, is rarely detailed in these reports (see Blom-Cooper, 1986; Butler-Sloss, 1988; Laming, 2003). Having fragmented services reliant on individual, atomised practitioners each responsible for covering an entire spectrum of provisions sets dangerous precedents for achieving maximum effectiveness in difficult and sensitive areas. The exclusion of practitioners from positions where decisions about policy and procedures are made exacerbates the problem of a lack of fit between formal policies and the realities of practice. Consequently, the politics of practice become skewed by bureaucratic exigencies at the expense of practice ones.

Besides institutional responsibility, there is personal responsibility. If prevention of future abuse and the rehabilitation of an offender are to be valued, individual case notes should contain information that identifies a particular individual who may have experienced sexual abuse and/or perpetrated it. Providing this information can conflict with not labelling people or placing them in a straitjacket from which they cannot escape. Even though it may be shared among only the few who need to know, so as not to label a child unnecessarily, it can further stigmatise children or hinder future work aimed at promoting a capacity to relate to others in non-exploitative ways. Such situations are potentially difficult to manage and become sources of considerable pressure for individuals to resolve. Nonetheless, personal responsibility enables a practitioner to play specific roles in interventions with a given individual and take additional measures or precautions alongside the general ones initiated by the institution.

Issues of confidentiality are complicated in such scenarios. A social worker's commitment is to change individual behaviour in more socially acceptable ways. In pursuing this course of action, an offender's right not to have their past held against them in the interests of rehabilitation and change, or when serving their time if they have been punished, is no longer automatically assured. For sex offenders, one set of values –

protecting others from harm – supersedes a right to privacy. The Sex Offenders Act 1997 has enshrined this contradiction in law. This demonstrates anew that values cannot be practised in the abstract but in specific circumstances. Social workers have to make decisions that prioritise one value over another in particular ways. In such circumstances, most social workers must prioritise the rights of a vulnerable person.

Fine balances in judgement often have to be made. Sometimes, the weighting that a specific practitioner gives to a particular situation or factor turns out to be wrong, as Sarah Banks illustrates. Yet, the crucial question remains: How can social workers minimise the number of inadequate decisions made in such circumstances? Responding to this question requires discussion among employers, policy makers, trainers, the general public and the specific people involved in the case. Contemporary discourses on the subject seldom focus on holistic responses to the problem. Countless inquiries into the death of looked-after children or their continued sexual abuse indicate that the practice of an individual practitioner is usually scrutinised and held responsible when things go wrong more often than institutional practices.

Trust, or a belief in the goodness of others or the assumption that they will not cause a particular individual harm, is important when practising values that promote ethical behaviour among professionals. Although not often considered, trust is a value that underpins other values and must be evident throughout an entire operation if it is to permeate all social interactions in a given case. Trust is created (or not) in and through the interactions of the individuals concerned, although these may draw on an institutional context that may (or may not) support it. Trust is created through negotiations between people as well as being taken as a given in a supportive workplace. A social worker has to 'trust' that the organisation will facilitate their work and back it in particular ways. Clients 'trust' practitioners to do their job effectively and safeguard their vulnerability and interests. Trust is needed at many levels, none of which can be presumed in practice. Trust should be there as part of the taken-for-granted context in which helping relationships occur. As I show in Chapter 6, the climate in which reproductive rights are being simultaneously extended and curtailed both betrays and draws upon trust.

Understanding power relations and the roles these play at different levels in people's interactions in client–worker relationships is essential in a framework that appreciates the political and contested nature of values. Power relations can be practised as a zero-sum game that divides people into those who have power and those who do not. I argue for a more refined consideration of these. Following Giddens (1987), power can be conceptualised as a negotiated reality in which neither party is either completely powerful or powerless. The interaction between them is one that can either reproduce or challenge existing power relations (Dominelli, 1986; Dominelli and Gollins, 1997). Practitioners can respond to clients as agents who can take responsibility for their behaviour rather than being treated as passive victims who have everything done for them by experts. Thinking about power as multifaceted allows for more empowering practices that enable clients to voice their own opinions and views, and participate in shaping the outcomes of intervention. Reinforcing client agency ties in closely with putting substance behind the value of self-determination, even when practitioners have an eye on clients' potential to engage in further abuse, for example sex offenders.

Each situation is affected by a number of different and sometimes competing values. Audrey Mullender (Adams et al., 2009c, Ch. 3), when discussing domestic violence, demonstrates how what is valued or prioritised can change over time. For example, feminist actions to safeguard the interests of women and children who have been at the receiving end of domestic violence have demanded that this form of cruel and degrading treatment is taken seriously in and through practice and so ensured that it has risen up the social work agenda. This issue reveals how diverse client groups are valued and treated differently. Being treated differently does not result in better or more appropriate responses, as the experiences of lesbian women (Arnup, 1997) and black women experiencing sexual and domestic abuse (Wilson, 1993; Mama, 1996) show. For this to occur, being treated differently has to be accompanied by valuing or seeing the worth of a person undergoing that experience. Being treated with dignity as human beings whatever the circumstances is where humanism as a value comes through.

Values in critical practice

Critical practitioners have an important question to answer. In doing critical practice, are they practising different values? Do professional values for critical practice differ from professional values for other paradigms of practice? In my view, there are overlaps between the two. In critical practice, professionals are considered as moral agents engaging in a moral activity. That is why the value of social justice is so important to practice. Promoting this value may constitute the key difference between traditional practitioners and critical ones.

Critical practice can be about a variety of different positions, and, as this book demonstrates, its definition is a matter of continuous dialogue and examination of different points of view. There appears to be some agreement about the importance of reflexivity in the processes of critical practice, and in defining social work as both a moral and technical activity. This delineation of what counts in social work does not deal with difficult situations such as those where social workers or carers abuse those they care for, as occurred during 'pindown' (Levy and Kahan, 1991). Caring for someone does not necessarily mean caring about them. The latter implies a different sort of relationship. It conveys the idea that a non-exploitative arrangement can be expected. What happens when these associations go wrong and the opposite is delivered? Do we say that a person was not a carer, only an abuser? Or has the person been both? The depiction of each of these values as discrete and separate entities does not help to clarify this situation. This is because it covers both life-affirming and life-destroying values. An individual or organisation can espouse both simultaneously. It is through their behaviour and its outcome that a firm judgement can be made about what values the person has prioritised (a decision about which value was more important to them personally).

The dichotomous thinking that divides behaviour into either one or the other may help us to establish the harm that has been done to the victim-survivor of the abuse. It does not help us to understand the position of abusers who claim to endorse life-affirming principles through their behaviour, as sex offenders do when they claim they are demonstrating 'love' for their victims and not abusing them (Snowdon, 1980). Although practitioners tend to dismiss their comments as cognitive distortions if not outright lies, the sex offender may genuinely believe his statements. The challenge for practitioners is to get these men to revise their views. Practitioners tackle this if they believe in an absolute value that supersedes that of starting where the client is at, have knowledge that enables them to discount an offender's story, or use powers vested in them through legislation, social approbation or professional codes to entitle them to define what constitutes acceptable behaviour and what does not. This may mean that social workers have to hold uncertainty and ambiguity as defining characteristics of their work, even when called upon to act with certainty in difficult situations.

Critical practitioners would engage in these situations by trying to assist both the carer and the cared for, but in different ways. They may insist that different practitioners each undertake a particular piece of work. A traditional practitioner would struggle with similar issues and might find that except for a critical practitioner's overt commitment to social justice they have more in common than they expect. Their practice with individuals may be remarkably similar. This possibility guides claims that, at the end of the day, all practitioners are about good practice and explains why the Central Council for Education and Training in Social Work, when it lost the battle over anti-oppressive practice in the mid-1990s, claimed victory on the grounds that social work's value base had been retained intact.

Conclusion

Values provide tools for determining merit or worth. An important contribution of postmodernism to debates about values is its capacity to make explicit what has been implicit in the 'practice wisdoms' that practitioners draw upon in their practice. However, this contribution has been less about innovative insights into values than about presenting previously known ones in new ways. This has articulated the contingent and contextualised nature of values and highlighted the difficulties encountered in putting them into practice.

Critical practitioners need to start where clients are at. This, like other values, is contingent, not absolute. Its conditionality still leaves power in helping relationships in the hands of professionals. This is not in itself an undesirable feature. It depends on how this power is used by the professional and for what purpose. At this point, reflexivity in process and a commitment to social justice and client agency differentiate a critical practitioner from a more traditional one. Reflexivity leads critical practitioners to expect their practice to evolve constantly. Their practice development is always unfinished. A social worker is always in the process of becoming a critical practitioner even when acting as if they were one already.

For discussion of values, ethics and practice, see Adams et al., 2009a, Chapter 4, and for anti-oppressive practice, see Adams et al., 2009a, Chapter 5.

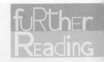

Banks, S. (2006) *Ethics and Values in Social Work,* 3rd edn, Basingstoke, Palgrave Macmillan. Comprehensive consideration of the issues and dilemmas that practitioners encounter in implementing their values in practice. Makes some international comparisons.

Barker, G. (2005) *Dying to be Men: Youth, Masculinity and Social Exclusion,* London, Routledge. Explores marginalised youths' attempts to become men in difficult surroundings. Masculine identity proves a powerful force in the transition between adolescence and adulthood for socially excluded young men seeking to become self-defining adults.

Dominelli, L. (2002) *Feminist Social Work Theory and Practice,* Basingstoke, Palgrave Macmillan. Examines the difference that feminist values make to work that is undertaken with clients at the centre of the helping relationship. Arguing for a reconceptualisation of power relations between service users and practitioners, it considers how social workers can work in empowering ways.

3 Professional values and accountabilities

Chapter overview

This chapter explores the concept of accountability and its implementation in social work practice. Although accountability is not a new concept, concern with accountability is currently a high priority. This chapter considers the implications of this for critical practice in social work, drawing on interviews conducted by the author with social work managers and practitioners to illustrate the wider issues.

The importance of accountability

A social work team manager, being interviewed about ethical issues in her work, made the following statement:

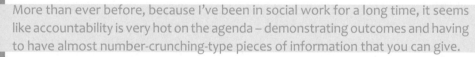

More than ever before, because I've been in social work for a long time, it seems like accountability is very hot on the agenda – demonstrating outcomes and having to have almost number-crunching-type pieces of information that you can give.

This interviewee made two important points. First, concern with accountability seems greater than previously. Second, she referred to a particular type of accountability, which she later described as especially onerous – the production of quantifiable outputs and outcomes in response to demands by employers and central government.

Accountability has always been important for professionals. According to Tadd (1994: 88), it is 'the sine qua non of any professional group'. But the kind of accountability stressed by professional bodies is that owed to service users. Service to clients is the essence of professional practice; and any professional, whether a doctor, lawyer or social worker, must be prepared to account for their actions to people using their services. Although we may dispute how well professionals have implemented it, accountability to service users is integral to the core values of social work of respecting service users' freedom of choice, promoting their welfare and challenging discrimination and oppression. In addition to professional accountability to service users, social workers have always had a duty of public accountability to the wider political community (Pratchett and Wingfield, 1994: 9; Clark, 2000: 78–9). They often work directly or indirectly for public bodies, with a role to promote the public good by, for example, protecting the vulnerable and treating or controlling dangerous people. Social workers and their employers are therefore accountable to the public for the effectiveness of the services they deliver. So, notions of professional and public accountability are at the heart of social work, and in both areas demands are increasing. The two are interconnected, as employers are introducing quality standards, standardised assessment forms, contracts and complaints procedures, partly in response to demands from service users for their rights to more effective services, to participate in decision-making and to complain. However, the accountability demands of different parties may also conflict, and one of the themes of my interviews with social workers is that, in striving for organisational and public accountability, the voices, needs and rights of individual service users and their communities may get lost.

The nature of accountability

Accountability is an integral feature of everyday as well as professional life. The eighteenth-century philosopher Reid suggests it is a distinguishing feature of humans: 'that which makes them moral agents, accountable for their conduct, and objects of moral approbation and blame' (Reid, [1788]1977: 69). It is not just that we must be prepared to describe, explain or justify what we have done in order to be apportioned moral praise or blame, but 'giving an account' is an essential feature of our means of communicating with others, being understood and establishing our identities (Heritage, 1983; Buttny, 1993). What I have called professional and public accountability are part of this wider system of moral and social accountability.

To be accountable is literally to be liable to be called upon to give an account of what one has or has not done. The account may include all or some of descriptions, explanations, excuses or justifications. Frequently, giving an account is associated with the occurrence of a problematic situation and the apportioning of blame. Indeed, Holdsworth (1994: 42) defines accountability as 'the obligation to lay oneself open to criticism'. Buttny's concern in his sociological study of accountability is with 'talk used to transform pejorative ascriptions and resolve problematic events' (1993: 16). Hence, the main types of accounts tend to be excuses and justifications. Buttny (1993: 15) acknowledges that accounts can be 'descriptions', 'ordinary explanations' or 'self-reports' which would also include unproblematic situations, but his main concern, along with other sociologists, is with accounts as attempts to mend a social breach resulting from a problematic situation. Accountability is linked with laying oneself open to blame and criticism, and trying to counter any negative evaluations that might be placed on one's action. As Buttny (1993: 2) comments:

> This distinctively human capacity to be blamed and to be held responsible for actions creates the practical necessity for the communication of accounts.

This suggests an important relationship between accountability and responsibility. Being held responsible for my actions means that I am able to make rational choices and decisions and should therefore 'own' my actions. If something goes wrong, if I am accused of making a bad decision or causing a bad outcome, then I may be asked, or I may wish, to give an account of what happened, my reasons for acting as I did, perhaps pointing to circumstances of which others may be unaware.

Although some commentators treat accountability and responsibility as synonymous (Clark with Asquith, 1985: 40), and others just use the terms interchangeably (Tadd, 1994; Clark, 2000), this is unhelpful. Fairbairn (1985) lists four senses of responsibility, only one of which means the same as 'accountability'. The first relates to causing a state of affairs. For example, when we talk of someone having 'responsibility for an accident', we may mean that they caused the accident. Another sense of responsibility is that of having a duty to someone or to do something. For example, we might say: 'you have a responsibility to look after your daughter'. We may also use 'responsibility' to describe a person's character or behaviour, for example 'she acted with responsibility', in the sense that she was trustworthy and reliable. In none of these three usages of 'responsibility' could 'accountability' be substituted without changing the meaning. The final sense of responsibility is being liable to explain or justify action, that is, accountability. Accountability, therefore, is just one sense of 'responsibility', and is not always synonymous with it.

Accountability and blame

A senior social worker being interviewed on ethical issues in practice described a situation for which the worker had been 'called to account', held responsible and blameworthy.

CASE EXAMPLE

One of the really bad experiences that I did have last summer, and it was because I was working – I had too much work to do. I said I had too much work to do, and it was perceived as a kind of weakness on my part, it wasn't responded to positively at first. And also I had various personal problems. My son was ill at the time and one thing and another. I placed a 15-year-old young man with learning disabilities in a group care home. I was told to do so by my team manager. I'd written a comprehensive case conference report, in which I had alluded to various sexualised behaviours that this young man had exhibited in the past. I was pressurised by the people who were currently looking after the young man to move him within a very short space of time, so I took the young man to the care home and did an introductory visit. I completed the essential

> information pack that we have from the Department of Health – the essential information. There is no question in that pack: 'Has this child exhibited sexualised behaviour?' So the information, the documentation that you fill out is flawed anyway, because it doesn't contain the essential information. The young man then went on to sexually abuse one of the young women living in the home. And then there's a big enquiry about it and I'm to blame.

We will now analyse this account, also bringing in information given later in the interview, to elucidate what is involved in giving an account in the context of a problematic situation in social work.

Contextualising the worker

First the worker situates herself. Not only is she a social worker with the standard skills and responsibilities expected of all social workers (her professional identity), she is also a person with events happening in her personal life that affect how she feels and performs. Later she also locates herself as 'part of a system' – particularly the decision-making system that includes a team manager, care home manager and members of the case conference. The worker feels it is important to contextualise herself partly because she felt exposed:

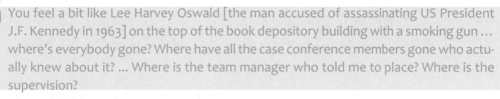

> You feel a bit like Lee Harvey Oswald [the man accused of assassinating US President J.F. Kennedy in 1963] on the top of the book depository building with a smoking gun ... where's everybody gone? Where have all the case conference members gone who actually knew about it? ... Where is the team manager who told me to place? Where is the supervision?

Descriptive narrative

The worker tells the story of what happened: she placed the young man in a care home; she completed the forms correctly and handed them over; the young man then abused another resident. Obviously this is not 'pure description', but a selection of what she thinks is the most relevant information to construct the case.

Explanations, justifications, excuses

Some of the descriptions may be serving as explanations, justifications or excuses – it is not always clear which until later in the interview. Explanations are about giving reasons for action. Justifications involve accepting responsibility for an action, but denying it was wrong. Excuses deny full responsibility for action, but admit that it was wrong or inappropriate (Scott and Lyman, 1970: 114). The fact that the worker was suffering from stress and that she followed the procedures and completed all the required documentation may serve as excuses for not informing the care home manager about the young man's sexualised behaviour. The fact that she was responding to orders from her manager and family pressure explain the rapidity of the placement. There are no obvious justifications in this extract, although later in the interview, the worker considers whether she could reasonably have been expected to regard the boy's previous behaviour as a danger signal, important enough to have communicated it to the care home manager. If she could not, then although she might accept responsibility for not passing on the information, and accept that the outcome in this case (abuse of a young woman) was bad, it could be argued that her action (not passing on the information) was not wrong.

Ascriptions of moral responsibility

The worker says 'I am to blame.' At this point in the interview, it is unclear whether she accepts blame, or is merely reporting that others are blaming her. Later, when referring to the care home manager's comment that had she known about the sexualised behaviour then she would have taken protective measures, the worker adds 'quite rightly'. This implies that the worker agrees that the care home manager had a right to this information. Although clearly taking some of the blame for not informing the care home manager, the worker later suggested in the following statement that she was not sure that workers can always be expected to spot a danger signal:

My mind would have had to be more like a computer than something created by God to draw in all that information and see it. You can see it instantly now that an abuse has happened.

This case illustrates the kind of account this worker chose to give in a research interview. It will not be the same as she gave to the others who requested accounts from her, but it is likely to be informed by the kinds of questions she had already been asked, and her view of what counts as a plausible or acceptable account in this context. I would suggest that the kinds of accounts expected and given in social work tend to be in terms of:

- *Technical accountability:* with reference to commonly accepted knowledge and skills about what works (evidence-based practice) and how to do things (such as a risk assessment). One of the questions at issue here was whether the type of behaviour exhibited by the young man previously was a likely predictor of his potential to commit sexual abuse. In this case, the social worker suggests that, although a computer might predict this risk, the technical competences of the human mind are limited.
- *Procedural accountability:* with reference to a set of rules or protocols about how to do things. In this case, the worker had completed the relevant *Looking After*

Children documentation (see Chapter 22) and passed it to the care home manager, so she could justify her actions in terms of following the required procedures for cases like this.

- *Managerial accountability:* with reference to orders or requests from a senior manager. In this case, the team manager had sanctioned the rapid placement in the care home.
- *Ethical accountability:* with reference to commonly accepted values about what is right and wrong. These may be personally held values, the stated values of the profession or prevailing societal values. The extract given above does not contain any justifications or excuses for actions in explicitly ethical terms. Later in the interview, the worker affirms the care home manager's right to have had the information about the young man in order to protect other residents. This implies that the worker thinks that the rights of service users to protection are important and are a material ethical consideration in this case. The social worker later reports being questioned about exactly what she knew about the boy's sexualised behaviour. The implication is that if she had had this information, she should have passed it on to the care home manager. Had the information not been in the worker's possession, then the outcome might be regarded as regrettable, but the worker might not have been held blameworthy. (See Banks, 2006: 20–5 for a discussion of the distinction between blameworthy and regrettable outcomes.)

Multiple accountabilities

This case illustrates the many different people and organisations to whom social workers are liable to give accounts of their actions. The social worker in our example first learned of the incident of abuse from a colleague. As she put it in retrospect: 'the residential care manager came running down the corridor saying "I'm so annoyed with you. You should have realised …".' An internal investigation followed, also drawing in people from outside agencies. Senior managers were calling the worker to account to them and to 'impartial' outside experts representing the 'profession'. The care home manager was also asking for explanations, as was the father of the young woman who had been abused. Finally, after the father persisted with a complaint, the ombudsman was called in. The local authority complaints officer sought explanations in order to respond to the ombudsman.

Clark (2000: 83) claims that 'complex accountability' is an important feature of social work, with workers having accountabilities to many different parties for a range of different and often conflicting responsibilities (in the sense of duties). Social workers are constantly faced with conflicting duties, for example to respect parents' rights as well as to protect children, to promote the wellbeing of service users and to distribute resources in accordance with the rules and regulations of the employing agency. The kinds of accounts expected by the different parties may often be in terms of these different duties. Often a decision is made to give one duty priority over another, for example protection of children over parents' rights to care for their children. In such a situation, parents might seek an account in terms of their rights and competences (a focus on ethical accountability). The employing agency will expect technical and procedural accountability. If the social worker gives an account of her action to the parents with reference to procedures and rules, it is quite likely that the parents will remain dissatisfied, not just with the unwelcome decision, but the explanation or justification given.

Buttny (1993: 127–41) discusses a transcript of a 'welfare interview' featuring a white American caseworker and a mother and daughter of African-American origin seeking financial assistance. The caseworker justifies her decision to refuse assistance with reference to institutional procedures (an application to court must take precedence). The mother and daughter put their case in terms of obvious needs and the fact that all other channels have failed. Buttny comments on the asymmetry in this interview and the impossibility of the applicants successfully challenging the caseworker's decision without a specialised bureaucratic knowledge:

> Decision-making involves not only explicit institutional rules and procedures, but also tacit conventions and criteria based on cultural assumptions of the situation, appropriate ways of structuring information, and preferred ways of speaking. Those ignorant of such conventions and criteria are put at a disadvantage in attempting to attain their goals. (Buttny, 1993: 128)

Accountability, transparency and critical reflection

So far we have stressed the importance of accountability in the context of problematic situations, its role in apportioning blame, and accountability to the employing organisation in terms of procedures. If we consider accountability from a critical practice perspective, we might pay more attention to routine accountability in everyday situations, collective responsibility for untoward events, and transparency of communication with service users.

In social work, routine accounting is very important – making recordings of everyday unproblematic encounters with service users. Of course, social workers always have an eye to the case going wrong, having to answer a complaint, to appear in court, to justify a decision to a team manager or a case conference. As one of the social workers interviewed by the author put it:

> One of my clients hung himself in the garage, yesterday afternoon. The first thing I was asked was: 'Is the file up to date?' Because it's so important that the file is up to date and that nobody can be held to be responsible.

Nevertheless, at the time they are made, these routine recordings are primarily descriptions and opinions rather than excuses or justifications. They may enable the social worker to engage in reflective practice, to clarify the nature of the situation and her role within it, and to reflect on possible courses of action. She may also go beyond this to critical reflection or reflexivity, which involves developing awareness of the political context of social work, the role of the social worker as a political actor, and the potential for social and political change (Fook, 2002; Fook and Askeland, 2006; Banks, 2007).

Supervision in social work (see Adams et al., 2009c, Ch. 15) is also a routine way in which social workers give accounts of practice. Certainly, these accounts can be framed in such a way that workers present their practice in a good light and demonstrate that they did the right thing so they cannot be blamed if things go wrong. But accounts in supervision can also be about sharing mistakes and uncertainties. Supervision should be a process that allows workers to reflect on and learn from their mistakes. The worker in the abuse case described earlier felt her supervision was inadequate and commented that a new policy was now being established requiring supervision to occur free from interruptions and to involve 'thinking things carefully right through'. In relation to the abuse case she commented:

> I think that if I had thought carefully about ... [the sexualised behaviour], I might have remembered, as it were. I hadn't even forgotten. It just hadn't been in my mind.

Unless workers trust their supervisors and are clear about what information is confidential between the two of them, and what is on record for the organisation, then the potential for reflective learning and hence the value of supervision is considerably diminished. In a climate of blame and defensiveness this can be difficult to achieve, as can any 'safe space' within a team or agency where open dialogue can happen. Rossiter et al. (2000) note the importance of 'ethical deliberation' as a vital part of developing a critical awareness of the political and ethical context of social work. It is also an important step in moving beyond the individual worker as the locus of responsibility and blame. As McNamee and Gergen (1999: xi) point out in their exposition of relational responsibility: 'the tradition of individual responsibility – in which single individuals are held blameworthy for untoward events – has a chilling effect on relationships'. The abuse case is an example of this, where, during the course of the investigation, the worker reported feeling as if she was 'some kind of pariah, a child abuser by proxy'.

The importance of honest and open dialogue and sharing responsibility both among social workers and between workers and service users is one of the key features of critical social work. In the relationship with the service user, the emphasis is on transparency, which means acknowledging the power of the worker and sharing that power when possible (Healy, 2000: 30). It requires giving clear accounts to service users of why a social worker is involved, what her powers are and what might happen. It involves listening to service users' own views, hearing the stories of their lives, cultures and identities, recognising their experiences of racism or homophobia, responding in language that is comprehensible and with a commitment to challenge the structures in society that perpetuate their negative experiences. Such an approach to relationships with service users reflects the commonly accepted values of social work (see Chapter 2), which are about respecting and promoting the rights and choices of service users, promoting their welfare and working for social justice.

So why do we need to restate these values? Surely all social workers believe in them and act on them? They may certainly believe in them, as most of the social workers I interviewed evidenced, but the difficulty is in interpreting and implementing them. To do this, debate, dialogue and discussion are needed (Banks, 1998). In the past, the stumbling block may have been 'paternalism' or parentalism – the belief that social workers know best and should be trusted by service users without question to work in their best interests, or the best interests of society, whichever was the most important. Trust in the professional meant there was little need for detailed, 'user-friendly' accountability. Today, according to many social workers, one of the main threats to user-friendly accountability comes from a certain type of overzealous accountability demanded by employers and central government. Although aspects of this accountability may be about improving the standard of services and giving users the right to complain, its development is often largely in terms of organisational language and needs.

The team manager quoted at the beginning of this chapter referred to the ongoing accountability required of individual social workers to their organisations and of social work agencies to central government. This is creating demands for massive documentation to demonstrate that the work is being done to prescribed standards. This requires not just the collection of statistics, the inspection of practice, but changing the way the work is done in order to facilitate the accountability process. Many of the procedures and protocols that have been developed to aid social workers in conducting a fair and comprehensive assessment, reviewing and monitoring needs and outcomes for service users are designed both to improve practice and demonstrate that good practice has occurred. The extensive *Looking After Children* documentation (DH, 1995b; see Chapter 24) referred to in the abuse case is a good example. The documentation was devised to standardise practice, improve the outcomes for young people, and give more information to all the parties involved (Jackson, 1998). Since the forms are prescribed, they also facilitate social workers in being able to demonstrate, when asked, what they have done. But social workers report spending so much time filling in the forms that they neglect to develop a relationship with the people with whom they are working. As one social worker commented: 'You can spend so much time ticking boxes that you can actually forget that there are people who need to be helped.'

Although the forms may ask questions about ethnic identity, use of language, health needs and preferences, this does not guarantee that the social worker will behave in an ethnically sensitive way, will spend time communicating and getting to know the person, and helping them to express the hopes, fears and desires that cannot be accounted for on the form. Reliance on the forms can also cause workers to neglect to reflect more broadly on factors that are not covered on the comprehensive forms, as the abuse case detailed above demonstrates. Having completed them in full, the social worker may be lulled into a false sense of security. Many of the practitioners interviewed were cautious about overreliance on set procedures. One group leader in adult care summed this up:

> Procedures are guidelines, and not tablets of stone. You've got to use your intelligence, you've got to look at them in the context of people, and in the context of situations, and procedures can't cover every eventuality. There are times when you just have to use your brain and judgement, and people say: 'Well, what if I get it wrong?' and I say: 'Well, you get it wrong then'. If we're not paid for our judgement, then what are we paid for?'

Conclusion

Much of the literature on accountability focuses on problematic situations, where something has gone wrong and there is a desire to allocate blame. In social work, routine accountability in the form of recordings has always been important, as has supervision as a learning process. It is important not to lose sight of the potential for reflective learning and the development of critical practice through these traditional means, rather than focusing excessively on ever-more bureaucratic and detailed procedures and forms. The association of accountability with problematic situations and with criticism and blame can lead to defensive practice and a reluctance to take risks, and to a focus on public accountability (to the employer, the public at large) at the cost of professional accountability (to the service user). Critical practice involves a refocusing of attention on the importance of the communication with the service user, a recognition of and honesty about potential conflicts and powers, and a striving to change the organisational culture of social work agencies through shifting the focus from individual to collective responsibility.

For further discussion of the complex, changing nature of social work organisations, see Adams et al., 2009a, Chapter 9 and Adams et al., 2009c, Chapter 19.

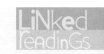

Banks, S. (2004) *Ethics, Accountability and the Social Professions*, Basingstoke, Palgrave Macmillan. Explores the impact of changes in the organisation and practice of social, community and youth work in Britain on ethics in professional life, including a research-based chapter, 'The new accountability and the ethics of distrust'. Offers further details of the interviews on which this chapter is based.

Banks, S. (2006) *Ethics and Values in Social Work*, 3rd edn, Basingstoke, Palgrave Macmillan. Overview of social work ethics, including discussion of blame and responsibility, the role of codes of ethics and analysis of practice dilemmas.

Buttny, R. (1993) *Social Accountability in Communication*, London, Sage. Exploration of the use of accounts in everyday and professional talk, with analyses of a variety of examples of conversation, including a 'welfare interview'.

Chadwick, R. (ed.) (1994) *Ethics and the Professions*, Aldershot, Avebury. Includes useful contributions by Holdsworth and Tadd on accountability.

Hall, C., Slembrouck, S. and Sarangi, S. (2006) *Language Practices in Social Work: Categorisation and Accountability in Child Welfare*, London, Routledge. Examines language practices in social work with children and families, using a discourse analysis approach, including useful chapters on 'Categorisation and accountability' and 'Justifying action in a public inquiry'.

Acknowledgements

I am grateful to the practitioners who gave interviews, to Robin Williams for references to sociological studies of accountability and to the Leverhulme Trust for a research fellowship in 2000–1, during which the first version of this chapter was written.

Identity, individual rights and social justice

4

This chapter deals with questions of rights and justice and shows how these seemingly abstract ideas are of immediate concern to social workers. It examines how five different ways of conceptualising the state affect policies, people's identities, rights and obligations to each other in society. The view we have affects how we define and label the 'client' of social workers. As critical practitioners, we need to manage the tensions between people's individual rights as citizens and what principles of individual and social justice regard as due to all people.

Chapter overview

Rights and justice in social work

Social work is committed to individual rights. Every prescription for good practice holds that the client has the right to respect, autonomy, proper consideration of their interests and so on. Bad practice is often described as a failure to satisfy the relevant rights. We say, for example, that a young person who was abused in residential care was denied their legitimate right to a safe and wholesome upbringing conducive to proper growth and development.

Social work is equally committed to justice. Every plausible conception of social work builds in some ideal of social justice, such as the belief that individuals experiencing the effects of structural inequalities in society are entitled to fairer treatment because a morally wrong state of affairs needs to be corrected. Justice is a large and complex aim and, like rights, can seldom be perfectly achieved; but like the denial of rights, manifest injustice in service practice is always a priority concern. Nowadays, it is widely felt, for example, that requiring older people to sell their assets in order to pay for care is unjust.

The different faces of rights and justice can be illustrated by thinking about policies for the welfare of children. In Western countries, nothing attracts more popular outrage than the violation of children's rights in publicised but isolated cases of gross abuse and murder – especially when the social services are seen to have failed in their job of protection. In other places, social leaders may be more concerned about the systematic injustices and wholesale damage to human rights perpetrated on entire populations of children who do not have access to clean water and adequate food.

Rights and justice are not necessarily opposed in principle. Justice can be defined precisely as the satisfaction of rights, and the satisfaction of rights as the necessary outcome of truly just social arrangements. However, in the situated reality of service practice, there is a tension between the pursuit of social justice – with the emphasis on collectivity – and the fulfilling of individual rights – with the emphasis on individuality. The tension can be illustrated between two contrasting fields of practice: community development (see Chapter 11), and community care assessment under the NHS and Community Care Act 1990 (see Chapter 28).

Community development workers in social work, adult and community education and other related fields work in an enabling capacity with members of local communities to address issues of local concern. Community development differs from the mainstream of social work (with which it has had a lifelong ambiguous relationship) in that the primary focus is on the needs and aspirations of communities as a whole, rather than on the individuals who comprise them. Thus, it comes naturally in community work to cast its objectives as the pursuit of social justice. For example, a community may argue that the lack of effective and accessible public transport constitutes for its members a systematic injustice in comparison with the privileged position of car owners – who benefit from hidden subsidies denied to public transport users. Community workers tend to judge their efforts in terms of improvements in social justice brought about by global changes in that community; their concern for justice in the lives of particular individuals is secondary to their concern for systemic improvements in social justice. As a rule, community workers give priority to working with groups on local public issues over working with individuals and their private troubles, although in practice the distinction is often difficult to see and harder still to adhere to.

Community care assessment is the cornerstone of social work responsibilities for disabled adults since the 1990 Act. On behalf of the local authorities, social workers carry out assessments of adults who may have difficulty in managing the ordinary demands of everyday life. Social workers, and their clients, may well see this process as aiming to satisfy individual rights, for example someone's right to choose to continue living in their own home despite disabilities, and their entitlement to receive the publicly funded services that would make it possible. For social workers in community care, the individual service user's rights are at the top of the agenda. While it might be expected they should be concerned for social justice in the wider arena of publicly sponsored social care, that concern is secondary to securing improvements in the rights of the individuals with whom they are actually working. They will advocate for their client, whose interests in a world of scarce resources may be in competition with others. The possibility that successful advocacy in a particular case may actually decrease the justice of the system as a whole is not an issue that the case manager can afford to consider.

Practising rights and justice: five models

Rights and justice are both indispensable in social work (Clark, 2000; Jordan with Jordan, 2000; BASW, 2002; Jones et al., 2004; Connolly and Ward, 2008), but seem to be in tension and perhaps even contradiction. Critical practice demands, at the very least, a provisional answer to this tension. This section discusses several different models of the identity of the client or service user (to use two of the common terms). From these follow a number of ways of understanding rights and justice in social work practice. It will be seen that the appropriate term for 'client' itself depends on the understanding of the client's identity. I shall argue that it is by seeing the participant (as I prefer to say) as citizen that the tension between rights and justice is best addressed.

In his discussion of the 'imaginary relations' between the public and the state in the sphere of welfare, Hughes (1998) argues that the postwar, social democratic idea of the welfare state has disintegrated under attacks from both the political Left and Right. He proposes three models that might replace it: 'consumerism', 'community' and 'citizenship'. This typology will be adapted here and expanded by adding a further model based on feminist ethics of care. We begin with the social democratic model that some presume is obsolete.

The social democratic welfare state: clients

The social democratic welfare state assumes that it is the responsibility of the state to guarantee certain standards of conventionally defined welfare, especially in the traditionally recognised areas of income protection, health, education, housing and – to a more limited extent – social care. The public as clients are treated as largely passive recipients of services devised by an expert elite of policy makers and delivered by professionals or lower grade staff working under professional supervision. Rights are fulfilled and social justice is served by ensuring that the public actually receive what policy is supposed to provide; the public are deemed not sophisticated or knowledgeable enough to need any substantial influence over the content of services or policy aimed at them.

While nostalgia for the old social democratic dream of comprehensive, socially provided, expertly administered welfare services is by no means extinct, it entails a model of professional authority that is no longer tenable. The public have lost faith in the promises and purported expertise of professionals – perhaps more in social work than in some other areas of welfare. In the public mind, rights to welfare can no longer be restricted to what experts decide is good for us. Moreover, the social democratic notion of justice is biased by the working assumption that all members of society who share a particular condition of need – say, for example, help with childcare – should be satisfied with a similar choice and level of services – say, institutional daycare from a certain age. However, in a multicultural society, this is insensitive to differences arising from personal and cultural background or different social values.

Critical practice must therefore be dissatisfied with the old social democratic ideal of welfare. Its concept of rights is too limited, since the selection of rights identified by experts as the proper targets of welfare policy is apt to seem essentially arbitrary. Its notion of justice is biased towards a universalism that misfits the pluralism of postmodernity. The social consensus essential to the social democratic model of welfare has disappeared, or perhaps it would be more accurate to say that the voices that were suppressed during the dominance of social democratic welfare are now being heard, and they reject it.

The consumerist welfare state: consumers

The consumerist welfare state supposes that welfare needs are no different in principle from the other needs that individuals look to satisfy in the market. The essentials for welfare have always been partly supplied by the market even when, as for example in health, it was the aim of policy to insulate recipients and beneficiaries from the fortunes of markets. Marketisation of what were previously areas for direct public provision was crucial to the policies of the so-called New Right in the 1970s and 80s. For libertarians, it is a prime right of citizens to participate freely in markets. The effects of markets are in themselves neither just nor unjust, but interfering with markets is an infringement of liberty and therefore a source of injustice.

While there is now little support for distribution based on pure libertarian market principles, there is a more pervasive general reliance on contrived and regulated, rather than free, market mechanisms. Thus, for example, transport, communications and public utilities are regulated markets in which private and public organisations compete on terms controlled by state agencies. In social work, these principles are increasingly being adopted in all areas of service provision.

In the consumerist welfare state, the client is a consumer and professionals become primarily oriented to customer relations. For at least some user groups, this new consumerism may bring what they have long sought, for example, in the case of service users with disabilities, the possibility of becoming their own care managers, or their relatives undertaking the care management, instead of being forced to depend on the discretion of service professionals.

The consumerist welfare state promises some improvement in rights. On the other hand, it is founded on a meagre and unsatisfactory concept of justice. To regard citizens as no more than consumers ignores the wider contexts of social living and public responsibility. It is widely argued that the consumption of community care can never be equivalent to the consumption of groceries. This is partly because market mechanisms do not, in reality, function adequately to deliver social care. The consumers of publicly supported social care are in an inherently weak position and their power as consumers is highly circumscribed. Furthermore, giving and receiving social care is a qualitatively different activity from buying groceries; the complex issues of social relationships and social value are not understood within the functional commodity transactions of the market.

The communitarian welfare state: community members

The social democratic and consumerist welfare states are familiar from recent history and current experience. The remaining models are more tentative and exploratory. The communitarian welfare state is represented in the protests and proposals of a number of minority interests who have not so far greatly influenced the mainstream of welfare policy and practice.

For communitarians, it is fundamental that people's very identity is created in the statuses and relationships established and continually renewed in the communities to which they belong. Communitarianism rejects the abstract autonomous individual of liberalism, who – once basic human needs are satisfied – is considered to have no values and no projects beyond those he freely chooses for himself. For communitarians, the point is that no meaningful identity and no life worth living are conceivable apart from the concrete obligations and benefits entailed by one's own particular tradition, culture and involvement in a particular set of relationships. Communitarians stress the mutual responsibilities of community members and their shared duty and right to participate in the daily political processes (Tam, 1998).

There is no single or leading project for a communitarian welfare state. Indeed, that would be fundamentally incompatible with the community focus and pluralist principles of communitarianism, which expects and entitles communities to develop their own particular versions of welfare. Reflections of communitarianism are found in several versions of community social work. The locally based and personally committed approach to working with individuals and groups in areas of high social deprivation, long advocated by Bob Holman (1993), bears many of the characteristics of communitarianism. The Barclay Committee (1982) proposed a reformation – or reaffirmation – of social work that would widen its focus to address the social functioning of communities, and its first minority report (Brown et al., 1982) argued that the way forward was patch working. Similar approaches continued to be advocated for some two decades after Barclay (Smale et al., 2000).

In the communitarian welfare state, it hardly makes sense to speak of the 'client' at all. Instead we should think of community members who from time to time may need particular support, which should primarily be provided by other members of the community on a basis of reciprocity and in a spirit of common membership or fellowship. This does not preclude the employment of professionals, but where they are employed, they should be subject to the active governance of involved community members. Of course this is a far cry from the bureaucratic state services that currently dominate welfare provision.

Despite some affinities between communitarianism and the Third Way particularly favoured by the first New Labour government (Jordan with Jordan, 2000), there is apparently little prospect of communitarian models being adopted as the favoured template for social work services in the UK. To do so would involve a renunciation of power and financial control from central government to local communities that runs altogether contrary to the centralist tradition and practice of British politics. Nevertheless, there are elements in communitarianism that merit a place in the wider debate about reforming welfare.

Feminism and the welfare state: partners in relationships

The feminist critique of welfare is many sided and far-reaching (see, for example, George and Wilding, 1994, Ch. 6). Everyone knows that feminists have demolished the presumption that caring ought to be primarily a female activity, provided by mothers, wives, daughters and low-paid female servants. Many feminists have argued that it is the state, not female family members, that we should look to when care is needed for children and dependent adults. In some ways, the argument has been won, in theory if not yet in practice. It is no longer tenable that women should be systematically disadvantaged in the many areas of social life where men's interests have traditionally been dominant, and the public roles and private behaviour of men and women have begun to shift as a result.

There is another aspect of the feminist critique that is perhaps less widely appreciated. In the liberal tradition, persons are seen in the abstract as moral agents and bearers of universal rights. In this view, rights are not affected by one's specific obligations to the particular, real individuals with whom one happens to have actual, ongoing relationships. Some feminists argue that women think differently, choosing instead to give priority to their real primary relationships over abstract theoretical obligations. They hold that our understanding of moral responsibility has been unbalanced by universalist models of human relationships that are excessively abstract, impersonal and decontextualised – products of essentially masculine thought. Other feminists have wanted to celebrate the virtues of subjectivity without abandoning the rights that feminism has hard won out of liberalism, such as a woman's right to control her fertility. They resist giving way to any new essentialism about gender as false as the ones that feminism has spent so much energy repudiating (Sevenhuijsen, 1998).

Feminism provides no single, coherent answer to the question of how best to understand the identities of the givers and recipients of care, whether in the private sphere of personal relationships or in the public domain of welfare services. What feminism does put irrevocably on the welfare agenda is that users of formal services are, among other things, individually known persons to whom professionals as well as their own kin are bound by partly subjective ties of partnership in actual human relationships. The relations of welfare, therefore, are not accurately described or properly prescribed by the abstract role obligations favoured in the traditional discourse of the human service professions.

Citizenship

The identity of the participant in welfare services is most fruitfully addressed through the idea of citizenship (Coote, 1992; Clark, 2000; Powell, 2001; Dean, 2004; see also Adams et al., 2009c, Ch. 11). Citizenship invites us to think of the rights and duties of the individual as supported, enmeshed and realised in society. Civil and political rights are promised under the law and the constitution. Formal social, or welfare, rights reflect the rising expectations of human living that follow from prosperity. However, citizenship does not end with formal legal provisions and duties: it acknowledges that the individual's identity is realised in relation to innumerable informal filaments of social obligation and trust, and it requires citizens to recognise each other as mutually obligated and equally responsible. Citizenship thus incorporates the valuable attributes of the four preceding models, while offering checks on their less desirable features.

Social rights rest as much on the informal expectations and commitments that members of the community have in relation to each other as on the agencies and professions that constitute the formal services. In social services, it is convenient to speak of service participants – a term that deliberately dims the traditional distinctions between professionals, clients and the wider community. We should think, first, of professionals, participant/recipients, their carers and dependants, and the wider community as fellow citizens; as commonly protected and obligated by the shared rights and duties of citizenship. The policy papers of the 'modernising' New Labour government and the writings of its intellectual mentors (Commission on Social Justice, 1994; Giddens, 1998a) suggest one interpretation of citizenship rights. Critics of social services who advocate greater user involvement and participation in the provision and evaluation of social care have a different and more radical emphasis. But it is the discourse of citizenship that best contains the debate over rights and justice.

Critical practice and citizenship

The pursuit of individual rights may lead to the neglect, if not the contradiction, of social justice. How should critical practice address this tension?

A critical approach combines reflective and sceptical observation with positive and committed activism. Critical practice is alert to flaws in the veracity of observation, to defects in the basis of alleged evidence, to faulty inference and deduction and other common types of empirical and logical error. The critical observer accepts the reports, explanations or teachings of others only after attempting to subject them to some degree of independent scrutiny and evaluation. Moreover, the critical observer treats received knowledge and doctrine as matters to be questioned, as embedded in ideology, whereby the content of knowledge is necessarily formed by its conduit.

The critical activist or practitioner, however, knows that the scope for mere scepticism is infinite, and that no practical progress is possible without accepting the risks of committed action under conditions of inescapable empirical uncertainty and moral doubt. Critical practice is thus engaged in the world as well as contemplative of it. Critical practice embodies a theoretically informed vision:

> Theory … helps practical actors deal with social change by helping them see beyond the immediacy of what is at any particular moment to conceptualise something of what could be. (Calhoun, 1996: 436)

A mentality of critical practice accepts the tension of the perpetually irreconcilable demands of reflection and action.

Conclusion

The five conceptions of the identity of service recipients or participants – as clients, consumers, community members, partners in relationships or citizens – are all powerfully (but unequally) influential in the contemporary world of welfare. Critical practice teaches that each perspective has its value as a particular interpretation of rights and justice. But critical practice is sustained by having a common language within which conflicts of value can be articulated. Indeed, it is arguable that without such a common language, the attempt to improve rights and justice will necessarily fail, since we should have, in the end, no mutually intelligible way of judging progress. The dialogue on citizenship provides the best route to a resolution. In the pursuit of rights and justice, critical practice must embrace the concept of citizenship, yet remain somewhat dissatisfied with every reading of it.

For further discussion of rights and mental health work, see Adams et al., 2009c, Chapter 8, and for ethical aspects of researching practice, see Adams et al., 2009c, Chapter 20.

Asquith, S., Clark, C. and Waterhouse, L. (2005) *The Role of the Social Worker in the 21st Century: A Literature Review*, Edinburgh, Scottish Executive, www.scotland.gov.uk/Resource/Doc/47121/0020821.pdf. Study commissioned to guide policy review of the role of social workers in Scotland.

Brechin, A., Brown, H. and Eby, M.A. (eds) (2000) *Critical Practice in Health and Social Care*, London, Sage. Useful collection of essays on problems of welfare practice.

Campbell, T. (1988) *Justice*, Basingstoke: Macmillan – now Palgrave Macmillan. Clear textbook on theories of justice.

Clark, C.L. (2000) *Social Work Ethics: Politics, Principles and Practice*, Basingstoke, Macmillan – now Palgrave Macmillan. Provides a general ethical and political theory for social work, and develops the idea of social work as welfare citizenship.

Dean, H. (ed.) (2004) *The Ethics of Welfare: Human Rights, Dependency and Responsibility*, Bristol, Policy Press. Combines theoretical analysis, policy review and empirical research findings to look at welfare rights and citizenship obligations.

Hughes, G. (ed.) (1998) *Imagining Welfare Futures*, London, Routledge. Focuses on changing ideas of the place of welfare in contemporary societies.

Jordan, B. (2004) 'Emancipatory social work? Opportunity or oxymoron', *British Journal of Social Work*, 34(1): 5–19. Critical review of social work's current professional project and identity from a leading author.

Sevenhuijsen, S. (1998) *Citizenship and the Ethics of Care: Feminist Considerations on Justice, Morality and Politics*, London, Routledge. A particularly reflective application of feminist insights to the provision of care under official auspices.

Pushing ethical boundaries for children and families

5

This chapter explores the complex territory of balancing the core ethical tenet of confidentiality with transparency and openness in child and family policy and practice. It draws on Indigenous and asylum seeker examples as a challenge to the erosion of social work values by employers and the state.

Chapter overview

Introduction

At different times and in different contexts, social work is faced with new dilemmas and challenges and confronted with the need to interrogate and adapt its philosophies and practices. This is nowhere clearer than in the field of child and family welfare, where social workers have been compelled to move beyond their comfort zones to embrace 'new' approaches that appear in different guises. In many ways, social work has adapted well. In other ways the profession has lagged behind. This chapter explores some of the dilemmas facing the social work profession in clinging to traditional tenets in the wake of change. The chapter uses two examples from the Australian context: Indigenous peoples and asylum seekers. The term 'Indigenous' is the preferred term to describe the Aboriginal and Torres Strait Islander peoples of Australia. The chapter explores the specific issue of whether concepts of confidentiality are oppositional to increasing pressures for transparency in policy and practice. This issue is one that challenges to the very core some of the fundamental values of social work, particularly as framed within codes of ethics, and exemplifies the contradictions inherent in the contemporary context of social work practice.

Changing conditions in which social work is managed and practised

In the policy context, social work is increasingly working within a managerialist framework, where corporate planning processes have been transplanted from the private sector into the human services (Hough and Briskman, 2003). No longer is social work practice based primarily on need, but effective practice is often conceptualised organisationally as meeting the demands of funding bodies where financial accountability and certainty evolve as key driving principles. This is happening at the same time that the profession is grappling to include human rights and social justice concepts in its everyday practice, concepts that do not sit easily in a managerialist climate. Managerialism creates a closed environment where the principles of privacy, containment, mainstreaming and competition thrive, constructs that are antithetical to social work's engagement with postmodern concepts of diversity and context. Managerialism pervades both the government and non-government sectors where child and family welfare are located. This results in social workers experiencing a gap between their ideals and the realities of practice (Lymbery and Butler, 2004).

Social work has also had to adjust to new family forms, with the increased acceptance of single-parent families, gay and lesbian families and newly arrived migrant and refugee families with varying cultural mores. The profession has been required to discard Western views of family, acknowledging a range of child rearing practices and adopting new forms of intervention. There has been pressure for social work to respond to media criticism of child protection practice, taking the relatively privatised realm of the organisation into the public sphere. In addition, social work has had to adapt itself to interdisciplinary ways of working, accelerated by increasing deprofessionalisation and the claim by others that social work does not hold the keys to effective human services practice in its own right. In so doing, it has needed to re-explore its conceptual frameworks as the world of the caseworker/client is opened to new methodologies that combine advocacy and critical reflexiveness in its endeavours.

Despite continually emerging questions and contradictions, the social work profession largely resists major reforms. Although there are new theories, methodologies and pressures, social work traditionalism prevails, guided by competency-based practice and codes of ethics that are largely individualistic. These are vexed issues for a profession that is, at least in its rhetoric, endeavouring to reinvent itself.

The pervasiveness of notions of confidentiality reflects its importance in maintaining client interests, and there would be little justification for arguing for its abandonment. But maintaining confidentiality uncritically conflicts with notions of transparency, social change goals and advocacy, and has the potential to distance social workers from others working for social and political change. With increasing challenges to concepts of confidentiality, there is a revisiting of accusations of the social control function of social work and the view that social work, as it is still practised, emphasises power differentials. This is exacerbated by work environments and a broader political context where human rights may be eroded through adhering to narrow tenets of confidentiality that impose limits on the capacity to expose practices that violate human rights.

Social work with children and families in the new era

Social work with children and families takes a number of forms, but in many Western nations, including Australia, the emphasis is on 'protection' at the 'hard' end of the scale, rather than prevention and support. To a degree, social workers have colluded with the media line that exposes child deaths and publishes photographs of damaged children. Public inquiries continue to reinforce the notion of protection in a narrow sense. In Australia, as elsewhere, child protection offers employment opportunities for social workers. Social work with children and families creates confusion and ideological conflicts for many. Social workers are confronted with a barrage of rules, procedural manuals and a lack of support structures. The turnover of social workers in these positions is high. Many do not have opportunities to question 'the system' and provide alternatives. In addition, they are usually restricted from speaking out or publicly challenging policies. The demand to meet performance targets means that there is little time, energy or opportunity to work for social reform.

The centrality of confidentiality to child and family practice is reinforced by privacy provisions, including in legislation which specifies penalties for those who breach them. In some settings, social workers may also be required to sign confidentiality agreements. In addition to constraints on freedom to speak, there may be limits imposed on community engagement that are seen as a 'conflict of interest'. This contributes to the silencing of social workers and an inability to advocate for the interests of groups with whom they work. We need to question in whose interests these provisions are introduced and enforced. For, as Humphries (2004) expounds, social work has choices to make about a new moral effort to engage its knowledge about sources of inequality with a new sense of imperative and urgency.

There have been challenges to confidentiality and privacy around the 'right to know' in spheres such as adoption, artificial insemination and IVF. The freedom of information provisions of governments in Australia have partially paved the way for an openness not previously contemplated. Social work also has to be mindful of debates and developments in other spheres. This includes the 'confessional' where Catholic priests are being challenged about maintaining secrecy in cases where the confession involves criminal offences including child sexual abuse. Social workers are aware that they may be commanded to appear in court to give testimony, or for their documentation to be compulsorily acquired for evidence.

The language of 'risk management' that has now entered the social work domain is a constraint to openness, flexibility and collaborative approaches for change (see Adams et al., 2009c, Ch. 4 for further discussion of risk management). Although the intent is seemingly directed at reducing the potential for harm to the people with whom we work, much of the discourse is underpinned by fear of risk to governments or organisations. The concern of a backlash against harm to children results in increased regulation and procedurally driven practice. This has the effect of increasing organisational restrictiveness and creating a climate where there is little scope for responsiveness and transparency through open debate by social workers. Rather than exposing the irrationality of many of these directives, social workers may inadvertently collude with repressive policies. Terms such as 'competences', 'risk assessment' and 'case management' are now accepted in social work practice frameworks (Ward, 1996: 152).

Questions arise as to how social workers can identify the consequences of their actions when endeavouring to adhere to policy and practice directives. This requires a great deal of reflexivity and analysis on the part of a social worker in determining a course of action, an approach that requires time and sometimes courage. Problems can particularly arise in settings where social work is not dominant.

The two examples outlined in this chapter – Indigenous children and asylum seeker children – will hopefully resonate with others in their own practice domains. Underlying the issues explored is a plea for social workers to move beyond the immediate pressures in their practice in order to speak out, support alternative voices and join with activists. There is a pressing need for a changing accountability beyond the profession and the organisation to accountability based on relationships with the range of groups with whom social workers interact. To do so requires courage, reflexivity and a constant analysis of complex boundary questions that pervade social work practice.

The boundaries of confidentiality

The question of confidentiality raises ethical, legal, moral, organisational and professional issues. One of the ways forward in trying to apply or limit tenets of confidentiality is for social workers to always pose the question as to where their basic accountability rests. From a human rights perspective, the answer should be the powerless and the most vulnerable and not with the professions and the powerful.

Arguably, there are some circumstances where confidentiality is clear, whether prescribed or not. But in their daily work social workers confront problems of many kinds, demonstrating that confidentiality is neither absolute nor sacred, but is contingent on a range of factors that need to be taken into account in specific situations. What is one's obligation if a client's partner does not know they are HIV positive? What does a social worker do when a repeat child sex offender is living in a household with young children after serving a sentence? What is the right course of action when a young adolescent does not want their whereabouts disclosed to family members? What of the diversity of cultural understandings about confidentiality? And even though the primary responsibility is to the client, there may be other competing responsibilities, including to the wider community.

Government and community service organisations purport to have high degrees of confidentiality. Yet once a record and file-keeping system is established, the likelihood of total secrecy is diminished. With the advent of computerised records and email, this is compounded. Over and beyond the technology, there has always been an informal sharing of client information between workers and between agencies, creating an artificial barrier between private information and public space. Social workers do not operate in a practice vacuum, they are generally consultative and the 'social' in social work lends itself to practices that involve a large group of stakeholders. This collaboration is usually seen as meritorious, but it can also result in breaches of legal and policy standards and is justified 'in the interests of the client' and the 'duty of care'. In fact, it becomes normative and is not questioned. Yet this can constitute a clear violation of the rights of the individual client. As clients begin to form themselves into 'consumer' organisations, these questions are likely to arise further.

The ethics of confidentiality

In my experience as a field educator, I found that when social work students and practitioners were asked what they knew of social work ethics, most said they never used
them. They were, however, able to refer to confidentiality as a key element of the code
of ethics. Few students or their supervisors talked about influencing or even subverting
policy. Many did not see the link between maintaining secrecy as a form of control and
perpetuating a system that can act against the interests of families and communities.

A fundamental problem is that social work is still basically viewed as an individual
rather than a collective activity. This is reinforced in codes of ethics and adherence to
the concept of confidentiality per se reinforces this. Transparency, multiple accountabilities and critical and transformative practice remain elusive. An exploration of social
work codes of ethics in a range of countries uncovered an emphasis on individual
choice, minimising structural disadvantage and social dependency (Briskman and
Noble, 1999).

Confidentiality is clearly enshrined in various social work codes of ethics throughout the world. For example, the codes of the British (BASW, 2003), US (NASW, 1996)
and Australian (AASW, 1999) social work associations all contain clauses that refer to
client confidentiality and/or privacy. However, it appears that the concept is under some
challenge. A draft document on ethics, formally adopted by delegates to the 2004 AGM
of the International Federation of Social Workers (IFSW, 2004) in Adelaide, states:

> Social workers should maintain confidentiality regarding information about people who
> use their services. Exceptions to this may only be justified on the basis of a greater
> ethical requirement (such as the preservation of life).

It is unclear what the full gamut of 'exception' might be, and to date there has been little
exploration of issues of transparency, human rights, social justice and advocacy and how
these might relate to confidentiality principles. This chapter is work in process in
endeavouring to understand the limits to confidentiality and the ensuing boundary
issues. The following examples highlight some key tensions.

Indigenous children

In a number of countries, including Australia, the US and Canada, children were
removed from their families in what was considered their 'best interests'. Although these
policies and practices took different forms in each country and within each jurisdiction,
children were often placed far from their families in institutions, or with foster care or
adoptive families. This practice is no less than institutionalised and systemic abuse of
children (Thorpe, 1986), and was usually assimilationist in intent. Assimilation in these
contexts can be defined as endeavours to eliminate Indigenous peoples and cultures
by ensuring that children, particularly those of 'mixed race', were absorbed into non-
Indigenous life ways and that their own cultures, languages and families were discarded.
When the Human Rights and Equal Opportunity Commission (HREOC, 1997) in

Australia released the findings of a national inquiry into what is now referred to as the 'stolen generations', there were many in the wider community who expressed astonishment and denied knowledge of the practices. The public disclosure was drawn from more than 500 oral testimonies from Indigenous people and the practices they describe have been referred to as 'evil' (Rintoul, cited in Garrett, 1996), 'an Australian holocaust' (Katona, cited in McLean, 1996), 'genocide' (HREOC, 1997) and as attempts 'to take the Aboriginality out of Aboriginal children' (Dodson, 1997).

In 1997, research was conducted on the role of church agencies in the removal and placement of Aboriginal children in the state of Victoria. To their credit, the three participating churches – Anglican, Catholic and Uniting – saw this new openness as a form of reconciliation and apology to Aboriginal people for past wrongs. But their openness was restricted by a legacy of past practices, practices that remain hidden from public scrutiny. Examination of the records revealed that in the interests of assimilation, Aboriginal identity was not referred to in the files. It was sometimes only by racist comments contained within the documentation that Aboriginality was evident. It was even more disturbing to realise, as a researcher, that many of those who had been in the children's homes were probably unaware of their Aboriginal origins, the ultimate betrayal of confidentiality.

Part of the collusion in maintaining the secrecy has been a dominant discourse that privileges the views of professionals over those affected by the policies and practices. Since the time of European colonisation, policy-making has regrettably always been a 'white' activity in Australia. As historian Peter Read (1981: 20) notes: 'white people have never been able to leave Aborigines alone'. This does not bode well for Indigenous groups who still struggle to have their voices heard on policy agendas. Despite the existence in legislation and policy throughout Australia of an Aboriginal Child Placement Principle that advocates for keeping Indigenous children with their families and communities, this has not been fully adhered to in practice (Briskman, 2003).

Powerful advocacy by Indigenous peoples in Australia and elsewhere ensures that alternative ways of changing hearts and minds are in the public arena. The confidentiality that shrouds the activities of social workers is in stark contrast to the songs, autobiographies and films that tell personal stories in order to paint a picture that touches hearts and minds in endeavours to expose the 'locked cupboard of history' (Hartley and McKee, 2001: 1) and prevent ongoing oppressive practices. Storytelling has the potential to be healing and influential. Indigenous groups have united in many ways to ensure that their experiences reach the public domain. In research on stolen generations advocacy, Indigenous people told of how they 'had the same stories' throughout Australia, stories of the horror of child removal that were only exposed when Indigenous people united to form national organisations to advocate for their causes (Briskman, 2003).

Indigenous organisations lobbied long and hard for an inquiry into the stolen generations to bring out the truth and determine how many children had been taken away and how this had occurred (Briskman, 2003). This was in part to counteract what Aboriginal writer and historian Jackie Huggins (1998: 120) describes as being 'fed on a diet of lies and invisibility about the true history of this country from a very young age'. This amounts to what was described by anthropologist Stanner as the 'great Australian silence' (cited in McGrath, 1995: 366).

Many of the practices involving the removal of Indigenous children from their families and communities were shrouded in the utmost secrecy. With many Indigenous children enslaved in missions, reserves and children's homes, the practices were hidden from public scrutiny. In some institutions, the names of children were changed and their origins were not recognised (Minajalku, 1997). Yet the extent of the 'success' of the secrecy of these practices has been challenged. Newspapers reveal stories of public indignation at removal practices (Haebich, 1998), as well as evidence emerging of campaigns and public opinion against Aboriginal child removals (Paisley, 1997). Yet these endeavours did not reach the public sufficiently to bring about change.

EXaMPLE

The practices of policy imposition and lack of transparency continue. This was exemplified by the federal government of the deposed Prime Minister John Howard, which, in June 2007, declared a national emergency in the Northern Territory. Ostensibly to deal with child abuse, the interventions announced by the federal government were monumental, including sending in the military and the police, widespread alcohol restrictions, welfare restrictions, enforced school attendance, compulsory health checks for all Aboriginal children and the acquisition of townships (Hinkson, 2007). The announcement was made just before a federal election in which the conservative coalition was losing support and many Indigenous people and their supporters were highly suspicious of the underlying motives for the intervention. The measures were introduced abruptly, astounding many including social workers who were among those who spoke out against what was happening. The most powerful opposition was from the National Coalition of Aboriginal and Torres Strait Islander Social Workers Association. This is not to deny existing problems, but myriads of quality research reports were discounted by the government in policy formulations. On the other hand, media reporting rampaged to expose problems in a sensationalist way, with an emphasis on family 'dysfunction'. In this scenario, social workers employed in such settings needed to step outside the client–worker relationship and organisational restrictions, both of which were inevitably at risk of breaking down after such actions, and to speak publicly of the harms created, the ineffectuality of the policies and the devastating impact on the families and children with whom they work.

There is now talk of a 'constructed silence' in Aboriginal affairs, not just based on mere ignorance of Australian history but an exercise in actively reconstructing known history to remove the crimes of white colonisation (Indigenous Social Justice Association, 2003: 1). Yet some social workers have refused to collude with the silence or cooperate with the authorities. Bill Jordan (1990: 6) comments that social workers do participate in isolated acts of banditry, although there is limited engagement in a systematic manner to challenge systems that continue to oppress. One Indigenous activist, Mary Graham, speaks of how in the early days of Indigenous people organising to control the future of their children, some social workers met with Indigenous organisations after hours and under cover, as they were not legally allowed to talk to them. She tells of car chases in the streets because the government department suspected that such meetings were occurring (Briskman, 2003).

Asylum seekers

There is a view, somewhat contested, that Indigenous child removal practices are of the past and based on 'good intentions', 'standards of the time' and a high level of community ignorance. There is no possibility for anyone to express such views about asylum-seeking children, in the light of information constantly before the general populace in a number of countries including Australia and England (Cemlyn and Briskman, 2003).

In Australia, there is no clearer evidence of the systemic abuse of children than in the treatment of asylum seekers. The practices of immigration authorities are shrouded in secrecy, masked behind the political rhetoric of border protection, people-smuggling containment and controlled immigration. Through closed processes, the federal government has gone to great lengths to mask the abuses of children, even presenting false images of children being thrown overboard on their way to Australia, and refusing to respond to allegations of complicity in the tragic drowning of 353 asylum seekers, including many children, on their way to Australia in 2001. Despite intense advocacy from community groups, including legal challenges, children remained incarcerated in detention centres until 2005 in Australia and Nauru, which was part of the so-called 'Pacific solution'.

Despite a wall of silence in detention centres, many people endeavoured to expose the injustices of the system of mandatory detention of asylum seekers who arrive without authorisation. These include journalists, church groups, actors, activist organisations and professional bodies. They circulated information about individuals that the government hid in the name of confidentiality. Social workers have taken a lead, with the Australian Council of Heads of Schools of Social Work convening the People's Inquiry into Detention, which held public hearings and received written submissions in an endeavour to influence policy and ensure that the stories of detention are on the public record (ACHSSW, 2006). In detaining children, Australia flouted UN conventions, including the UN Convention on the Rights of the Child, which it has ratified. The ongoing damage to children of these practices is being continually exposed by professional groups. Barbara Rogalla, a former nurse in a detention centre, is among those with insider knowledge who have spoken out about how the policies of the government placed children in conditions of pain and suffering. She argues that this could amount to torture as defined by the Convention against Torture and other Cruel, Inhuman or Degrading Treatment or Punishment (Rogalla, 2003). I have personally observed children behind the razor wire and electric fences, and have heard stories of self-harm, despair and loss of hope. An inquiry conducted by the Human Rights and Equal Opportunity Commission in 2002 spoke of the effects of institutional living on parenting, the exposure of children to adult disturbances, the harsh and restrictive environments and the dehumanisation. The federal Human Rights Commissioner Sev Odowski says that the treatment of refugees in detention centres is the harshest of the world, pointing out that by April 2003, 50 children had been detained for more than two years (Gallagher, 2003).

CASE EXAMPLE

The much publicised case of a small boy, Shayan Badraie, exemplifies the harms of locking up children. In his time in detention, Shayan became totally withdrawn and refused to eat. The harms inflicted were recognised through government compensation in a later out of court settlement (Briskman and Goddard, 2007). Ways to publicise information about detained children and to circumvent the privacy within occurred in a number of ways. In 2001, the Australian Broadcasting Commission programme, *Four Corners*, aired a video secretly recorded in the Villawood detention centre about the then six-year-old Shayan. The video explained that Shayan would not eat or drink and had become mute after witnessing acts of violence and self-harm, including discovering a man who had just slashed his wrists. He was admitted to hospital and rehydrated eight times and later diagnosed with post-traumatic stress disorder (Australian Broadcasting Commission, 2005).

The secrecy that veils detention has been described as an 'information lock-up'. This statement was coined by the *Business Review Weekly*, which revealed that the contents of a damning report on detention centres were kept secret (Washington, 2003: 18). The newspaper gained access to the contents only after a long-running Freedom of Information request. Other groups have spoken out with information they have gleaned in various ways. This includes some former staff of detention centres who, despite having signed confidentiality clauses, have publicised the plight of children and other detainees through the media, published articles and by speaking to the People's Inquiry.

Social workers have little contact with detention centres. They may, however, have some contact with those released into the community on much criticised temporary protection visas. A combination of overwork and fear of losing funding prevents many social workers from speaking out about what they see and hear. Yet recent research revealed extensive barriers to services and found prolonged suffering and "time torture" associated with temporary protection', with many refugees living in 'secondary detention' (Marston, 2003: 3).

A range of professional groups presented submissions to the national inquiry into children in detention. Submissions were received from former professional staff employed in detention centres, demonstrating the courage of some to speak out. Similarly, with the People's Inquiry, psychiatrists, nurses, GPs and psychologists have spoken about the ill-treatment of children and the long-term impact. More importantly, former detainees, including parents and their children, spoke out.

In 2002, the boundaries were tested by social work academics Chris Goddard and Max Liddell, when they reported systemic abuse of all the children in the Woomera detention centre to the South Australian protection service. Yet the South Australian government relinquished its authority for investigating such reports to the federal immigration authorities (Cemlyn and Briskman, 2003: 175). In a newspaper article, two social work academics called for an inquiry into the stolen childhoods in detention centres so that those complicit in this 'organised and ritualised abuse' be held personally accountable (Goddard and Briskman, 2004: 17). In another newspaper article, Goddard wrote about what he saw during a visit to a family in detention:

> I have seen an infant behind grey wires and electric fences, in a high-security prison on the edge of Australia's dead heart. I have seen her parents found guilty, without trial, of wanting freedom. I have seen parents so proud of their first-born, but so close to despair. I have seen an infant given a number. I have seen a baby girl kept in a cage. (Goddard, 2004)

As detention facilities are run by private prison operators, what are known as 'commercial in confidence' principles further diminish public knowledge on policies and practices. This was nowhere clearer than in a scenario I experienced at my former university, when, following fear of exposure, the university's public relations arm was forced to admit that a group of education faculty academics had participated in a tender with a private prison operator to provide education within Australia's detention centres. Together with another social work academic, Heather Fraser, and with the support of wide sections of the university including the staff and student union, some NGOs and immigration detainees themselves, a newspaper article was written to publicly outline the opposition (Briskman and Fraser, 2002), bringing some transparency into what had been a secretive process in the interests of commercial profit. In addition to the secrecy of the proposed venture, a range of ethical issues were identified, including the inappropriateness of financially profiting from people's misery, collusion in the government's propaganda war against asylum seekers and an implicit fatalism that mandatory detention was here to stay. The university withdrew the bid, established and resourced a refugee project to offer ethical and transparent assistance to asylum seekers and refugees, including the provision of free places to people on temporary protection visas. In taking our stance, as social workers, we saw our allegiance beyond the organisation in the interests of what we saw as a greater ethical good.

Interrogating accountability

One of the inherent contradictions in social work practice is that of competing account-abilities, some of which are vested in the scrutiny around professional practice. In delivering social work services to clients and families, social workers are confronted with contradictory expectations. Social work is very much an organisational activity (Jones and May, 1992), and there is strong pressure on social workers to work within the guidelines of their employing body, which usually has to comply with government funding agreements. Moreover, there is the accountability to the social work profession, with much of this framed by ethical codes.

Powell (2001: 129) reminds us that a dual mandate defines the role and task of social work as promoting the interests of both the state and the service users they purport to help. By definition, this dual mandate makes social work a politicised activ-ity. For some, this has involved a high degree of sensitisation to avoid the implications of the use of professional power. However, many social workers avoid the implications of the dual mandate by adopting an individualised therapeutic approach that locates social work in the apolitical world of psychology and the personalisation of social prob-lems. In Australia, the Human Rights and Equal Opportunity Commission (HREOC, 1997: 584) maintains that welfare departments continued to pathologise and individ-ualise the needs of Indigenous children. Jordan (1997: 219) talks of how many social workers have a stake in a style of work that is power laden, formal and individualised.

In South Africa, there has been some exploration around dual loyalty and human rights in the health sphere (Physicians for Human Rights, 2002), something from which the social work profession could learn. The Physicians for Human Rights note that dual loyalty becomes problematic when the professional acts to support the inter-ests of the state or other entity instead of those of the individual, in a manner that violates the human rights of the individual. One example they raise is where under a repressive government, pervasive human rights abuses combined with restrictions on freedom of expression render it difficult to resist state demands and report abuses. They comment that closed institutions and detention centres would come under this category, as they demand allegiance from health professionals even in the face of common human rights violations against those held there. The Physicians for Human Rights' analysis can extend further to asylum seekers and refugees in the community where violations of people's rights of access to services can arise from government-imposed policies, where professionals may be called on to withhold services from certain groups in discriminatory ways.

Conclusion

Opportunities for transformational social work
Social work is less able to hide behind the confi-dentiality mask as social workers become increas-ingly aware of human rights abuses, breaches of international obligations and practices that are antithetical to the values of social work. Although social

workers are unlikely to be direct perpetrators of current abuses, their knowledge, skills and espoused human rights and social justice values should result in using their voices to join others in advocating for change, adopting what Payne (1998: 127) refers to as the 'transformational potential of socialist-collectivist views'.

Ife (2001: 1) points out that human rights is one of the most powerful concepts in contemporary social and political discourse. Yet, it is a framework rarely embraced by social work in a rigorous or applied manner. Although a somewhat contested concept, particularly because of legalistic underpinnings and Western-driven approaches, more relevant human rights discourses are increasingly finding their way into a range of forms of practice, including with Indigenous peoples and asylum seekers. This presents challenges to social work's focus on the micro-elements of practice, and provides opportunities for more transparent practice. It can help to move practice away from the narrower accountabilities and create a more robust engagement with the politics of social work.

If social workers are to be committed to social change, justice, inclusion, diversity and participation, they must develop theories and practices that foreground social, political and economic power relations, as well as cultural relevance (Quinn, 2003). The profession needs to guard itself against co-option by a prevailing discourse that privileges individual rights and responsibilities (Briskman, 2001).

Fook (2002) talks about what counts as legitimate knowledge and whose knowledge is privileged. This is one of the issues with confidentiality, drawn as it is on professional tenets and acted on in specific ways that maintain professional 'integrity'. Fook (2002: 89) further explains that dominant discourses are powerful often because they are unquestioned. She explains that by pointing out the contradictions, there is scope to challenge and change dominant meaning systems. Social work could rise to the challenge presented by Adams (2002: 87) for the critical practitioner, who, he argues, 'offers the prospect of transformation by not being bound by the status quo'. He sees the critical practitioner as bringing to bear on a situation the contextual, theoretical and conceptual understandings of social work, and incorporating political engagement for a broader good.

Instead of seeing alternative voices as irrelevant to social work, there are opportunities for the profession to advocate for their inclusion in policy and practice decision-making. For Ife (1997: 181), social workers have a particular responsibility to allow the voices of the marginalised to be heard, by working alongside marginalised people and not taking it upon themselves to define the needs of the oppressed. Experience has shown that even those whose voices have been largely silenced through intentional government isolation, such as asylum seekers, are able to exercise agency, utilising other groups as vehicles to help in gaining access to the public sphere.

A revisiting of social work codes of ethics is warranted, with less concern for professionalism and a greater articulation of social work's unique positioning for advocacy and social change. In so doing, social work codes need to shift from their more individualistic positioning to embracing collective issues, framed around a sense of justice and rights. As with other codes, the Australian social work code of ethics does not push for activism on the part of its members (De Maria, 1997), and hence is being left behind as other professions engage with collective action.

If social work is to be truly inclusive and contribute effectively as a social change agent, it must continually reinvent its practice. The sphere of child and family welfare is a critical area for ongoing critique, analysis and engagement. A review of some of social work's basic tenets, including confidentiality, in the light of the ongoing challenges, is an urgent task for social work academics, professional organisations and practitioners.

For further discussion of risk and work with children and families, see Adams et al., 2009c, Chapter 4, and for work with asylum seekers and refugees, see Adams et al., 2009c, Chapter 9.

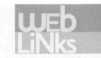

www.snaicc.asn.au Secretariat of National Aboriginal and Islander Child Care

www.hreoc.gov.au Human Rights and Equal Opportunity Commission, Australia

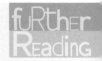

Briskman, L. (2003) 'Indigenous Australians: towards postcolonial social work', in J. Allan, B. Pease and L. Briskman (eds) *Critical Social Work: An Introduction to Theories and Practices*, Sydney, Allen & Unwin. Discusses how social work can respond to Indigenous families by not replicating the ideologies and practices that saw the removal of Aboriginal children from their families and communities. The problematic nature of dominant social work theories provides a useful reference point that can be considered in other fields of practice.

Briskman, L. (2007) *Social Work with Indigenous Communities*, Sydney, Federation Press. Useful in its exploration of how social work can engage with Indigenous peoples, avoiding the tensions associated with applying Western social work paradigms. Theoretical and practice leads are provided.

Briskman, L. and Noble, C. (1999) 'Social work ethics: embracing diversity?', in B. Pease and J. Fook (eds) *Transforming Social Work Practice: Postmodern Critical Perspectives*, St Leonards, Allen & Unwin. The challenge of making social work codes of ethics relevant to diverse communities is the subject of this chapter.

Drawing on research conducted by the authors, it endeavours to assist social workers and students to adopt a reflective and critical approach in their application of the codes to their practice.

Briskman, L., Latham, S. and Goddard, C. (2008) *Human Rights Overboard: Seeking Asylum in Australia*, Carlton North, Victoria, Australia, Scribe. Account of the brutal treatment of asylum seekers in Australian immigration centres, including children and their families. The harrowing testimonies are the work of the People's Inquiry into Detention conducted by social work academics in order to publicly expose malevolent policies and practices.

Hough, G. and Briskman, L. (2003) 'Responding to the changing socio-political context of practice', in J. Allan, B. Pease and L. Briskman (eds) *Critical Social Work: An Introduction to Theories and Practices*, Sydney, Allen & Unwin. Assists social workers to contextualise the constraints that limit the enacting practice that is coherent with social work frameworks and a social work value base. Presents emancipatory challenges for social work.

Ife, J. (2008) *Human Rights and Social Work: Towards Rights-based Practice*, 2nd edn, Cambridge, Cambridge University Press. Delves into how a human rights perspective can guide social work practice. Presents a clear analysis of the dimensions of human rights approaches and the paradoxes that exist.

Women's reproductive rights: issues and dilemmas for practice

6

Women's reproductive rights, linked to their roles as wife and mother, sexual expression and bodily integrity, are contested within patriarchal social relations. I explore their contradictions for practice around women's choices of adoption, the use of reproductive technologies and abortion. The new reproductive technologies offer women opportunities as mothers, but challenge our understandings of family relationships.

Chapter overview

Women's reproductive rights, associated with women's roles as mothers and wives, are central to society's notion of womanhood and the right of a woman to control her own body, particularly her entitlement to express her sexuality, take contraceptives to control her fertility and give birth to children that she wants. They are also embedded within cultural practices that raise profound ethical and moral questions about women's bodily integrity and their relationships with partners in intimate relationships with either men or other women. Women's rights to sexual expression and freedom are often configured in opposition to their obligations in the continued reproduction of their nation and men's rights to control women's bodies within patriarchal relationships that favour men's choices over those of women. These diverse social expectations have meant that women's reproductive rights are also contested rights. Women's right to sexual expression has been constrained within a marital relationship involving heterosexual men and women rather than women's enjoyment of sex for its own sake. This construction of their reproductive life and sexuality has reduced opportunities for women to engage in either extramarital relationships involving men other than their husbands or lesbian relationships. In circumstances affecting her capacity to give birth, the rights of the fetus or child can contradict those of the woman to decide whether she wishes to become a mother or not.

In contemporary societies, tensions around a woman's choice to have or not have children are further compounded by the new reproductive technologies. These have expanded women's capacities to give birth in situations where this

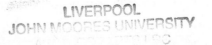

option might otherwise not have been possible and at the same time created new sites for the expression of patriarchal relations. Consequently, new sites of struggle for women who wish to control their bodies on their own terms have been produced. Steinberg (1997) argues that this area of practice has been cloaked in silence because technical and gender-neutral language hides the gendered bodies that are centre stage in the medicalisation of women's reproductive rights and disempowers women as active participants in life-giving processes.

Social workers are drawn into women's reproductive lives primarily in their roles as mothers and to protect the rights of the fetus or child. Child protection procedures can be central in addressing both concerns. Social workers can help women to become mothers through fostering and adoption processes ,whereby they assess women's capacity to be 'good enough' mothers or parents to children who may already be in or are about to enter the care or 'looked-after system'. They can support birth mothers, foster mothers or adoptive mothers discharge their childcare responsibilities more effectively through various forms of practical assistance. Social workers can be drawn into resolving conflicts involving women's rights to control their own bodies and act as autonomous agents who can choose whether or not to have children and those of a baby pre-birth and post-birth. For instance, a learning disabled mother may seek social work support both during pregnancy and after the birth of a child. The support of a non-judgemental practitioner may be central to ensuring the wellbeing of the disabled mother, especially if she is facing hostility about her right to become a mother. Social workers based within health and voluntary settings can be involved in advising a young teenage woman about contraceptives to avoid teenage pregnancy. If she does become pregnant, social workers may have to support and monitor the child's long-term welfare. The social worker who has to take a child away from a mother with serious drug problems illustrates a situation in which the practitioner's responsibilities towards ensuring the safety of the child supersede those of the mother.

In this chapter, I argue that it is important for social workers to understand women's reproductive rights, especially those involving childlessness, adoption and abortion if they are to support women accessing services. Crisis intervention and preventive work are both relevant in addressing issues involving women's reproductive rights. In practice, this is likely to entail working in health settings with other professionals in multi-agency relationships. I cover the new reproductive technologies because these challenge practitioners' assumptions about work with women and children alongside their notions of families being rooted within the nuclear family and kinship based on blood ties. I also urge practitioners in statutory settings and social work educators to address women's reproductive rights as a normal part of both the academic and practice curriculum.

The social construction of women's reproductive rights

Women's reproductive rights are socially constructed within cultural relations about women's role and place in society. Women's identities are embedded in these, often endorsing women's role as mothers and/or transmitters of a nation's culture. Religious views, as part of cultural relations, can be crucial in defining what women can(not) do with their bodies. Traditional femininity revolves around women's status as wives and mothers, with children being seen as the product of loving relationships between men and women. Framing women primarily as mothers has instituted social controls to encourage women to give birth even when they would rather not and prevent the termination of pregnancies that women do not want. Women are expected to become mothers and devote their lives to raising and caring for children. Social workers have recognised that these expectations idealise women's lives and created the idea of 'good enough' mothering. This concept indicates that caring for children is ultimately linked to the realities in which women live. Today, support for a range of family styles in the West includes single-parent families and those led by same-sex couples.

Women in the UK have sought to access good prenatal and antenatal care and support for children from birth and until they grow up. They have also struggled to have control over their bodies:

- birth control to give them choice in when they have children
- abortion to terminate unwanted pregnancies
- adoption when they were unable to give birth
- and, recently, being assisted in becoming mothers through the new reproductive technologies.

The broadening of the options open to women as a result of the new reproductive technologies may place them in conflict situations with wider sociocultural expectations, particularly religious ones that endorse women's existence as mothers above all other choices, and with their partners, especially if men wish to have children when women do not, or if a woman wishes to terminate a pregnancy when a man would rather not.

Choice as central to women's reproductive rights

'Women's right to choose' has been central to a woman's reproductive rights. Feminists developed this slogan to support women who:

- wanted children to have them at a time of her choosing through access to safe contraceptive devices
- sought to terminate pregnancies to do so without risking illegal backstreet abortions that might have endangered her life as well as risking imprisonment
- demanded an end to enforced sterilisations, an issue of great importance to black and/or disabled women.

Social workers seldom engage women in discussions about their experiences of infertility and childlessness and attempts to overcome it except in counselling relationships. Social work practitioners in mainstream agencies, including hospital settings, seldom deal with the issue. This is due partly to lack of time to take on further work and partly to lack of specific skills in this area. In Britain, services, including counselling distraught women, are now mainly provided by health professionals and voluntary agencies. This indicates that this is a site of changing practice routines and there is a blurring of the boundaries between health and social care so that other professionals begin to undertake social work activities. Below, I consider key points in women's endeavours to secure reproductive rights that they chose and defined as appropriate to them. These often involved women in sustained campaigns and networks that engaged them in public education initiatives and finding allies to support their demands for the right to choose in a variety of settings. The right to choose remains fragile.

Birth control

Women have sought to control their fertility through a range of contraceptive devices that have placed them in charge of their bodies. Ensuring that these were reliable, easily accessible and unstigmatised by associating these with health provisions was key to women being able to decide when and under what conditions they became pregnant. Crucial to establishing these rights was women's endeavour to disassociate having sex with marriage and labelling women who had sex out of wedlock as whores or disreputable women. In Britain, the efforts of Josephine Butler and later Marie Stopes in enabling women to become sexual agents in their own right by accessing contraceptive devices were an important part of this struggle. So were scientific developments that ultimately produced 'the pill' that gave women the freedom to choose when to become pregnant and inaugurated the sexual liberation of the 1960s.

By delinking pregnancy from sex, access to contraceptive devices ranging from interuterine coils to the pill liberated women's sexual agency and capacity for sexual fulfilment. It also exacerbated existing social conflict over women's 'right to choose' as contraception reduced men's ability to control women's bodies in ways previously endorsed by social custom and traditions.

Health social workers, especially those attached to GP surgeries, birth control clinics, or hospital settings, can assist women, including adolescent women, in making these choices and in promoting sexual health. Women often prefer that health professionals handle these issues because seeing a social worker can be stigmatising. Women's choices become important if birth control is not practised or it fails. Their opting for a universal service illustrates how, in areas of overlap between social workers and health professionals, the residual nature of social work can deny women support during emotional crises, especially if there are no child protection concerns. In child protection cases, the rights of the child, even at the fetus stage, can supersede those of the mother. This can happen if women misuse substances like alcohol or drugs, where concern about damage to the fetus can lead to child protection procedures being invoked either at the point of birth or during pregnancy. A mother can be ordered through a court to look after her health and that of the fetus, with the threat of losing her baby as an ultimate sanction. Social workers apprehended Baby G in Canada because the mother, a First Nation (indigenous Canadian) woman, was misusing substances, especially alcohol, and not eating properly during the pregnancy (Rutman et al., 2000) and health professionals were worried about the health of the fetus. Social workers initiated care proceedings to 'protect the unborn child' and thereby solve the dilemma between a mother's right to choose what to do with her body and her responsibility to feed the growing fetus by looking after herself.

Social workers also participate in sex education initiatives in the drive to reduce teenage pregnancies, an issue of particular government attention in the UK (SEU, 1999). These have not proved to be effective and the UK continues to have the highest teenage pregnancy rates in Europe. Research and youth work with young mothers reveal that young women often choose motherhood as a way of validating their existence in difficult social situations where social disadvantage often deprives them of other opportunities to self-fulfilment. In the global South, high fertility rates are more prominent among poor women with limited educational achievements than richer, more highly educated women and raise questions for social workers in how to support poor women in carving out better social existences for themselves and their children. The lessons learned overseas may have implications for social work practice in the West. For example, encouraging women to continue with their own education well beyond the basic minimum and finding funds to enable this to take place can be one of the ways in which women can be helped to make their own choices about their fertility, when to become sexually active and with whom and when to marry or not.

Adoption

Adoption is a possibility for childless women, particularly those in stable relationships. Adoptions can occur within a country or from outside it, when it becomes an international adoption. Both are subject to social work investigation to determine parental suitability for adoption. Until recently, same-sex parents were discriminated against as prospective parents, as were black minority ethnic groupings, especially for white babies, even though black children are disproportionately represented in the care system (Barn et al., 2006). Parents' desire to bypass social workers' scrutiny in adoption negotiations has led significant numbers of Westerners to initiate direct contact with parents in low-income countries and privately contract adoptions. This can include so-called 'celebrity adoptions' like Madonna's adoption of a Malawian child, David Banda. In this case, British social workers eventually became responsible for monitoring her mothering capacities once David entered the UK. The desire for children has led to a market in adoptions. For example, 46 babies and young children intended for the US American market were found in an illegal foster home in Antigua, Guatemala (Rosenberg, 2007). Zoe's Ark, a charity based in France, was accused of trafficking children from Chad (Chrisafis, 2007). These illustrate the significance of social work scrutiny of international adoptions and convincing prospective parents of the importance of promoting the interests of children, including their cultural heritage and identity, rather than defining them as being 'rescued' from a life of poverty.

Abortion

Women's efforts to secure the right to safe abortions have been a site of continuing struggle because they challenge socioreligious views about the point at which a fetus becomes a child with rights accorded to human beings who are capable of living an independent existence. Social workers were involved in securing women's right to choose whether or not to end unwanted pregnancies at both structural and individual levels. On the structural level, in Britain in the 1960s and 70s, women argued for legislation that legalised it and insisted that their trade union, NALGO (now part of UNISON), endorsed it as an integral right of women workers in a society that was hostile to these ideas. Once the 1967 Abortion Act was passed, social workers were able to support individual women by explaining their rights and choices in this area, including offering counselling to address the varied emotions that women experience in making a choice and implementing it, often in distressing circumstances. These responses remain relevant today. Women's reproductive rights, particularly those linked to the 'right to choose', continue to be vulnerable and there have been numerous attempts aimed at undermining them. The most recent of these in the UK occurred in 2008 when Parliament debated the issue. At that time, a coalition of those seeking to curtail women's rights in this area, including the Roman Catholic Church and pro-lifers, lost the vote to reduce women's right to demand abortion from 24 weeks to 20 when Parliament refused to concede to their views. Despite losing the vote, this coalition vowed to continue to fight for their demand, and another attempt at lowering the time limit to 20 weeks is forecast in the near future.

The new reproductive technologies: forces for changing thinking and behaviour

The new reproductive technologies now offer another avenue out of childlessness to the traditional one of adoption. The 'the new reproductive technologies' cover hi-tech interventions like *in vitro* fertilisation (IVF), artificial insemination by donor (AID), surrogate mothering, and human tissue transplants. There have been 2,200 children born through sperm or egg donation and 100 surrogate births (Inman, 1998), but the number is growing. Medical interventions have seriously eroded women's right to be active participants in the process of giving birth (Klein, 1989), while increasing possibilities for women to have children and reaffirm their mothering roles (Steinberg, 1997). Professional treatments for childlessness and infertility have become medicalised processes that usually exclude social work (Stanworth, 1987). The power of and roles played by doctors, particularly consultants with research interests, have shaped discourses in this area and privileged their voices over others in multidisciplinary teams. They have promoted this as a highly scientific medical enterprise or capital-intensive venture of benefit to childless women (Winston, 1987). As commercial businesses controlled by hi-tech medical experts and pharmaceutical companies, they provide services with an eye on making profits for shareholders (Burfoot, 1990). They can lose the focus on women's experiences within these technologies and operate at women's expense, often as an unintended consequence (Steinberg, 1997).

A woman I interviewed poignantly described how confined and confining her choices were. She said:

> I felt glassed-in. Just like my babies on those petrie dishes. For years, I came and went, came and went, with nothing to show for it. It got so I dreaded the next appointment. But I couldn't talk to anyone about it. And the doctors never asked. (Dominelli, 2002b: 72)

Lay discourses – as debates carried out either in the popular media or by the general public in their interactions with each other – now encompass the cloning of babies, the substitution of human body parts by those of animals, artificially created ones, and the 'purchase' of babies via the internet. The question 'Who am I?' no longer has a straight-forward answer, if it ever did. Tracing one's genealogy becomes an identity puzzle that would exercise the mental agility of a Sherlock Holmes. Finding one's ancestors can become a traumatic quest that challenges existing legal and practice definitions of parent-hood, whether motherhood or fatherhood, and what or who constitutes the family, extended or nuclear. One health practitioner I met claimed that a child could have as many as six parents. Reproductive technologies also raise difficult questions about differ-ent if competing and irreconcilable rights to information or anonymity of the different parties involved in the processes from conception to birth (Blyth, 1998). These are tough questions that social workers have traditionally addressed in their practice.

The question of who is a fit parent is a major concern of social workers, although the focus is usually on the mother. This was addressed in debates about the regulatory framework to control clinicians and putative parents. Who could be a 'donor' or a 'recipient' was aired in a media that endorsed stereotypes of able-bodied heterosexual couples in their youth. The outrage when newspapers revealed that new reproductive technologies had enabled a 60-year-old woman in Italy to give birth exposed the gendered and ageist character of these discourses. Little sympathy was given to this woman's right to choose motherhood at this age. This contrasted with the lack of comment in the media shortly afterwards when men in their eighties were reported to have become fathers.

IVF validates the continued viewing of disability as a medical rather than socially created condition (Oliver, 1990; also Chapter 30). Ultimately, the medical approach feeds into desires for 'designer babies', as the media labels them, that conform to racist, sexist and ablist stereotypes. This issue was aired when Molly Nash's parents used genetic screening and IVF techniques to produce an embryo that was 'disease-free and a perfect match' in terms of providing blood cells from the forthcoming baby's umbilical cord to substantially increase her chances of surviving Fanconi's anaemia (Thompson, 2000). This procedure, lawful in the US where it was performed, is illegal in Britain. This did not prevent Alan and Louise Masterton in Scotland from demanding this treatment to 'restore the "female dimension" of their family' because they had lost their daughter in a tragic accident a year earlier (Thompson, 2000). Few people would argue against this technology's beneficial potential, although the eugenicist dimensions of these 'choices' are worrying. These examples also demonstrate the ethical minefields that these technologies can produce. RADAR and Mencap have been vocal in raising these concerns (Fletcher, 1999).

The 'designer baby' fallacy was exposed by a group of attractive women models using the internet to sell their eggs to the highest bidder. This turned out to be a spoof perpetrated by jokers at the end of the last century. It was followed by a 'tug of love' between two childless couples, one British and the other American, who 'purchased' the same set of twins through the internet. The commodification of children thereby acquired new twists as national boundaries became blurred at the same time that problem-solving based on solutions rooted in national jurisdictions revealed their inadequacies. The racial and class dimensions of this saga are not commented upon, although obvious. The two sets of 'adoptive' parents were white; the twins and their biological parents were poor African-Americans. Social workers were called upon to take the children into custody and find legal ways of solving the dispute. The 'best interests of the children' was advocated as the way forward. And, while important as an issue, an equally troubling set of questions, implied in the affair, received little considered attention. The needs that the two sets of parents were trying to fulfil, their motivations in choosing an unorthodox manner for becoming parents and their suitability for such a role were sidelined. The problem that the twins' biological mother was trying to resolve was also left as an unaccompanied apostrophe in the air. How important were poverty, racism and sexism in her decision? Did the internet offer a vehicle for decision-making that she could control? In another instance, social workers had to assist in a dispute involving a surrogate mother who refused to give up 'her baby' to the contracting father in the US.

Issues for social workers to consider

Social workers have traditionally held key roles in working with children and families, where questions about fertility, pregnancy, childbirth, childlessness and family networks have been discussed in the context of social problems to be addressed. Their absence from most interventions involving the new reproductive technologies means that their expertise in handling complex moral and ethical dilemmas is being/will be lost. It is not being made available to social workers in the voluntary sector who are replacing statutory ones. Research in this area reveals that the medical profession is not meeting women's needs as individuals who have their own specific interests that merit attention as well as those of the subsequent implanted embryo or child to whom she gives birth (Sewpaul, 1998). In my view, social workers should become an integral part of the multidisciplinary team that deals with women undergoing fertility treatment of whatever kind, and they should be involved in responding to women's needs at all points in the process. This includes helping a woman examine the meaning of childlessness for her, including acknowledging the acceptability of being childless. This is crucial, given the low success rate of fertility treatments like IVF (Sewpaul, 1998). If she decides to go ahead with treatment, its invasiveness should be considered carefully and the difficult moments a woman might encounter explored. Medical practitioners are too busy and lack training in handling the complex emotions and dilemmas that women experience when treatment does not work or demoralisation sets in when after years of trying they are unable to have a child.

The issues that women face depend on whether they are considering fertility treatment or surrogacy arrangements. Women undertaking these will share some concerns but not others. Points of convergence include worries about:

- someone else's gametes being involved
- whether the child is hers and her partner's
- her partner's willingness to become the ensuing child's father
- how to explain genetic differences to the resulting children.

Another difficulty is whether these concerns can be left to one side until the child grows up and makes demands in their own right. Addressing these concerns may be avoided for a while, or be unproblematic if they arise while a woman is in a stable relationship. However, her situation can deteriorate rapidly and she may find that she is unsupported and isolated when she needs help most. Not having considered these matters during the good times can intensify her feelings of vulnerability. Appropriate and sensitive social work intervention before this dilemma arises and afterwards can ease a woman's transitions between these different states.

Surrogacy arrangements raise moral and emotional dilemmas alongside contractual and legal ones for all parties in a transaction. They have the added complication of having to deal directly with people other than the surrogate mother. This can exacerbate conflict if their motivations for engaging in surrogacy relationships differ. This can occur if the surrogate mother wants to retain contact with the commissioning family while her partner does not. Alongside a conflictual relationship, the woman may be deprived of urgently needed support. The commissioning or social mother may form a relationship with the baby and want to end contact with the surrogate mother. She may reach the same conclusion if she decides that she does not want her mothering capacities to be qualified by constant comparison with the surrogate mother as her presence could evoke evidence of her incapacity. Where the 'best interests of the child' lie in such situations and how this can be ascertained remain relevant if problematic. Social workers may not have all the answers for these occasions, but they can provide practical and emotional support or refer women to other agencies or professionals for assistance. They can also support children and adults who have been adopted or those born through the new reproductive technologies to find their parents where legislation enables them to do so.

A woman who acts as a surrogate mother also feels a range of, and at times conflicting, emotions. These include mood swings during pregnancy and uncertainty about whether or not she is doing the 'right thing'. Whatever contract she has signed, she may wish she had not agreed to part with 'her baby'. These feelings may be intensified after the birth and lead to serious depression. Or, despite careful legal crafting of its content, she may refuse to comply with the contractual agreement and have expensive legal proceedings initiated against her. Careful exploration of her motives and feelings before entering such agreements could be provided by a supportive social worker. If available, this service is currently provided by voluntary or non-profit organisations, which operate networks that put women who want to become mothers in touch with women willing to act as surrogates. Childlessness Overcome Through Surrogacy (COTS) was an organisation begun in 1988 by Kim Cotton, a surrogate mother. It has a nationwide network that includes counsellors as part of its services. Systematic research into these counsellors' qualifications to practice is lacking, as is an analysis of which women seek and which act as surrogates. COTS claims to promote responsible surrogacy, carries out police and HIV checks and provides counselling before matching intending parents with a surrogate mother and afterwards (Inman, 1998). The latter function is now conducted under the auspices of its offshoot, Triangle. COTS follows the British government's code of practice that sets out minimum standards for surrogacy arrangements. This code declares that the interests of the children must guide professional activities in these situations. COTS has standards of openness that require prospective parents to tell their offspring about their origins. COTS had arranged 600 surrogate births by 2007.

Cotton strongly defends women's rights to choose whether or not to become mothers or act as surrogates. Steinberg (1997) suggests that focusing solely on choice issues ignores the context in which women make their choices. And, from their practice in other areas, social workers are aware that the context is often central in determining what women do. In this case, it could affect which women would use the new reproductive technologies and which would not. Questions about 'race', sexual orientation and age can intersect with views about persons fit for these treatments. The unavailability of money can constrain women's decisions. Even fertility treatment funded by the NHS can be a 'postcode lottery', where getting treatment for a period sufficient to yield results can vary according to residential location and clinical discretion. The literature suggests that donors and surrogates will be either poor 'black' women in low-income countries meeting the needs of wealthy 'white' women in the West, or poor 'white' working-class women doing the same for their wealthier sisters in high-income countries (Steinberg, 1997).

Relationships between all those involved in these transactions can become complicated after the birth. The child may be disabled. An American experience demonstrates that commissioning parents may refuse to accept delivery of their disabled baby and set the scene for an expensive legal battle. Arrangements for minimising or maintaining contact between the contractual parties may break down. Keeping the origins of 'donors' a secret may be extremely difficult, as some adoptive parents have discovered. Despite earlier assurances of anonymity in New Zealand, for example, sperm donors can have their offspring turn up on their doorstep because legislation now permits children access to information about their genetic parent (Blyth, 1998). Similar arrangements are being considered in the UK as part of the review of existing legislation governing these activities.

Another strand of argument endorses the child's right to know by focusing on 'the best interests of the child'. In Britain, the Children's Society, COTS and Barnardo's, for example, support openness on these grounds. The Human Fertilisation and Embryology Authority collects this information, but offspring are currently unable to access it. Some non-identifiable information such as height and medical details and whether or not an applicant is related to an intended partner can be provided. This data can remain beyond reach if parents do not tell children that they are the product of donor gametes. Identity is a crucial area in which social work intervention could be supportive. One argument in favour of a child's right to know has been tinged with eugenicist overtones, namely, to identify a rogue or disease-carrying gene for medical purposes or actuarial reasons for insurance companies. Such information can be devastating to the unprepared person who simply wants to find out who a 'parent' was. Social workers assist people through difficult decisions that may profoundly alter their lives as they have previously understood them and this area can be one of them. The review of the Human Fertilisation and Embryology Act of 1990 may alter existing limitations around donor anonymity.

Conclusion

Women have had to struggle to obtain rights of sexual expression and reproduction independent of men. The new reproductive technologies have opened new doors for women wishing to become mothers alongside the more traditional one of adoption. At the same time, some technological developments have eroded the scope for women to decide for themselves how they want to treat their own bodies and approach their own fertility. In the case of deciding whether or not to have children, technological advances can intensify the pressures of using these instruments to solve a problem that might not be solvable through such means. Additionally, increased scientific input into human reproductive processes has remedicalised a normal activity for women, reaffirmed the powers of male medical practitioners and researchers to make decisions affecting fundamental aspects of women's lives, and reinforced patriarchal relations in favour of men. The legal framing of these opportunities and the media's involvement in public discourses of women's reproductive rights have reinforced conventional ideologies and norms regarding motherhood and family life.

Social workers have been in the background in these debates, even though they cover ground with which they are more than familiar, and for which they hold the skills and knowledge for responding sensitively. As a result, their expertise in dealing with complex matters has been largely inaccessible to women undergoing fertility treatments or engaging in surrogacy arrangements. Social workers have had little to say about women's roles as either women or mothers in these discussions. It is time for social workers to find their voice and provide the critical reflexive practice for working in anti-oppressive ways with and for women in an area of crucial importance to them. It also requires social work educators to include this subject on the academic and practice curricula.

For further discussion of social work with families, see Chapter 25, and for aspects of sexuality, see Adams et al., 2009c, Chapter 6.

www.wgnrr.org   Women's Global Network for Reproductive Rights

Bywater, J. and Jones, R. (2007) *Sexuality and Social Work*, Exeter, Learning Matters. Explores the significances of sexuality in social work practice, including in the promotion of parenting rights.

Jordan, J. (2001) *Josephine Butler*, London, John Murray. Tells the story of Josephine Butler's struggles to ensure that women had sexual and reproductive rights in Victorian Liverpool.

Rahman, A. (2000) 'Emerging issues in women's reproductive rights', *International Journal of Gynecology and Obstetrics*, **70**(1): 6–16. Sets out key issues that women face in exercising their reproductive rights.

Steinberg, D.L. (1997) *Bodies in Glass: Genetics, Eugenics, Embryo Ethics*, Manchester, Manchester University Press. Providing a comprehensive examination of the new reproductive technologies, this book explains what these technologies are and considers their contradictory potential to both expand and limit women's choices because the medical model prevails.

Ethical tensions and later life: choice, consent and mental capacity

7

Chapter overview

While social work is based on the values of self-determination and empowerment, in the best interests of the person who receives services, there are situations where the goals of social work and the interests of the person apparently do not coincide. This chapter explores some of the main tensions arising in such circumstances and how the critical practitioner may develop ways of living with, that is, managing, them.

Considering choice and consent

There are three main circumstances in which tensions are likely to arise between the goals of social work and the goals of meeting the needs of the person who uses services in the least restrictive way, that is, offering them the fullest choice to consent:

1   When people are judged capable but, because of family circumstances, social work intervention is judged by professionals to be necessary.
2   When people are judged vulnerable and social work support services are partly imposed and partly agreed with them.
3   When people are judged vulnerable but lacking the capacity to agree to the services that are assessed as necessary to meet their needs.

In each of these circumstances, professionals are making judgements about people's capacity and are deciding whether or not to intervene or provide services.

When intervention is judged by professionals to be necessary

Social work services may be involuntary, in that they may be focused on people in poverty and those excluded in various ways from participation in many aspects of life. As a result, they may grudgingly accept social work without real consent or silently resist interventions. Another aspect of the involuntary nature of social work is the way in which it often intrudes into what are usually the private lives of people – into their homes or personal relationships. Moreover, social work is often stigmatised by potential users, because it deals with people perceived as having 'social problems' and because needing social work services may be thought to imply that a service user is dependent on others for the normal activities of daily life; this dependent status is disapproved of and avoided by many people.

Many users of social work services are involuntary; they are forced to receive the attentions of a social worker. This may be because they are children who are considered to need protection, or they have a physical or learning disability and so are thought to need protection and care because they are not always intellectually able enough to look after themselves. Alternatively, they may have been an offender or are perceived by some social agency as having a problem that requires social work intervention, even if they do not accept this. Social workers also have responsibilities to enforce the law, taking children away from their parents and organising compulsory admissions to mental hospital. Even if social workers try to consult and involve service users, it can be hard to explain what their role is, and lack of public acceptance of their work may lead people who need their help to avoid or reject it.

◊◊◊◊ CaSE EXaMPLE ◊◊◊

Using compulsory powers

Clancy, a social worker who is an approved mental health professional, is called by a GP to consider an emergency compulsory admission to a psychiatric hospital, which is prepared to admit the patient. Clancy visits and talks to John (53), who was found by his wife, Harriet, having taken an overdose of prescription drugs during the morning, but had come round without apparent physical damage, according to the GP, by the afternoon when she returned home from work. John had been increasingly depressed, having been unable to find a new job in their rural area after he had been made redundant by a transport company, where he was a manager. They were thinking of moving to a nearby town to improve his chances of finding a job, but Harriet would have to give up her work, which she enjoys, and their two children would have to move school. John refuses to consider admission to hospital, at least partly because he thinks this will have an adverse effect on his chances in the job market but partly because of the stigma of hospitalisation for mental illness. Clancy talks to the consultant psychiatrist, who is prepared to offer an appointment for assessment at a clinic in four days' time, after the weekend. In the meantime, Harriet is prepared to stay home from work to be with John all the time.

Clancy thinks about the decision she has been asked to make. She follows her agency's protocol of questions to ask to see if someone is at serious risk of committing suicide. Doing this brings her to the conclusion that, while this attempt was serious, John is not now actively planning to take his life. He is prepared to try to do something about the situation. Indeed, in spite of his depression, he has remained active in trying to resolve the family's position, and a lot of his feelings are about feeling a failure in supporting his family and the possibility that their lives will be disrupted by his redundancy. Clancy comes to the conclusion that he might be helped by a more realistic attitude to the situation, and that this could be achieved fairly quickly by cognitive-behavioural therapy, which both she and her colleagues could offer. A psychiatric assessment would be possible soon, John in not in danger now, and until he has that assessment, his wife will stay with him, and he will have a period with his family, rather than being alone at home brooding. She decides therefore not to take up the GP's recommendation of a compulsory admission. The GP is angry that his judgement has been questioned and complains to the mental health team that the decision puts John's life in danger.

In this case, Clancy has been able to manage the risk, and provide an alternative that meets the user's and carer's wishes; this has been achieved at least partly because some resources are available from the family and the psychiatric clinic.

When people are judged vulnerable and professionals make conditional decisions about services

Sometimes situations arise in which people are assessed as vulnerable to an extent, but as still having the capacity to maintain a certain level of lifestyle. The professionals decide to an extent to follow their wishes but to an extent override them, for example, with a view to managing risk or allocating scarce resources.

CaSE EXaMPLE

Carers' and users' consent

The daughter of a frail older woman rang the adult social service department (ASSD) to refer her mother, who has been coping with increasing frailty and loss of memory, but her mother has not agreed to the referral. When the social worker visits, the mother is courteous, but does not want to be involved with the social services, yet she is clearly in difficulties.

This fairly commonplace situation faces the practitioner with the need to balance a wish to protect the older woman from risk, and support the daughter in caring for her mother. These positive aims also need to be balanced against the possibility of acting without the mother's consent. Ideally, the practitioner might work to develop a relationship with the mother, so that her help is more acceptable, or support the daughter to help her to decide on other ways of helping her mother. Often resources are not available to offer social work time to achieve such outcomes, and the best we might expect is a watching brief by checking with the GP and referring the daughter to a carers' organisation.

When people are judged by professionals not to have the capacity to assess for themselves what is in their best interests

Sometimes people are referred to social workers without accepting or knowing about the referral or having a clear idea what will happen to them when they are referred.

In contrast to this general picture of uncertainty about how much service users really consent to receive social work services, social policy has focused on service users in all public services having a wider range of choice in what services they receive and how they receive them. Public choice policies are a neoliberal political strategy to increase the citizens' collective influence on how the services they receive are delivered. This idea is partly derived from consumerism, an ideology that purchasers of goods and services should be protected from failings in the market that may lead to them being unable to make a rational decision about the best purchase at the best price. This has been extended into public services, even though in market economies, government regulation is usually used to protect consumers, and there are difficulties in the government regulating itself. Inspectorates or independent regulators have increasingly been used to overcome this problem. In the public sector or in quasi-markets where there is rationing or restricted choice, ethical, legal and administrative controls on officials' decision-making maintains some semblance of public choice. This is because public choice and practices such as user participation in service planning, management and policy-making are used to limit official and professional discretion, and to apply economic pressures for cost containment and for quality management.

One of the ways in which neoliberal policies seek to achieve generalised public choice is by arranging for people to have individual choices when they use services. For example, one of the authors of this chapter recently needed to go for an outpatient's appointment at a hospital. His GP offered a choice of two hospitals and had no professional view whether the treatment team in one was better than the other. But the writer's previous experience of one was that it was inefficient and the other was slightly easier to travel to, so he chose that one. The combination of hundreds of thousands of people making such choices might mean that one of the hospitals would lose patients and the income that came with them, so they would either improve their performance to increase their patient numbers or would have to close services in that specialty. However, this may inconvenience people who cannot travel to another place, lead to insecurity in running the hospital that is losing patients, and may lead to inappropriate pressure and longer waiting times at the preferred hospital; there is only so much time and space. Generally, it will be poor and marginalised people who have less knowledge and support to make individual choices of this kind, and public choice policies are likely to force them to use less successful providers in the market, leading to an issue of social justice unless they are helped to make and enforce choices.

Public choice policies face practitioners with consent issues, while adult and child safeguarding policies face social care services with the need to intervene without clear consent. This often applies pressure to practitioners to use professional or social power to enforce 'safe' decisions, when consent does not exist.

CASE EXAMPLE

Consent and risk

A blind man is admitted to hospital and his GP is anxious that his very frail wife will not be able to manage at home; he persuades her to go to a care home, but they need a social services assessment. When the social worker visits to carry out a community care assessment, the woman will not let her in and refuses to have any services. The GP is irritated with the social worker for not pressing on with the assessment, and feels that his patient is at risk. He has told the woman that it will only be a short admission, while her husband in is hospital, but the doctor judges that this will become permanent, because the husband is unlikely to be able to care for her again. However, he has not told the woman this, because he knows it will encourage her to refuse to be admitted; the social worker feels unable to ally herself with this tactic, because it will lead to mistrust of professionals and carers later.

A common response from ASSDs is to refuse to act unless there is consent; however, as with the daughter and her mother, there is a wish to help in a difficult situation and minimise risk. Also, to take the easy option of refusing to help may be an administrative convenience for the agency, but it does not accept a legitimate professional responsibility to respond, the duty of a profession to the community. Again, resources may not allow for an engagement to develop the necessary relationships to be able to achieve personal influence in the situation.

CASE EXAMPLE

Want, need and eligibility

Helen, a hospital social worker, visits the bedside of Mrs Morris, 93, who has been in hospital and then in intermediate care receiving rehabilitation after a serious fall. Her daughter has been caring for her, visiting regularly, doing the shopping, cleaning and other household tasks. She is in her sixties, caring for a husband with advanced cancer in his seventies and visits her husband's mother, also in her nineties, living in a care home in another town. Mrs Morris will be much less mobile after her fall and will need help in her home with getting up, washing and other personal self-care. As an adult social services care manager, Helen is arranging a package of care. But Mrs Morris will not agree to this; her daughter will give her all the help she needs. Helen's discussion with the daughter suggests that this amount of help will not be possible. She arranges a family meeting in the intermediate care unit to discuss the options. Faced with the impossibility of her demands, Mrs Morris says she will go home anyway, although the professionals involved and the family are appalled by the risk that she accepts in doing this. However, they do what they can.

Some weeks later, Mrs Morris has another fall, another period of rehabilitation, and, realising that going home is impossible, agrees to move to a care home. She is shocked to realise that she will be charged for this, but does not want to give up her home. Instead, she comes to an agreement to the local authority to defer charges; they will sell her home to clear the debts when she dies.

Two years later, now seriously disabled after a further episode and also ill with cancer, Mrs Morris is eligible for NHS continuing care funding for a nursing home. She and her daughter prefer an expensive, good quality one, but the primary care trust, which will make the payments, says that her needs can be catered for in a perfectly good home near her family that is much less expensive. The continuing care procedures do not allow her to 'top-up' the NHS payment with her own money, as the local authority allowed with community care funding. She has no choice about where she will go.

Promoting the idea of user choice implies that people may have what they want. But in the early stages of Mrs Morris's care, when she wants her daughter's care, this is not possible because of her daughter's other commitments. In receiving continuing care, she can have her needs met, but provided they can be met, she cannot choose where or how they are met. Social workers constantly deal with tensions between care needs, user preferences and eligibility for public help. They mediate between the needs and wishes of all the people involved, recognising that help paid for by the public purse will sometimes mean charges for or limitations on what can be provided. Working in these situations means being clear about legal responsibilities and aware of the Human Rights Act 1998 and related legislation, which may confer general rights that may sometimes be relevant, such as a right to family life and not to be treated inhumanely. Within legal limitations, practitioners need to be clear when a user's needs and wishes conflict with a carer's needs and wishes or the preferences or rights of another person. They must also distinguish between needs and wishes, and, where public responsibilities are involved, the limitations of eligibility for public funding.

Mental capacity legislation: tensions between safeguarding and independence

Important procedures in cases of mental illness, learning disability and where gradually failing faculties among older people may lead to difficulty in their deciding on their course of treatment derive from the Mental Capacity Act 2005. This Act, which came into force in England and Wales in 2007, offers increased protection in the interests of people who may become vulnerable or incapable of making their own judgements. It allows people to express their wishes about their formal care, and give directions where medical and other forms of treatment may be foreseen. For example, someone with motor neurone disease, who will lose their physical faculties but retain mental capacity, can give an advance directive about the care to be provided where certain symptoms that are common in the final phases of the illness arise. It is increasingly accepted practice to help someone make these formal statements of preferences. If people need to have decisions made for them, there is a process, involving an independent mental capacity advocate, for someone to act on their behalf and in their interests.

Section 1 of the Mental Capacity Act sets out five principles:

1   The assumption should be made that a person has the mental capacity to make judgements about their best interests, unless there is clear evidence otherwise.
2   All practicable steps to help the person decide should have been taken.
3   Inability should not be inferred from unwisdom.
4   A decision must be in the person's best interests.
5   A decision must be least restrictive of rights and freedom of action.

The point about unwisdom is that simply because someone behaves unwisely, in a practitioner's judgement, does not mean that they are incapable of making their own decisions, but simply that their decisions are not the same as ours. We can see a number of practice tensions in the following example.

CaSE EXaMPLE

Belief, professional practice and advocacy

Haley, a hospital social worker, is approached angrily by Selina, the daughter of a woman on the geriatric ward. The doctor has told Selina that her mother has agreed to a 'do not resuscitate' (DNR) instruction, which means that if she is dying of an infection or coronary thrombosis, no effort will be made to revive her. Selina protests against this; it is helping her mother to commit suicide, and contrary to their Roman Catholic religion. Haley talks to the mother's primary nurse, who says that the patient has advanced cancer and resuscitation would not be effective. She understands this and wants to die comfortably. Haley interviews the daughter, who argues strongly that as a family member she is entitled to demand that treatment is continued. She was surprised to learn from a nurse that her mother has been placed on the Liverpool Care Pathway. This is a widely used protocol for the care for dying people, which means that the tubes that have been providing hydration (water) to her mother have been pulled out from her arm and she is not now being fed. Selina feels that this is a process that is actively killing her mother. The consultant oncologist joins them and explains that it is unethical to act in a way that increases the likelihood or speed of someone's death; these decisions aim to provide the best care for Selina's mother. He explains that the DNR decision will prevent unnecessary discomfort to her mother if she does suffer a sudden organ failure, and that feeding and hydrating her mother will lead to additional discomfort and is not physically necessary for her mother, whose body cannot absorb nutrition. Selina says this is taking the chance of life away from her mother; she is her mother's next of kin and the doctor should do as she wants. The doctor explains that her mother is the only one with the right to decide on how she is treated and has given informed consent. The daughter says she would never have agreed if she had really understood what she was doing. The doctor says that in any case nobody, even the patient, can require a doctor to provide treatment that research has shown will cause damage or danger to a patient. Hydration and artificial feeding are medical treatments in this kind of situation; they are intended to help people over a crisis, not be maintained in the long term. After he goes, the daughter asks the social worker to help her stop the withdrawal of treatment to her mother and to make a complaint.

There are a number of factors to think about here. First, the different professions involved have different roles and knowledge. Haley knows about the usual treatment of cases in her specialty and the arguments that support them, but unlike the nurse and doctor involved, she will not have studied the evidence that supports them. She is expected to support and help to implement team decisions that have been properly made, so she feels that she cannot help Selina in making a complaint. On the other hand, Selina is her client and needs help in dealing with the position she is in. By arranging the meeting with the oncologist, Haley has acted as an advocate, in allowing Selina to put her views and for colleagues to explain the reasoning behind their decisions; Haley might also need to go over those explanations with Selina again to make sure that she has understood them. She can go further, by helping Selina to meet nurses and other professionals to explain what they are doing and why they are making decisions. She can also facilitate Selina's participation in her mother's death by interpreting her feelings and beliefs to colleagues, so that they can respond to her concerns. This is a situation in which Selina has limited choices and influence, but can be helped by a significant involvement, which the social worker may facilitate and if necessary advocate for. It is also appropriate to help Selina make a complaint, and by helping her understand the rationale behind the decisions, she can facilitate the framing of the complaint in ways that will ensure that it is heard properly. On her own, feeling strongly as she does, Selina could probably only complain in ways that would be dismissed; instead, her legitimate feelings and beliefs can be recognised by helping her with a complaint. Although it is appropriate for Haley to do this, to avoid team conflict, it is also important for her to have established the advocacy role of a social worker in a healthcare team, and to explain to colleagues why she is doing this work and how it will benefit Selina in dealing with her bereavement if she feels she has been able to act strongly on her mother's behalf.

A second area of difficulty is the position of family members of a patient; this is one of the areas that often puts social workers in healthcare in a different place from their colleagues in other professions. Social workers work with the impact of illness on the whole family, while healthcare professionals have a primary responsibility to the patient. Only patients can give consent to treatment or to decisions not to treat a condition. This right may only be bypassed if the patient lacks the mental capacity, according to the criteria set out in the Mental Capacity Act 2005, to make a decision. While social workers are encouraging the involvement and support of family members, who may have given up a lot of their lives to provide most of the care over many years, their colleagues cannot include family members in medical treatment decisions; they may be informed but not obeyed. By understanding this, Haley can facilitate Selina's involvement to the extent that it is possible.

A third area of difficulty is views about hydration and artificial feeding, which are controversial (, 2005). While in law and healthcare practice, they are medical treatments, aimed to achieve healthcare objectives, pro-life campaigners regard them as natural extensions to the human right to receiving food and water as means of survival. People have a right to their beliefs, and again understanding the debates fully enables Haley to help Selina present her views fully and appropriately. It is important not to be seduced by the team or professional conventions into suppressing alternative perspectives.

A fourth issue for a social worker is often to disentangle genuine emotions associated with bereavement or other important life experiences. Anger is a common emotional element in dying and bereavement. Professionals or administrators faced with a complaint may be tempted to feel that the emotions of grief are being displaced into the container of some administrative difficulty. However, the emotions are genuine, even if they seem disproportionate or misplaced, and need to be treated with respect, valued and responded to.

A fifth issue is consent, and the extent to which someone is informed about the decisions that they must make. In healthcare, partly because many procedures involve physical touching that in some circumstances might be a legal assault, careful explanation is made and a written signature obtained from patients; however, consent for less invasive involvement is assumed unless there is protest. Many social work procedures use an informal discussion followed by a spoken agreement about what the practitioner, user and carer will do, but community care plans are written and incorporate legally binding agreements to provide service. Many social work processes, however, assume consent, without testing it. A more explicit focus on consent often permits practitioners to raise and deal with uncertainties in service users and carers transparently and form more effective relationships as the basis for their work together.

Self-determination, ethical tensions and resources

The case examples discussed above examine a number of quite commonplace situations in which social workers are presented with issues about the degree to which users and carers have agreed to social work intervention, and tensions between different family members about decisions. Obtaining written consent from service users for social work involvement is not a common procedure, as it is in healthcare agencies, since physical violations are not usually involved in social work.

As a consequence, the social work profession has often focused on ethical principles such as self-determination, which require social workers to permit and encourage service users to decide the aims and form of social work interventions and manage their own affairs to the maximum extent possible. There are inherent complexities in this position, because, as we have seen, people's own preferences or needs may conflict with the preferences of others around them. Also, the right to make decisions about our own affairs is not absolute, since in any society, we all have to conform with social expectations and rules, and legal and administrative requirements. The social worker has to consider the extent of the self-determination possible, balancing this with other factors relevant to the decision.

Some social work practice theories, such as task-centred practice, require practitioners to establish agreements or formal written contracts for the social worker's intervention. Administrative procedures such as care management and looking after children require formal written care plans to be prepared and reviewed regularly. However, these are often produced in situations where service users feel that they have little power and influence. This question of the power differential between the practitioner and the person who uses services brings us back to the core tension between how far the professional or the person should have the right to determine how and where they live. This final example illustrates this.

CASE EXAMPLE

Anton is 78. He is physically frail and lives alone in a ground-floor flat. His neighbour, a retired doctor, telephones the social work department to say Anton is at risk and needs to be in a home as he is not keeping the flat clean, looks to be in poor physical condition and from the way he walks when leaving and re-entering his flat, seems not to be able to look after himself.

A social worker visits Anton, who admits that increasing frailty means he finds it physically hard to continue maintaining the lifestyle he has enjoyed for many years. Even with domiciliary support, the social worker assesses Anton's independent lifestyle as able to be maintained only with a significant level of calculated risk.

The question is whether Anton is at risk and even if he is, whether he has the right to remain at home. There is a tension between the goal of professionals, which would be to ensure that Anton maintains his quality of life and his preference to remain independent. Respecting Anton's wish to remain independent and living at home does not necessarily correspond to managing the risks and having him admitted to residential care. These two goals exist in tension with each other and the more vulnerable Anton is, the greater the tension between them. The best option could be that the practitioner respects Anton's wish to remain living at home by providing sufficient domiciliary services to enable the risks to be reduced significantly.

Anton's situation is typical of the case where intervention to minimise the risk could be against the wishes of the person and should not take place. The wishes of the vulnerable person should be respected, provided they are capable mentally of deciding on the basis of their best interests. The principle guiding this decision should be whether the person is judged to have the capacity to take decisions in their best interests. The judgement about whether the person has this capacity rests on two criteria:

- the extent to which the person is in good physical health for their age
- the extent to which the person is mentally competent.

Anton's case highlights the necessity for the practitioner to distinguish between a person judged unwise and a person judged irrational, incompetent or incapable. A person should be free to make unwise decisions, but decisions of an irrational, incompetent or incapable person should be considered differently. This raises further complexities for the social worker, in that no objective test exists to distinguish between value judgements of unwisdom and incapacity.

Conclusion

The above case examples indicate that it may be better in many practice situations to acknowledge the tensions that often exist by making explicit what the practitioner's responsibilities are and seeking explicit consent for intended actions. This would transparently place more control over care and intervention with service users. Adaptations of formal procedures such as the Mental Capacity Act process for stating preferences in advance (Henry and Seymour, 2007) might also offer opportunities to social work practitioners to be more open about their work, gain greater confidence and understanding from the people who they work with and greater public respect than social workers currently achieve.

Another important issue to identify in the case examples discussed above is the reality that many of the difficulties are made worse by lack of resources. The most useful resource in many situations in which practitioners find themselves uncomfortable in applying pressure to users to accept care or intervention is time to make an appropriate trusting relationship, in which the practitioner's influence and protection can be accepted by the service user as valid and welcomed. Haste is the enemy of ethical practice.

For further discussion of mental health aspects, see Chapter 29, and for work with frail, older people, Adams et al., 2009c, Chapter 7.

Bowles, W., Collingbridge, M., Curry, S. and Valentine, B. (2006) *Ethical Practice in Social Work: An Applied Approach*, Maidenhead, Open University Press. Chapter 6 offers a useful discussion of issues about autonomy, paternalism and self-determination in social work practice.

Department for Constitutional Affairs (DCA) (2007) *Mental Capacity Act 2005: Code of Guidance*, London, TSO. Contains much useful help in dealing with situations where there is concern about people's capacity to make decisions.

Henry, C. and Seymour, J. (2007) *Advance Care Planning: A Guide for Health and Social Care Staff*, London, DH. This guidance on helping people to express their preferences in advance is practical and sensitive.

Holloway, M. (2007) *Negotiating Death in Contemporary Health and Social Care*, Bristol, Policy Press. Provides a comprehensive, sensitive and practically informed analysis of many of the decisions about dying and bereavement made in healthcare settings.

Part 2

THEORIES FOR PRACTICE

Social work theories offer organised views of social relationships and behaviour that help social workers to both identify the issues that service users need help with and decide what action to take. This second part of the book surveys the major theoretical approaches to social work in a way that makes them accessible to the student, using practice illustrations where appropriate.

We begin with counselling, which though a separate profession with its own standards, shares many aspects of values, knowledge, understanding and skills with social work (Chapter 9). Groupwork is a distinctive, though somewhat minority, area of practice (Chapter 10). Community work contributes uniquely to the 'social' dimension of practice (Chapter 11). It is helpful to understand psychosocial work from the perspective of attachment (Chapter 12). Cross-cultural and black perspectives provide a critical view of the mainstream of practice (Chapter 13). Cognitive-behavioural approaches are increasingly popular (Chapter 14) and task-centred work provides an important resource (Chapter 15). Empowerment and advocacy contribute to a wide range of practice settings (Chapter 16). Many strands of radical and critical practice (Chapter 17), feminist (Chapter 18) and anti-oppressive (Chapter 19) approaches have their roots in critical social sciences, social constructionist and postmodernist perspectives (Chapter 20).

Critical reflection and social work theories

8

Reflective practice and critical reflection are methods of inter-preting social knowledge, professional and social values and agency and policy aims into practice actions. The reflective cycle and processes of critical reflection enable practitioners to use ideas from practice theories to develop and renew their practice.

Practice theories and critical reflection

Each chapter in Part 2 of this book examines an example of an important and well-known practice theory that seeks to explain in an organised way how social workers may usefully act, using their knowledge about the social world in which they operate. Practice theories are important because good practice requires theory in order to be critical. In Adams et al., 2009a, Part 2, we introduced social work practice as a process, in which social workers progressed through a sequence of actions: assessment, planning, intervention and eva luation and review. The three different forms of intervention presented suggest that there are alternative ways of intervening from which practitioners might choose. Practice theories extend this analysis to help practitioners to decide between the different courses of action that are open to them. Whenever we act, as a social worker, we are operating according to some sort of theory, which says: 'If you do this, you will achieve that.' Even where what we are doing seems commonplace, or common sense, an informal theory lies behind it. However, if we are going to be effective, consistent in our actions, and accountable to the people we serve and our agencies, we need to be able to understand why we are taking the particular actions that we choose and to be able to explain this according to an organised system of thought: a practice theory.

Part 1 of this book has shown that we need to approach ideas about social work critically because many of them are in debate. Understanding the purposes and context of our work does not, therefore, give us any easy answers. To apply the knowledge and understanding of society, policy and people explored in Adams et al., 2009a with the actions we will take as social workers, we need practice theories as systems of thought. Figure 8.1 shows how this works. We build up our understanding of society and humanity, social work values and aims and our agency's policies and objectives. Pawson et al. (2003) suggest that this will include:

- *organisational knowledge*, about government and agency organisation and regulation
- *practitioner knowledge*, drawn from experience of practice
- *user knowledge*, drawn from users' knowledge of their lives, situation and use of services
- *research knowledge*, drawn from systematic investigation
- *policy community knowledge*, drawn from public and academic debate about policy options.

These contribute to forming aims that we are required to achieve by our agency and profession. What users, carers and their communities want interacts with these aims. Practice theories convert the aims into interventions, again in partnership with users, carers and their communities. I have presented this as a linear process in Figure 8.1, but the interaction of all these factors means that practitioners have to balance and negotiate them throughout their interventions. Practice theories provide a structure within which we may negotiate the processes of intervention.

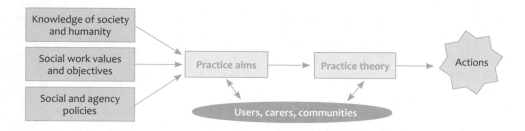

Figure 8.1 Practice theories apply knowledge and values to practice actions

Connections to ideas of reflexivity, important in research and feminist thinking, make links to current ideological concerns and offer interesting insights into implementing reflectiveness (Healy, 2000; Taylor and White, 2000; Finlay and Gough, 2003).

Critical reflection helps practitioners to handle the range of practice theories available. Research by Marsh and Triseliotis (1996) has shown that social workers are confused by the profusion. Morgans (2007) suggests that this is because theories are often presented competitively, that is, they seem to be in competition to be the 'correct and complete' theory. Reflection offers a way of thinking through the application of ideas in particular circumstances. Another attraction of reflective practice is the hope that it seems to hold out for personal professional development and the transfer of learning from one setting to another (Cree and Macaulay, 2001). Martyn (2001) argues that reflection can help people to make sense of the circumstances presented to social workers in complex situations, relating them to agency requirements. For similar reasons, reflective practice has become influential in healthcare professions (Jaspers, 2003; Bulman and Schutz, 2004; White et al., 2006).

Reflective practice

Many hopes rest on critical reflection. Therefore we must ask if it can bear the strain. There are several different meanings of 'reflection' in social work and two concepts related to the idea of 'reflective practice'. Each of these has their parallels in critical reflection, set out in Table 8.1.

Table 8.1 Reflective practice and critical reflection

Reflective practice	Critical reflection
Thinking things through carefully	Critical thinking
Reflective practice	Critical reflection
The reflective cycle: experience-reflection-action	Critical processes: reflexivity-deconstruction-critical social theory

Thinking issues through in all their complexity and acting towards clients and others in a considered, thoughtful manner is the common-sense meaning of reflection. It sometimes encourages a particular style of practice – slow, considered, thoughtful, thinking out all the angles, checking out all the details before taking the plunge. This has relationships with other important ideas in social work theory and practice, and with widely accepted views about the role of social workers. Reflection in this sense connects with study and diagnosis.

The idea of 'reflective practice', developed from the ideas of Argyris and Schön (1974; Schön, 1983), is a more complex way of understanding reflection, based on the ideas of pragmatic philosophies, which see education as concerned with practical problem-solving (Ixer, 1999). These ideas similarly influenced Perlman's (1957) problem-solving social work theories. Schön argued that some professions deal with work (such as building bridges), which uses 'technical rationality', that is, you can calculate through mathematics and scientific thinking exactly what the consequences of your decisions and actions will be (and so be sure that the bridge will not fall down when you have completed it). Schön thought that some kinds of work deal with such complex and variable situations that complete technical rationalism is impossible. Theories in this kind of work offer guidelines for action in the average daily situation, rather than complete rules about what to do. When we come across something out of the ordinary, we have to stop, think over and amend our guidelines. Thus, our guidelines (theories) grow every time we deal with a yet more complicated bit of human life, but they will never cover everything.

The implication of Schön's ideas are that people doing jobs such as teaching and social work, for example, should be educated to expect that their theories and guidelines will only help them so far. We should learn how to identify when existing theories are not helpful enough and should be trained in techniques of reflecting on situations and theory together so as to develop theories further. His particular concern is education for such techniques, and several of his examples use a supervisor, as in social work, for an exploring and questioning discussion. Schön (1983: 76–104) describes reflection as having 'a reflective conversation with the situation'. Issues in our work are reframed into different kinds of problems, so that an alternative way of dealing with them can be worked out. Gould (1996) describes this as 'imaginisation', that is, creating images in our mind of the problems with which we are dealing. In Schön's view, we argue out the implications of our new approach, leaving it open to rethink our rethinking if our new premise does not seem to work. We bring past experience to bear on new unique situations and try out a rigorous 'on-the-spot experiment' to see whether our ideas work.

Schön (1983: 157–62) emphasised that reflection takes place in a 'virtual world' of our own constructions about the problem and possible answers to it; it is not reality and action itself. These points of view and debates are represented by different practice theories, explored in Part 2, which suggest different ways in which social workers may interpret and react to the situations they face.

Mattinson's (1975) ideas about reflection suggest that social workers reflect their relationships with their clients in their behaviour towards their supervisor. So if a client is frightened of getting things wrong, and becomes dependent on their social worker, always coming for advice and guidance before doing the simplest thing, the social worker will start doing this, in an out-of-character way, with their supervisor, too. This is also common sense if you think about (reflect – in the first sense – on) it. The social worker is helping someone in a complex situation, and takes on the pressure of being worried, losing some self-confidence and passing on to the supervisor some of the pressure and also, probably unwittingly, some feeling of what the relationship with the client is like. Practitioners can use this idea. This view of reflection comes from the psychoanalytic idea of transference, which suggests that the nature of relationships with important people in our past influences current important relationships.

The 'reflective cycle' is a way of implementing reflective practice. Jaspers (2003) usefully presents three elements of reflective practice in sequence that she calls ERA: experience-reflection-action. First, we have experiences coming from interactions with our clients, their families and communities; we identify and describe these as clearly as we can. Then we reflect upon these experiences, applying theoretical ideas to them; this allows us to test out the relevance of particular theories in the situation we are presented with. Finally, we test out these ideas with various actions, leading us to have a further concrete experience about which we can reflect. To build this into a learning experience, we can identify possible alternatives and think through possible future guidelines for our own and colleagues' practice if the situation arises again, building on the knowledge we have created with this experience.

In summary, then, reflection takes place in our minds both as we act (reflection-in-action) and afterwards as we think about and try to understand the events we have experienced (reflection-on-action). Reflection implies attending to particular situations, and using observation, imagining alternative ways of understanding those situations ('imaginisation' and reframing). Reflection, then, leads us to experiment with alternative approaches that eventually become incorporated into our ways of thinking and acting in social work. Practice theories, such as those reviewed in Part 2, help us to express and identify those alternative approaches in models of practice that we might use when we act as social workers.

Critical reflection

Critical reflection has developed from reflective practice during the early twenty-first century; there is, as yet, less agreement than with reflective practice about precisely what it entails.

A starting point of critical reflection, set out in Table 8.1, is critical thinking. This includes the examination of arguments in theoretical debates to ensure that they are logical and well founded in evidence (Bowell and Kemp, 2002). It also includes searching for a range of alternative sources of information to test that we are not taking a particular point of view for granted. Glaister (2008: 8), for example, uses the term 'critical' to refer to little more than reflective practice: 'open-minded, reflective approaches that take account of different perspectives, experiences and assumptions'. She is mainly concerned to distance the term 'critical' from its everyday negative and destructive connotations, in statements like: 'he was very critical of the way I behaved'; certainly, critical thinking is more than this. Jones et al. (2008a: 286) are concerned to link criticality with the official UK government term, 'best practice', suggesting that this requires practitioners to 'focus in a sociologically critical way on what actually gets done well in social work, why and how it gets done and with what consequences'. This means, as Glaister argues, that practice improvements may be achieved by constantly examining and testing out the ideas and evidence we are using. Here, though, critical practitioners emphasise sociological ideas, because, as H. Ferguson (2008: 18) suggests, sociological critique involves asking awkward questions about the way in which society is structured and how power is used, and goes beyond immediate and emotional reactions to situations we experience.

In Table 8.1, therefore, critical thinking goes beyond reflective practice. This is because it proposes that we should not just draw on our existing knowledge, experience and reactions, but should actively seek alternatives that question present social structures and assumptions. This is particularly because of what Smith (2007) calls 'normative generalisation'. To make everyday life, service provision and policy development smooth and consistent, he suggests, we accept existing conventions about how things are done. We generalise from accepted standards because of the effort and complexity of thinking in new ways, echoing what Schön says, that mostly we follow existing guidelines and it is only when we come up against something that does not fit, that we reflect about how we can deal with it. Critical thinking argues that we should not accept these conventions and guidelines, but should be ready to look at alternative ways of seeing social situations all the time. Practice theories help us with this systematically because they provide clearly different alternatives. If we study them so that we understand the major differences between the alternative theories, we have ready-made ways of thinking critically.

'Critical reflection', developed in social work particularly by Fook and her colleagues (Fook, 2002; White et al., 2006; Fook and Gardner, 2007) provides a technique for doing this. They argue that there are certain kinds of theories that are particularly good for thinking critically; if we use them, we can help the reflection process. This is because these theories consistently question the existing structures and ideas in society. The aim is to be creative and have alternatives available. The various publications about critical reflection have alternative formulations as ideas have developed, but they usually:

- Start from reflective practice and follow the reflective cycle.
- Emphasise 'bottom-up' approaches to understanding situations, in particular focusing on the 'narrative' of the service user or client. This gives importance to their own understanding of their experiences, rather than putting people into administrative or service-providing categories.
- Use 'critical social theory', including the work of sociologists of the Frankfurt School, such as Habermas. These theorists make a link between people's personal and cultural experiences in society and the ways in which societies are structured and organised, in particular the way in which some people are unconsciously oppressed by economic, social and political organisation. Pease et al. (2003: 2) summarise these ideas as follows:

> Most critical theorists are concerned with emancipatory education that enables people to see the links between their experiences and the material conditions and dominant ideologies in society ... [emphasising] the capacity of critical theories to explain the sources of oppression in society in such a way as to encourage those affected by oppression to take action to transform it ... Critical theory also questions the place of existing institutions, such as the family, educational establishments and governance, with a view to constructing a more just society.

In this view, social work is a form of this emancipatory education, seeking to free people from personal constraints and limitations that have often been created by social structures that we do not think about on a daily basis. Because of this, it is easy to forget to challenge the accepted way of doing things.

- Use postmodernist ideas, in particular 'deconstruction'. Postmodernism suggests that societies are not rationally organised along scientific lines. Therefore, social life cannot be explained in one organised systematic account of the world, but reflects many different points of view interacting with each other. Deconstruction involves taking apart ideas so that we can see where the power of conventional assumptions and acceptance of normative generalisations are leading us to see as inevitable things that we could have a go at changing.
- Use reflexivity, the circular process by which our thoughts affect our actions, which affect the situation we are dealing with and therefore offer feedback through the reactions of others involved, which can affect how we understand and think about the situation. This sets off another cycle in which our thoughts affect our actions. Circularity is important because social work is active. We do not just think and assess but act on the situations we deal with. Reflexivity means that we constantly gain evidence about how effective or worthwhile our actions are, and we can change what we are doing according to the evidence of its value. To do so means being constantly alert to the possibility that what we are doing needs to change and we have to keep our minds open to changing according to the evidence we see about the effect we are having.

These are complex ideas, which are taken up more fully in some of the theoretical chapters in this part of the book, in particular Chapters 17 and 20 and the concluding chapter by the editors. However, here, we are looking at them as ways of constantly questioning what we are doing and they lead to a number of critical processes. Although these are similar to the reflective cycle, in that they are ways of thinking about our practice, they do not form a cycle, rather we use them constantly, and one interacts with the other. Practice theories help us to do this because they offer many different ideas about how to think about social situations and how to test them out with the people involved. Another important point about critical reflection is that it involves service users and the people around them; it is done jointly with them, by exploring their own 'narratives', that is, how service users jointly make sense of the story of the social issues that have affected them. Reflexiveness means using this to put yourself as a practitioner in their shoes, and understanding how they have reacted to the social pressures that have affected them.

Critical social theory helps with taking an alternative view, because it starts from the position that present social arrangements and structures have contributed to a feeling, and perhaps a reality, that everything is oppressing service users, bearing down upon them. It looks for the external social pressure, not just the personal responsibility of the user and their family and community. Moreover, even where they seem to be to blame, critical social theory is on their side, because it starts from the assumption that they may have come to accept the reality of social arrangements, when, with a bit of thought, we can see that there are alternative views. We came across this sort of idea in Adams et al., 2009a, Chapter 23 on adult and health-related social work.

However, Adams et al. (2009a: Ch. 1) also noted that critiques of this idea have said that we must nevertheless not police a questioning view like this so that it becomes a new orthodoxy, because we must always identify a range of different perceptions and experiences. Disabled people also experience pain, distress and limitations, which are very real for them. This is reflexive, putting yourself in the other person's shoes to understand a range of matters that affect them and reacting to the full reality of their situation.

All these ideas also deconstruct complex ideas, and identify possible alternatives. Deconstruction means looking at the components of everyday concepts to see where power is used to make problems seem impossible, when we can benefit from seeing them more flexibly. Coppock and Hopton (2000) do this with ideas about mental health. They also look at common social inequalities to see if these inform our understanding. Do poor people, women and people from minority ethnic groups suffer more from mental illness? If so, it might suggest that these groups differ in physical or mental differences from wider populations, but it might also show that social arrangements, the ways we treat poor people, women and people from minority groups affect whether someone becomes or remains mentally ill. Coppock and Hopton (2000) also look at the question of legitimacy: who is accepted as being able to say that someone is mentally ill and to help them? It might be doctors, or only specialist doctors, or people around the mentally ill person, or a multiprofessional group of staff. If we work in healthcare, the answer to all these things might be that mental health is an illness diagnosed by doctors and treated by specialists using medication; however, deconstruction through critical reflection offers other thoughts about possible interventions.

There are broader implications to reflexivity. In research, the idea is used to draw attention to the way in which the researcher's presence and involvement affects the situations being investigated. A researcher is never a neutral inquirer. Neither, of course, are social workers, because the whole point of social work is that their involvement helps to achieve change, individual or social or both. Taylor and White (2000) argue that by a detailed understanding of the evidence about how interactions with people have effects, we may build up a more flexible and broadly applicable base for understanding and action than specific evidence-based practice theories can offer. These ideas also help to emphasise how the experience of social work will change the worker, and how interpersonal practice experiences can help to build the knowledge to apply in broader social and political action, to make the personal become political.

'Praxis' is a Marxist term that takes this idea a little further. It emphasises that our thoughts and the circular reflexive process are affected by our ideology, that is, what we believe the social world is like and how we think it should be. Our ideology causes us to think and therefore act with particular objectives. This interacts with the world, and praxis proposes that we should allow the evidence of how the world is to reform and affect our beliefs. Marxist ideas emphasise the importance of using praxis to experience the inequality and oppression in the world that we deal with, so as to strengthen our ideology of opposition and desire to work effectively within the world to change it.

The ideas of reflexivity and praxis emphasise how our thoughts interact with practice to affect clients and service users, and how their reactions and experience come to affect our own view of the world and our thoughts. Critical reflection, then, is one of the processes through which clients participate in social work. We are forced by our experience of their world and problems to think carefully about their experiences and respond to them. Social work does not impose a set of prescriptions on clients. Instead, it reacts to clients and the world in which they live, and it does so through reflection.

Using critical reflection with practice theory

There are some aspects of using theory and knowledge in an organised way that the idea of critical reflection does not help us with. In the first place, reflection in 'critical reflection' takes place almost in a social vacuum, even where service users and their families are involved in our thinking processes. Practice theories help us because they suggest areas where we might focus our thoughts. Attachment theory suggests, for example, that we should examine people's linkages with others, how they learned to make such linkages and difficulties that they have experienced in building relationships. It also suggests certain common kinds of attachment behaviour that we can explore with people. Task-centred practice, on the other hand, suggests a focus on defining particular problems. What are the priorities? What tasks will help towards problem-solving? Empowerment theory pushes us to think what actions will be empowering and why.

Focusing on reflection may be oppressive, because it leads to a lack of clarity both for practitioners and the people they work with; we can seem to go round in circles or come up with unrealistic ideas that conflict with the aims of our service. It may be unclear to practitioners and service users what the process of reflection actually is and how it connects with taking action. Again, practice theories help, because they propose actions as a result of the direction that our thinking takes us in. Cognitive-behavioural theory, for example, suggests techniques that we can follow to get people working on their cognitions in a practical way. Feminist, anti-oppressive or transformational theory suggests an approach to engagement with service users that can help us to build a shared dialogue about what might help and what is practical in the circumstances that users face.

Theories are sometimes presented, as in the chapters in Part 2, as more or less complete perspectives on how we should try to understand the world or as models of how to respond to particular situations. Theories are said to explain and justify why particular perspectives or models are valuable to social workers. How do we identify which theory or theories to use, and how do we use them? We now explore how we can reflect on theories as we apply them in three different ways: selectivity, eclecticism and critical engagement. Each of these ways of reflecting on theory tries to answer the question of whether it is realistically possible to understand and implement a wide range of theoretical ideas.

Selectivity

This approach to using theory proposes that we should select just one, or one group of related theories, and apply that to all the situations that we deal with. The advantage of this approach is that we can go into the ideas of the theory in depth, become comfortable and assured in applying them and act consistently throughout our work. There are, however, problems with this approach, both practical and theoretical.

Among the practical problems are that most social workers operate in (sometimes multidisciplinary) teams with others who may not share the particular theory they use, and the theory may not make sense to clients either. Many workers who operate selectively are supported in doing so because they work in agencies, for example psychiatric units or specialist centres such as women's refuges, where workers share a theoretical position, often in a fairly small group of people who work together consistently, as in a day or residential care setting.

The theoretical problems with selectivity lie in the difficulty of one theory extending into a wide range of different situations. Many theories, such as psychoanalytic or cognitive-behavioural theories, claim this possibility and some, including these examples, are extensively developed. However, it is often enthusiasts who claim this, and observers often consider that such theories are overstretched, overcomplex and hard to follow, or ignore large areas of work that their theory does not fit. For example, both of these examples are primarily therapeutic in character and do not deal well with the practical problems of people in poverty or suffering from racist abuse in an inner-city housing estate.

Eclecticism

The eclectic approach suggests either that workers should select aspects of different theories and use them together, perhaps all at once or perhaps successively, in a case, or that workers should use different theories in different cases, depending on which is appropriate. Eclecticism enables different ideas to be brought to bear, helps to amalgamate social work theories when they make similar proposals for action, deals better with complex circumstances and allows workers to compensate for inadequacies in particular theories.

As with selectivity, however, there are theoretical and practical disadvantages. Workers may be unable to decide which set of ideas to select and how they should put them together. Also, it is difficult to know many complex theories well enough to take parts of them and use them appropriately. Social work theories may produce similar action proposals, but this often implies different ways of understanding issues. So, in contrast with the selective approach, eclecticism may confuse clients and workers by bringing together ideas in inconsistent patterns. Epstein (1992), therefore, proposes that eclecticism should be built up by continuing reflection, agreement and debate, and recommends doing this cooperatively in a team rather than encouraging individual flexibility from moment to moment in our practice. Approaches to reflective practice suggest using a mentor or supervision as a structure within which you can reflect carefully and critically (Taylor and White, 2000).

An important focus of eclecticism is systems theory (Pincus and Minahan, 1973). This biologically based perspective on practice emphasises working at different levels in society: the individual, the 'system' surrounding individuals, and the more extensive systems that form a context for lower level systems. This allows practice with agencies and other people and groups on behalf of clients to be theorised, and Roberts (1990) argues that systems theory was part of a trend in the 1970s to integrate many different aspects of social work into a generic form of practice. Systems theory's integration is at least partly eclectic, since it suggests that different theories might be used at different levels, for example therapeutic theories with individuals, radical theories with social systems, and with different systems, for example family therapy with a family, task-centred work with peer groups. Since it provides a model for analysing the different systems and levels with which workers might operate, it provides a basis for deciding which aspects of a case might have different theories applied to them. However, it does not help to decide which level or system to work on or which theory to choose and how it may be integrated with the other theories chosen.

Another way of thinking about eclecticism is to emphasise the basic approach of a theory: looking at how people's past experiences have affected their present relationships in attachment theory, for example, and how to solve problems in task-centred practice or change specific behavioural issues in cognitive-behavioural work.

Critical engagement

An alternative way of using theories to help in reflection is by using them critically against one another. Many social work theories offer criticisms of other theories. Differences between theories can help critical reflection in practice by enabling alternative and opposing theories to criticise practice that used a particular theory.

CaSE EXaMPLE

Mrs Jones is a single parent who was very depressed and unable to care adequately for her three preschool children. The social worker focused on her depression and found that this came from isolation and loneliness. Her GP supplied antidepressants and the worker thought through with her the life she had led so far and plans for the future.

Reflecting on this, radical and critical theory would criticise the individualised approach. It does not look at how single parents may be stigmatised, put in the worst housing and blamed for not bringing up a conventional family. Feminist theory would draw attention to the oppression of women by forcing them into caring roles and not validating their aspirations for the future. Cognitive-behavioural theory tells us that she might benefit from learning different ways of thinking that would enable her to cope better with the world, instead of our approach of being concerned with her feelings and responses to her present situation. By reflecting on these alternative views of the situation, the worker can criticise and develop her approach, even if she does not use them to guide her practice according to their own model of action.

Critical reflection on integration and dissent

So far, we have examined ideas about reflective practice and critical reflection and, following that, some of the difficulties that arise in reflecting on practice theories. The argument has been that the idea of critical reflection is often discussed in a social vacuum and that we need to reflect in a context of awareness about debates around the value of the practice theories we are considering. We have to incorporate into reflective practice and critical reflection an understanding of the interaction between the ideas we are using to guide our practice, and we have to have models for thinking out the interaction of ideas.

Our reflection must also include the material considered throughout these books, which gives us evidence about human beings and their social world. Critical reflection must integrate this into our thinking about action, because our action needs to use this knowledge. Complete integration is neither possible nor desirable, however, because there is no agreement about how we should interpret and act on much of this material. So, again, our reflection must incorporate the possibility of dissent and disagreement. We should not try to put everything together, but accept that many ideas will be in tension; this helps us to be creative.

Theory, the law and the agency

One of the difficult aspects of applying theory is understanding its role in relation to the legal basis of social work practice and agency requirements, factors that influence and constrain how social workers practise. Magistrates and judges reading pre-sentence reports and managers looking at our practice are not likely to concern themselves with which theory was used. Colleagues in a multidisciplinary team are interested in the results we produce, not explanations of how it all came about. Lay people are naturally entitled to have reports and explanations of practice presented in clear, non-technical language, and colleagues are entitled to expect our practice to be competent and success-ful. This does not, however, make theory irrelevant to our practice.

Everything we do implies a theory about the circumstances that we deal with. Obviously, as we undertake social work activities, we use theory, even if it is not one of the formally stated ones. Knowing about and using the formal statements of theory help to clarify and organise ideas about what we do. It helps report-writing and justi-fying ourselves to managers and magistrates if we can be clear about why we took this or that action. Occasionally, a particular case goes wrong and there is a formal inquiry. Even if this does not happen very often, our practice and everyday activity will display greater self-confidence and consistency if we have an organised view of what we are doing and why. Colleagues and clients will also have their own theories about the world, both formally organised and informal. Our own understanding of theory enables us to see where their theory is situated in the constellation of possible views of the world. We can also identify more easily inconsistencies and difficulties in deci-sions that they have chosen to make. Where colleagues' theories agree with our own, we can cooperate and work together on a more common basis and cement multidis-ciplinary work more effectively.

Theory, then, can be used for accountability to agencies and external institutions such as the law, because it clarifies our ideas about what we do. Moreover, applying, and being able to refer to, an established form of practice enables us to justify our practice to outsiders.

Theory in practice

Perhaps the most important group to whom we can justify our practice by using theory is our clients. They are entitled to know that we have an organised view of what we are doing and why and gain understanding and explanation of what we are doing, so that they can agree or disagree with it. This is one of the claimed advantages of approaches such as cognitive-behavioural practice and task-centred work, since a clear and often written agreement is made between worker and client. It is one of the essential features of radical, feminist and anti-oppressive theories, which require a dialogue between equals rather than an expert therapist helping a disempowered client.

Obviously, clients do not need to be involved in every technicality. However, Seck-er's (1993) study of social work students suggests that students who succeeded in applying theory with confidence had certain important characteristics. Their skills in using theory were not about intellectual ability, but about skill in working openly with clients. Their use of theory started from the clients themselves. They listened well and responded to what clients told them. They did not put clients in theoretical categories. Instead, they used theoretical ideas all the time in discussing matters with clients. As a client said something, they might say: 'That reminds me of an idea …'. They picked up ideas and talked them over with clients, they did not keep them to themselves. They worked together with clients to test out their ideas, first in discussion and then in what Schön (1983) calls 'on-the-spot' experimentation.

Using theory, then, does not require great intellect, rather it requires the application of exactly those social and interpersonal skills in working openly with people that social workers most like to claim. It involves reflecting theoretically with clients and also with colleagues, making reflection-in-action and reflection after the event an everyday part of what social workers do. Also, it means having the self-confidence to be open about your ideas and willing to experiment, alongside your clients, in putting your ideas into action.

Conclusion

This approach to theory suggests that we should be cautious and critical of all simplifications of the world. Indeed, it argues that we should be critical and reflective in all our dealings with other human beings. We should never use theory to pigeonhole and restrict the infinite variety of humanity and its possibilities for future development. Instead, theory should be a guide to be used together with clients to explore, understand and transform the social world in which we live together.

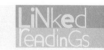

For further discussion of understanding critical practice, see Chapter 1, and for entering critical practice, see Chapter 21. Chapters 9–20, which comprise Part 2, offer a beginning in using social work's theoretical ideas.

Fook, J. and Gardner, F. (2007) *Practising Critical Refection: A Resource Handbook*, Maidenhead, Open University Press. The first and third part provide a sophisticated account of critical practice and its application in agency settings, the middle part offers a comprehensive training programme, which may also be useful.

Gould, N. and Baldwin, M. (2004) *Social Work, Critical Reflection and the Learning Organization*, Aldershot, Ashgate. Useful collection of articles on various aspects of critical reflection, focusing on how they may be applied in an organisation committed to developing its staff.

Payne, M. (2005) *Modern Social Work Theory*, 3rd edn, Basingstoke, Palgrave Macmillan. A more extended critical review of social work theories than is possible here.

Schön, D. (1983) *The Reflective Practitioner: How Professionals Think in Action*, New York, Basic Books. Classic, creative and easy-to-read book about how some professions benefit from learning how to use 'reflection-in-action' to inform their practice.

Taylor, C. and White, S. (2000) *Practising Reflexivity in Health and Welfare: Making Knowledge*, Buckingham, Open University Press. Thoughtful book directly based on research into practice and full of ideas and stimulating insights into social work practice.

Counselling 9

This chapter explores the relationship between social work and counselling, and the use of counselling theories, values and skills within social work practice. It covers the changing context of counselling within social work, the different theoretical underpinnings to counselling ideas and skills relevant to social work, counselling theory and skills within social work practice today and some current issues emerging from counselling and social work.

Chapter overview

Introduction

The current context of this chapter on counselling is radically different from that which gave rise to the Barclay Report of the early 1980s. The report argued that it was:

essential that social workers continue to be able to provide counselling and we use the word to cover a range of activities in which an attempt is made to understand the meaning of some event or state of being to an individual, family or group and to plan, with the person or people concerned, how to manage the emotional and practical realities that face them. (Barclay Committee, 1982: 41)

On the same page, Barclay argued that social workers have themselves seen counselling 'as the hallmark of their calling'. Brearley (1995) documents the social, political, legislative and policy changes that have impacted on social work since the mid-1970s and have altered social workers' relationship to counselling. Today it would be more likely that social workers would see their hallmark as brokerage or care management rather than counselling. Social work students are often resistant to undertaking direct in-depth work with service users, seeing 'counselling' as something they feel they are neither prepared for nor trained to undertake.

With a few exceptions, social work practice is located within a legislative context. Where counselling is employed by its practitioners, it will be alongside other interventions and within a legislative, procedural and organisational context, compromising it as a form of 'pure' counselling, its being instead one of several possible social work methods of intervention. Social work practitioners, in all their various manifestations, have traditionally had a complex relationship with counselling. Bringing together the separate enterprises of counselling and social work has posed theoretical, organisational, ethical, practical and practice dilemmas. They are two separate areas of helping interventions, governed by different professional bodies, underpinned by separate bodies of knowledge and offering different outcomes, while sharing many of the same values, intentions, processes, ideas and methods. They are both interested and engaged in the processes of change, and they are both predominately preoccupied with the psychosocial. It might well be difficult to distinguish some social work interviews from a counselling session. Social work training has traditionally drawn heavily on counselling methods when teaching social work interviewing skills. However, it is often argued that, despite the close relationship between social work interviewing and counselling, they are separate activities, one being the practice of counselling and the other the utilisation of counselling skills. Feltham (1995: 72) points to the different views of professional bodies in relation to this distinction; the British Association for Counselling and Psychotherapy arguing that social workers are employing counselling skills rather than practising counselling, whereas the Group for the Advancement of Psychodynamics and Psychotherapy in Social Work has occasionally argued that casework can be not just counselling, but also indeed psychotherapy. Historically, social casework, as practised by psychodynamically oriented social workers, would hardly have been discernible from counselling.

Social work students and practitioners now occupy the twenty-first century and are engaged in discourses different from those of the Barclay Report. One change has been the gradual de-emphasis on the 'collective' and the re-emphasis on the 'individual' and the individual's responsibility to facilitate change, whether that be social, economic or personal. The past 20 years have seen a corresponding mushrooming of personal therapies, increased professionalisation of counselling, growth in numbers of private counsellors and psychotherapists, and an explosion of related trainings. The same period has seen counselling, within the social work context, being relocated into the private and voluntary sectors, and a growing reluctance on the behalf of social workers to undertake counselling with service users, seeing it as outside their remit, outside their theoretical and skills base and outside the realm of the possible, because of time and resource constraints. A cynical observer might comment that one major development in the differentiation between counselling and social work has been that the former is now rarely used other than for the benefit of the bourgeoisie and the latter is used for the working class.

In its many different forms and contexts, social work practice today still needs to employ counselling as a possible method of intervention in specific and appropriate contexts, while drawing on counselling theory and skills to inform its knowledge and skills repertoire more generally. Social workers still have to 'do the work' with service users, whether it be in-depth, long-term work or as part of an assessment in order to devise a care plan. Without counselling theory and counselling skills, social work practice is likely to be ineffectual and inefficient.

Theoretical groupings within counselling

Before looking at some of the broad theoretical groupings of ideas underpinning differ-ent 'schools' of counselling, it may be important to say something about what counselling is. The word 'counselling' is often used interchangeably with the word 'advice'. For example, it might be more accurate to refer to careers 'advice' given in schools rather than careers 'counselling'. Emphasising the distinction between the spon-taneous giving of help and professional intervention, Dryden et al. (1989: 4, quoting from BAC, 1985: 1) write:

> Counselling is a more deliberate activity and in its definition of the term the British Asso-ciation for Counselling spells out the distinction between a planned and a spontaneous event. 'People become engaged in counselling when a person, occupying regularly or temporarily the role of counsellor, offers or agrees explicitly to offer time, attention and respect to another person or persons temporarily in the role of client.'

One of the most comprehensive definitions of counselling is offered by Feltham and Dryden (2004: 40), who describe it as:

> a principled relationship characterised by the application of one or more psychological theories and a recognised set of communication skills, modified by experience, intuition and other interpersonal factors, to clients' intimate concerns, problems or aspirations. Its predominant ethos is one of facilitation rather than of advice-giving or coercion. It may be of very brief or long duration, take place in an organisational or private practice setting and may or may not overlap with practical, medical and other matters of personal welfare.

This definition illustrates why there may be some confusion over what it is, precisely, that makes counselling and social work perceived as being so different.

What are the 'psychological theories' referred to within this definition? As it pertains to social work practice, counselling has two areas related to it that have been of signifi-cance to its practice and knowledge base: the theoretical underpinning of different 'schools' of counselling and their related skills application. There are many different counselling approaches built on a number of diverse theoretical perspectives. Only some of these have been influential upon social work and they may be grouped under four general headings: psychodynamic, humanistic person-centred, cognitive-behavioural, and eclectic and inte-grative. These headings represent whole sets of ideas separate from counselling, which can be traced in relation to their influence on social work practice, and the ideas related to each heading can be shown to have been influential upon both social work and counsel-ling at similar historical moments. For example, the interrelationships between psychodynamic ideas and social work and psychodynamic ideas and counselling are similar for both social work and counselling (Yellolly, 1980; Pearson et al., 1988; Payne, 1992; Brown, H., 1996; Fleet, 2000; McLeod, 2003: 23; Jacobs, 2004; Bower, 2005; Miller, 2006). Theoretical developments are part of an economic, social, geographical, historical, racial and gendered context; both social work and counselling have been subject to similar influences in their different processes of professionalisation since the beginning of the nineteenth century. Both professions developed in an often defensive relationship to their more orthodox and (often perceived as) intellectually superior relatives psychoanalysis and psychotherapy. Both social work and counselling have suffered from developing in their shadows, despite their undoubted enrichment as a result of their close liaisons. There is no clear, singular, linear relationship between psychoanalysis, psychotherapy, counselling and social work, neither in their historical development nor in their theoretical underpinning. However, the myth and to some extent the reality of their interdependency has had a powerful influence.

Psychodynamic ideas

Jacobs (2004) offers a useful account of the interrelationship between psychodynamic ideas and counselling. This is one of the most complex theoretical areas drawn on in counselling, utilising a whole range of evolving ideas developed by many different individuals – Freud, Jung, Klien, Bion, Fairbairn, Winnicott and Bowlby, to name just a few of the originators – over a considerable period of time. Key psychodynamic concepts relevant to counselling would include the unconscious, the structures of the mind (the id, the ego and the superego), the past being relevant and impacting on the present, psychosexual development (oral, anal, phallic (Oedipal), latency, adult sexuality), defence mechanisms, envy, depression, transference and countertransference, projective identification, ambivalence, attachment, separation, loss and crisis. It is beyond the scope of this chapter to detail the meaning and different interpretations of these concepts. McLeod (2003) offers a useful precis of their development and application to counselling. Psychodynamic and psychoanalytical ideas have had a profound impact on the way in which we view human development and have been integrated into our cultural heritages in ways that subtly influence our understandings about ourselves and others. These influences have also impacted on counsellors:

All counsellors and therapists, even those who espouse different theoretical models, have been influenced by psychodynamic thinking and have had to make up their minds whether to accept or reject the Freudian image of the person. (McLeod, 2003: 43)

Psychodynamic counselling has attracted much criticism, including its normative and potentially pathologising tendencies and the question of its efficacy. Questioning the outcomes of psychodynamic interventions has been raised alongside the problem of resourcing what was often long-term intervention that had no measurable outcome. The development of 'brief therapy', associated with people such as Mann, Sifneos, Malan and Davanloo, has been significant in relation to this (McLeod, 2003). The development of brief therapy has been highly significant to counselling, as by its nature it is about facilitating the mobilisation of the client's inner and outer resources to manage a particular life event or set of circumstances, circumstances where limited interventions are often appropriate, as opposed to, in the case of psychotherapy, often long-term intervention focused on personality change. This development has not just affected psychodynamic counselling, but has also had a general impact on counselling (Feltham and Dryden, 2006).

Both humanistic person-centred and cognitive-behavioural counselling developed partly, but not exclusively, in response to some of the perceived difficulties and limitations of the psychodynamic approach.

Humanistic person-centred ideas

The development of humanistic person-centred counselling has its roots within the broad developments of both phenomenological and existential influences within philosophy and psychology during the postwar period. Its inception is often associated with a talk given by Carl Rogers in 1940 (Rogers, 1942), in which he emphasised clients' potential to find their own solutions:

> The emphasis on the client as expert and the counsellor as source of reflection and encouragement was captured in the designation of the approach as 'non-directive' counselling. (McLeod, 2003: 63)

Coulshed and Orme (2006: 52) write that the:

> theory base and important concepts devolve from a philosophical background of the existential tradition which respects an individual's subjective experience and places emphasis on the vocabulary of freedom, choice, autonomy and meaning.

Although this approach can be associated with broad theoretical and philosophical developments outside psychology, it was also part of the so-called 'third force' (the first and second being associated with the work of Freud and Skinner) within psychology, person-centred counselling being one development within that 'force'.

As a set of theories and methods, the person-centred approach is associated with an optimistic view of human nature but tells us little about human development. Although Dryden et al. (1989) were right in seeing the necessity of contextualising these theories, with their emphasis on 'self-actualisation', within the Californian culture of the 1960s, they are still important in having established the central significance of empathy, warmth and genuineness as key to the effectiveness of counselling interventions. The emphasis here is on counselling intervention rather than explanation of human behaviour. This approach and its theoretical underpinnings have been highly influential in social work, particularly on ideas relating to social work interviewing skills. Egan (2006) is seen as a bridge between counselling and social work interviewing, and is still highly influential in social work training courses. He has also been seen as a bridge between the humanistic person-centred and behavioural approaches (Dryden et al., 1989).

Cognitive-behavioural ideas

Cognitive-behavioural ideas and their influence on counselling have been associated with developments within mainstream psychology, with its emphasis on scientific methods, and the growth of behavioural and cognitive psychology in the postwar period. These ideas built on work conducted earlier in the century that drew on animal experiments, associated with people such as Pavlov, Watson and Thorndike. From the 1950s onwards, these ideas were built on by Eysenck, Rachman, Skinner, Wolpe and others, who were chiefly interested in behaviour and learning, and with understanding how behaviours are learned and what interventions will enable behaviour to change. They were not interested in understanding the inner meanings of acts or causation other than how those acts were learned.

Feltham (1995: 83) noted that 'behaviour therapy is based on what can be observed, studied, measured and reliably changed'. These are a different set of criteria from psychodynamic or humanistic person-centred preoccupations. Within this tradition, there are numerous types of behavioural and cognitive counselling interventions, drawing on specific theories including respondent conditioning, operant conditioning, observational learning and cognitive learning to name but a few. These interventions are interested not only in behaviour, but also in thoughts and feelings, and how these then impact upon and affect behaviour.

There have been moments in the history of social work when it has been fashionable to be derisive about behavioural interventions, but their relevance to social work is important. Currently, cognitive-behavioural interventions are popular with government and research funding councils, and some specific interventions, for example multidimensional treatment foster care, are based entirely on social learning theory. These ideas are popular as they have been shown to be effective with specific conditions, for example enuresis, agoraphobia and anxiety. One strength is their capacity to be adopted and practised by ordinary practitioners, be they social workers or community psychiatric nurses, who have not had to receive such extensive training as would be expected of, for example, a psychodynamic counsellor in order to facilitate an effective outcome. Behavioural interventions are often seen as successful in the short term and focus on management, focused change, measurement and monitoring. In the current climate of social work, these methods might be seen as fairly closely matching the needs of the professional roles.

Social work has traditionally drawn on a wide range of counselling theories and methods, a combination of psychodynamic, person-centred and cognitive-behavioural approaches, often in a haphazard way rather than in a theoretically and therapeutically logical manner that considers efficacy and professional integrity.

Eclectic and integrative approaches

The eclectic approach, sometimes referred to as 'integrative', is where the theory and the corresponding method of intervention are chosen as the most relevant and appropriate to meet the needs presented by the client or service user's specific circumstances. It can be seen as a way of maximising the beneficial aspects of the three different schools. Thus, the practitioner could potentially have an underlying psychodynamic understanding, take a person-centred approach to the counselling relationship, one that is characterised by warmth, respect and empathy, while having the capacity, where relevant, to employ behavioural techniques. To many, this smacks of heresy, but there is a growing literature looking at the validity of integration. McLeod notes the difference between an eclectic approach, which is a more accurate description of the above, and one that is integrative:

> An eclectic approach to counselling is one in which the counsellor chooses the best or most appropriate ideas and techniques from a range of theories or models, in order to meet the needs of the client. Integration, on the other hand, refers to a somewhat more ambitious enterprise in which the counsellor brings together elements from different theories and models them into a new theory or model. (McLeod, 2003: 99)

For social workers, their approach is likely, more often than not, to fall within the eclectic category, one they are already overfamiliar with and one that is often used against them, reinforcing the perception that social work has a flimsy, incoherent theoretical base in practice, whereas, in fact, eclecticism can be a potential strength.

Counselling and social work

Within the statutory sector, social work comprises a set of activities and interventions that are primarily focused on assessment, administration, care management, risk analysis and monitoring. It can be argued that the focus social work did have, or was perceived as having, on the facilitation of change, whether it was at the level of the individual, household, group or community, has slowly been transferred out of the statutory sector and into the private and voluntary sector. Within this independent sector, social workers both practise counselling and employ counselling skills. In the areas of drugs and alcohol misuse, palliative care, mental health and family work, social workers will be negotiating a counselling component to their overall work with a service user. This counselling work will rarely be 'pure' counselling, as by definition it will, as with social work practice more broadly, be located in the context of a wider intervention context.

It can be argued, and the author is among those who do, that counselling has to remain an integral part of social work wherever its location or context. This is 'counselling' in its broadest sense, focusing primarily on the application of counselling skills and the use of specific or integrative counselling theories. If we examine the processes of assessment, be they in relation to family support and child protection, assessment and care management in community care or the assessment undertaken by the key worker under the care programme approach in mental health (DH, 1995c), these processes necessitate the social worker having the competence to deploy counselling skills to undertake a full and comprehensive assessment. This link is made explicitly by Smale et al. (1993) when they consider the skills needed to enable competent work to be done when assessment work is undertaken. From a counselling perspective, Pearson (1990) also explores what it has to offer to social support and care management.

Over a number of decades, Egan (2006) has provided social work educators with a relevant and applicable model for the application of counselling skills to social work interviewing. He developed his model utilising both person-centred theory and behavioural ideas. Coulshed and Orme (2006: 45) list seven qualities that counsellors (in the context of social work) should have, qualities that are often associated with person-centred counselling and are central to Egan's model – empathy or understanding, respect, concreteness or being specific, self-knowledge and self-acceptance, genuineness, congruence and immediacy. Egan's model can be summarised as having four components – exploration, understanding, action and evaluation. It is easy to see why Smale et al. (1993) built on and adapted this model for application with assessment and care planning in community care. It has real strengths, including its commitment to working with, and not for, the client. It is a model that fits well with ideas of, and emphasises the importance of, engagement, clarity, focusing, planning, prioritising, negotiating realisable and relevant goals, action and review, and evaluation, all aspects of competent social work practice whatever its context, congruent with a culture of increasing openness and practitioner accountability. While the Egan model has received much criticism for its focus, foundations and crises-free assumptions, it is a model that can be adapted and built on to enhance effective social work intervention.

It has been argued that in the current social work context, social workers are more likely to offer counselling only within the independent sector, which is made up of private and voluntary organisations. However, to be effective, social workers within all contexts need to apply counselling skills and be informed by counselling ideas to be effective. This remains particularly pertinent within the statutory sector, where the majority of assessment work is concentrated, the application of counselling skills being fundamental to the processes of assessment, care planning and review. The need to refocus on relationship-based social work intervention within statutory social work is being recognised. Seden (2005), Trevithick (2005) and Miller (2006) all write from the position of the importance of counselling skills and their theoretical underpinning being applied to all areas of social work practice.

Issues

Egan's model is one that draws on behavioural and person-centred ideas and methods. It largely ignores psychodynamic ideas, and that can mean that it has limited application. To focus on 'a problem', without an understanding of causation, may mean that the intervention has limited effectiveness. Also, to ignore the contribution of systemic ideas to social work could mean that 'the problem' is seen outside its context, again limiting the effectiveness of the intervention. For the model to be effective, it needs to be located within a familiarity with and understanding of both psychodynamic and systemic ideas.

Much has been written about the reflective practitioner (see Chapter 8; Schön, 1987; Yelloly and Henkel, 1995; Thompson, 1996). Thompson (1996: 222) wrote that the reflective practitioner is:

> a worker who is able to use experience, knowledge and theoretical perspectives to guide and inform practice. Reflective practice involves cutting the cloth to suit the specific circumstances, rather than looking for ready-made solutions.

Reflective practice also needs the practitioner to have what was earlier referred to as 'self-knowledge'. It requires the practitioner to be able, and be committed, to reflect upon their own perceptions, responses and feelings in any given situation, requiring an understanding of countertransference. Countertransference is a complex and fraught area of psychoanalytic and psychodynamic theories. 'Social work accessible' explanations of these ideas are available (Salzberger-Wittenberg, 1970; Jacobs, 2004; Bower, 2005). Without this theoretical base underpinning the application of counselling skills, we will not achieve reflective practice.

As ideas in counselling and social work have developed, so there has been a growing acceptance by both professions of their limitations in offering an appropriate service to a cross-section of all our communities. Not only have these two professional groups been unable to reach all communities, but they might also have been overtly and covertly, deliberately and by default, discriminatory and oppressive to individuals and specific communities. Inclusive practice has become an accepted part of the discourse of social work. Within counselling, there is a substantial literature developing, demonstrating a general acceptance that ideas and models may need to be adapted to enable inclusive practice that meets the needs of diverse groups at the receiving end of social work interventions (d'Ardenne and Mahtani, 1999; Atkinson and Hackett, 2004; Davies and Neal, 2004).

Conclusion

A key issue for counselling and social work is social work's gradual defensive rejection of and timidity towards its use of counselling and counselling skills. It has been argued that both are still and will remain central to the roles and tasks of social work. Counselling skills are integral to the processes of assessment and care management, and there will remain a need for counselling within the social work context, certainly within the independent sector. If we are going to achieve the goal of a profession that is made up of competent and reflective practitioners, we will need to draw on counselling skills and models that enhance effectiveness and make use of counselling theories that inform practice. This could enable professional reflection to take place when working with the needs of specific, unique individuals within their own context and lead to the deployment of sensitive, relevant and effective interventions that facilitate negotiated change.

For further discussion of cognitive-behavioural work, see Chapter 14, and for the importance of supervision, see Adams et al., 2009c, Chapter 15.

www.bacp.co.uk   The website of the British Association of Counselling and Psychotherapy is a useful source of information about developments in the profession, conferencesm courses and so on.

http://www.tcc.tv   The website of The Counselling Channel offers a range of audio-visual resources about counselling, including short interviews with leading academics about key theories and face-to-camera monologues from clients talking about their experiences.

Atkinson, D.R. and Hackett, G. (2004) *Counseling Diverse Populations*, 3rd edn, New York, McGraw Hill. Offers general coverage of inclusive practice issues in counselling.

Brearley, J. (1995) *Counselling and Social Work*, Maidenhead, Open University Press. Covers areas directly pertinent to the content of this chapter.

McLeod, J. (2003) *An Introduction to Counselling*, 3rd edn, Maidenhead, Open University Press. Helpful introduction to counselling theory and practice.

Miller, L. (2006) *Counselling Skills for Social Work*, London, Sage. Also covers areas directly pertinent to the content of this chapter.

Seden, J. (2005) *Counselling Skills in Social Work Practice*, 2nd edn, Maidenhead, Open University Press. Looks in detail at the application of counselling skills to social work practice.

Groupwork 10

Chapter overview

This chapter considers the changing nature of groupwork and, arguably, the lessening of its significance as a distinctive and skilled method in contemporary social work. Identifying core values and skills, the author argues, with examples, for a reassertion of the place of groupwork across social work practice.

Where has all the groupwork gone?

Although groups and groupwork are central to much that we do, in both our private and professional lives, 'groupwork' seems, almost without being noticed, to have faded from view. So, where and why has groupwork gone and what might be its future?

The late 1970s and 1980s saw an outpouring of British texts focusing on the generic basics of groupwork (for example Davies, 1975; Douglas, 1978, 1983; Brown, 1979, 1986; Houston, 1984; Heap, 1985; Whitaker, 1985; Preston-Shoot, 1987) and *Groupwork*, the first British journal devoted to the method, was launched in 1988. However, this output was failing to keep up with deeper changes that were taking place in society at large.

Little of this vibrancy and expansiveness is visible today. One or two of the established authorities continued to pursue the method (Brown, 1992; Douglas, 1993; Preston-Shoot, 2007), joined by a few others (Adams and O'Sullivan, 1994; Vernelle, 1994; Doel and Sawdon, 1999; Phillips, 2001; Doel, 2006), providing a continuing flow of outputs on the topic. However, I see little evidence of its take-up in field practice. *Groupwork* continues as a thrice-yearly publication. A scan of its contents since 1990 reveals that, of the papers published, many are by foreign authors. Few address groupwork practised in the statutory social services. Indeed, Doel and Sawdon (1999: 21) observe that groupwork is increasingly being practised by people who are not social workers, perhaps based on a view that groupwork is not appropriate for everyday statutory social work. While there are rich veins of practice experience and conceptual analysis in the journal, little of this is grounded in the mainstream of social work. Much of this literature must seem remote to social work students and social workers in statutory settings. As an external examiner to social work qualifying programmes, I have frequently commented on how the few students who do undertake groupwork in their practice placements rarely refer to the basic texts in their practice studies, but rather apply concepts and methods from non-groupwork sources to their work with groups. Doel and Sawdon (1999: 21) suggest that the real question 'may, therefore, be less of "where has all the groupwork gone?" and more of "why have all the social workers gone?"'

Since the 1990s, there have been tremendous changes in the vision and practice of social work as a result of pressures from several directions. In some respects, these forces are in conflict, but, in sum, they have had the effect of putting the notion of a social work organised around an agreed core of methods into terminal decline. These changes include:

- the drive towards specialisation, confirmed in the dismemberment of the unified local authority social services departments
- the emergence of the law as a central concern
- changes in the education and training of social workers
- the impact of 'new managerialism'
- the critiques of theory and practice from feminist, anti-racist and service user perspectives.

This list is neither complete nor exclusive, but will enable me to sketch the context within which I believe an identifiably different groupwork has come into position.

The 'demethoding' of social work

The child abuse scandals, starting in the 1970s and reverberating in the profoundly influential report on the death of Victoria Climbié (Laming, 2003), have had a profound impact. They cast doubt on whether social workers, who were managed, organised and trained generically, had the specialist skills to deal with complex childcare cases. Outcomes traceable to this are a concern for safety-first practice (DH, 1995a), and a trend towards specialisation, reflected in the splitting of social services departments into health and social care provision and children's services joined up with schools. The law, as the framework within which social work is practised and which provides legitimacy, is given great prominence in training and, manifestly, stands to the fore in the minds of social workers (Sanfacon, 2001).

In the probation service, another set of changes have taken place. A national survey (Caddick, 1991: 211) revealed that groupwork was being practised widely in the service, much of it 'providing developmental or enabling experiences for the members'. However, since 1992, a sequence of punishment-oriented criminal justice policies and legislation has established a new direction that has fundamentally changed the culture and practice of the service:

> an offence specific practice developed ... decreasing appreciation by practitioners of the dynamics of the groupwork process and concentration on the task in hand rather than the process. (Senior, 1993: 35)

Alongside these developments, and reflected in them, have been wider changes in the culture of Britain, developing momentum following the Conservative election victory in 1979, surviving the change in government in 1997 and duly institutionalised in social work practice. One element is 'new managerialism', with its focus on concrete and measurable outcomes, in a drive towards greater economy, efficiency and effectiveness (McLaughlin and Muncie, 1994). As Youll (1996: 39) argued:

> what is not directly observable and therefore easily measured and described gets left out: mindfulness, the process and nature of relationships, managing the affective component of the work, the 'artistry of social work'.

Inexorably, the attention moved away from the 'how' of the job. This was illustrated vividly in a probation text (Raynor et al., 1994), in which a chapter on 'a programme to reduce offending', which is predominantly group based, covers rationale, aims, content and evaluation but nothing on groupwork skills and methods.

Echoes of these developments can be seen in profound changes in social work education. Responding to accusations of inadequate training, most stridently made in relation to childcare practice, qualifying training has been reorganised around a competence framework. While there is much debate about the efficacy of a competency approach, the fact is that such an approach, consistent with the imperatives of new managerialism, concentrates attention upon precisely framed identifiable and measurable behaviour (Cannan, 1994/95). What is lost is the synergy of bringing skills together to form, collectively, a method.

The final factor I wish to note as influencing the 'demethoding' of social work has been a succession of radical critiques of traditional social work. These have interrogated not only the reactionary policies flowing from the Thatcherite New Right and New Labour's reform and modernisation agenda, but also how face-to-face social work, as experienced by service users, can be patronising, oppressive and damaging. It began with the radical social work movement in the late 1970s and early 1980s, and has continued with the trenchant critiques of feminist, disabled, gay and lesbian, and black and ethnic minority service users. I do not question the rectitude of the critiques – indeed, I have been an unashamed participant – but merely highlight their impact, alongside other factors, in moulding the current face of social work.

The four methods were a product of a time passed. They made sense as part of the knowledge base of an aspiring profession that confidently saw itself progressing to heightened status and security. Battered from all sides, those conditions no longer apply. Social workers' confidence in their identity is increasingly tenuous. It is not surprising that they have come to feel safer operating within instrumental but more clear and defensible frameworks, reflected in buzz phrases such as 'competences', 'risk assessment', 'care planning' and 'commissioning'.

Groupwork and work in groups

In contemporary social work, there is a good deal of evidence of a continuing interest in groups. Indeed, there is a considerable amount of work taking place *in* groups.

However, it is not recognisable as groupwork. It does not pay substantial attention either to the knowledge base of group dynamics or to the practice base in groupwork methods and skills. Nor does it incorporate the democratic and collective values that are, as we will see, at the core of real groupwork. It is to be found in cognitive-behavioural work, particularly with offenders; in residential and daycare; in voluntary action; in research and service evaluation; and, organisationally, in teamwork. In some cases, for example in so-called 'what works' practice with offenders (McGuire, 1995; Chapman and Hough, 1998; Underdown, 1998, National Offender Management Service, 2006), the guiding texts simply pass over groupwork knowledge and skills. In other areas, for example residential and daycare or management, the evidence is that groupwork is not taken seriously, although some theoretical work has highlighted its importance (for example Brown and Clough, 1989).

Work in groups involves moving away from a notion of the group as an 'instrument' (Douglas, 1993) or 'medium' (Whitaker, 1985) for help and change, where group members work together to explore and exploit group resources (Douglas, 1993: 31), to a greater emphasis on the group as 'context':

> in which a powerful and knowledgeable resource, usually one leader, operates ... in which all group members have a primary relationship to the group leader who works with each individual in turn in the context of the group. (Douglas, 1993: 33)

an orientation quite consistent with the changes in social work outlined.

Douglas (1993: 31) sees a close connection between groups as 'instrument' or 'medium' and 'concepts of equality and democracy', and for A. Brown (1996: 83), 'groupwork is anti-oppressive in its context, purpose, method, group relationships and behaviour'. Indeed, what has historically distinguished groupwork from forms of practice focused on the individual has been:

> an emphasis on the commonalities of problems and situations and the concomitant commonality of feelings to which they give rise. In groupwork each issue that is raised, even when that issue at first glance seems to have no relevance to others in the group, does have applicability for all. The worker who practises real groupwork draws out that applicability and elicits the commonalities and asks members to examine the issues of others. (Kurland and Salmon, 1993: 10)

According to Coulshed (1991: 161, summarising Yalom, 1970), at its best, groupwork can offer:

- a source of power for members
- mutual support
- an exchange of information
- motivation and hope
- opportunities to learn and test interpersonal and other social skills
- a sense of belonging
- role models

- feedback on behaviour and coping attempts
- a chance to help as well as be helped.

Furthermore, if affiliated to a purpose that explicitly rejects the splintering of public issues from private troubles and to a set of practice principles that stress the potency of self-directed action and non-elitist leadership, groupwork can be the preferred method for anti-oppressive practice. Bringing together people with common needs and problems to work on their own behalf represents the essence of empowerment (Mullender and Ward, 1991: 12).

Instead, in the mainstream, we find groups that are predominantly 'one-to-one treatment with the rest of the members acting as bystanders' (Konopka, cited by Kurland and Salmon, 1993: 8). Such groups are boring, suppressing and run by people who must maintain control. Process is used to enhance conformity, dissenters may be humiliated and revealing is required, with punishment if refused.

Although Kurland and Salmon are writing about the US American scene, British writers have made similar observations. Brown (1994: 45) notes a trend towards groups that are increasingly task-oriented, with decreasing emphasis being paid to process:

> reducing groupwork ... to a rather sterile exercise in which group members receive packaged group programmes of limited usefulness, making no real impact on them as unique individuals often caught up in oppressive social conditions of poverty.

Senior (1993) acknowledged that the individualised task focus had produced some high-quality training materials, for example the catalogue of 'accredited programmes' for use by probation and prisons (Home Office, 2000a), but was concerned that:

> unless groupworkers were skilled enough to use the group process appropriately, opportunities for personal development of clients were left undone. (Senior, 1993: 35)

As an example, Cowburn and Modi (1995) critically evaluated approaches, predominantly based in groups, to working with male sex abusers. In the then prevalent (and still popular) cognitive-behavioural programmes and, in particular, the practice of individual confrontation, they saw oppressive Eurocentric and heterosexist assumptions, grounded in conformity and obedience, which are potentially dangerous in reinforcing abusers' minimalist views of their own responsibility and the harm their actions have caused. Effective practice, Cowburn and Modi (1995: 204–5) argued:

> needs to help to develop a person's positive sense of identity as a firm base from which knowledge, skills and understanding about offending behaviour can be brought together to avoid re-offending ... it needs to be experienced within a context that is not oppressive.

Real groupwork may have become unfashionable precisely because it acknowledges that groups develop a life of their own over which the worker cannot ever have complete control. In a group, the agenda is likely to be holistic. Group members will raise what is important and significant to them, no matter what 'ground rules' and boundaries have been set. Such free-flowing characteristics are out of kilter with the current climate, emphasising, as it does, discipline, individual responsibility and, at an organisation level, preset objectives and audited outcomes. The outcome is many projects and workers for whom the ideas of real groupwork are unfamiliar and regarded with suspicion (Drakeford, 1994: 237).

However, there is a danger of throwing the baby out with the bath water. The drive for efficiency seeks, wherever possible, economies of scale, and this means gathering people together. Whenever this happens, group process and the need for groupwork skills will come to the fore.

A continuing need for groupwork

Sustaining Caddick's (1991) findings, work in groups has continued to develop as a vital activity across the probation service, but along the dimension of 'the modification of offending or offence related behaviour' rather than 'towards providing developmental or enabling experiences for members' (Caddick, 1991: 210–11). Cognitive-behavioural approaches developed in North America have provided the received model (Ross et al., 1989; Dowden and Andrews, 2004). Cowburn and Modi (1995) highlighted the risk of deconstructing fragile identities in such group-based work with sex abusers. Instead, they urge a groupwork approach which:

> allows offenders to feel power and consequently a strong sense of self ... [which] ... will allow them to develop non-offending ways of finding self-affirmation. (Cowburn and Modi, 1995: 205)

As noted, texts on 'what works' cognitive-behavioural practice pay minimal attention to group dynamics, group process and groupwork methods and skills.

Likewise, in residential and daycare, sometimes called group care, there is a dearth of literature with a groupwork base and practice examples. Exceptions have been Douglas (1986) and, particularly, Brown and Clough's (1989) *Groups and Groupings: Life and Work in Day and Residential Centres*. Brown and Clough built on the premise that better practice lies in understanding the complexities of the 'mosaic' of more or less formal groups which straddle the experiences of users and staff in day and residential settings. A particular contribution of this work was to extend attention beyond inter- and intra-group processes (Douglas, 1986) to the 'rediscovery' of the open and large group as contexts that require special consideration and skills (see also Ward, 1993).

In the organisation and management of social services, the problem is not the lack of literature on groups, organisations and management per se. Rather, it is the failure to apply the knowledge and understanding of group process, and to use groupwork skills, in the management of social work agencies as 'mosaics' and frontline teams as groups. The culture of new managerialism has led to a top-down style preoccupied with obedience, performance indicators and output measures, features that are an antithesis of groupwork. According to one former senior civil servant, this leads to a narrowing of vision, driving out initiative and distorting priorities, a flattening of the levels of performance leading to conformism, a reluctance to question received ideas and 'ultimately to secrecy and defensiveness' (Faulkner, 1995: 69). The capacity of groupwork, applying techniques of problem analysis, objective-setting, prioritisation and evaluation to enhance creativity and generate team spirit and enthusiasm for the tasks in hand, goes unconsidered in such a culture.

In the expanding field of voluntary action, much initiative takes place in group settings. There are two sides to voluntary action and the so-called 'third sector' more generally. Negatively, it can be seen as substituting for properly resourced, high-quality welfare services, providing an ideological smokescreen for rationing, contracting-out, privatisation and, at worst, the unpaid and unsupported care of the vulnerable by the vulnerable. On the other hand, self-help groups, besides providing the quality of empathy and support that only those in the same predicament can extend to their peers, have raised the profile of hitherto unmet need and brought about significant changes in policy and provision. Adams (1990, 2003) shows the importance of an understanding of group process if workers are to mobilise and empower, rather than stifle, the creativity and commitment of those involved. Crucially, Adams (2003: 117–18) explains how, in order to achieve these purposes, groupwork skills must be set within a paradigm of practice principles that is explicitly anti-oppressive.

Finally, I have come increasingly to note the use of groups in research and evaluation (Ward, 1996). This has come into public view with the prominence given to the use of 'focus groups' by political parties in devising their appeals to the electorate. While there is a technical literature on focus groups (for example Morgan, 1988; Krueger, 1994), there is little acknowledgement of group and groupwork matters in the research methods literature, even where participative, ethnographic, feminist and other anti-oppressive approaches are advocated. It is self-evident that the knowledge of group process and a measure of groupwork practice skill should be components in such methodologies. Indeed, the potential impact of research on groups studied and, indeed, its capacity to empower or oppress should be central ethical considerations for all researchers (Fleming and Ward, 1996; Taylor, G., 1996).

Re-establishing groupwork

A. Brown (1996: 90) identifies three key considerations for the future of groupwork that still hold good: values, practice-based model-building and sustaining groupwork and groupworkers into an uncertain future. Up to this point, I have identified forces that have undermined the presence of groupwork in mainstream social and probation work and how this may be counterproductive from both ethical and practice perspectives. What I would like to propose now is a practical reassertion of groupwork that can encompass the three considerations set out by Brown. A briefing by the National Institute for Social Work (1996) highlighted that a major cornerstone for social policy and the challenge for social work is the fight against social exclusion. The briefing argued that:

The challenges of reducing social exclusion through working with those individuals and groups currently denied access to employment or services demands new approaches and envisaged:

> the role of social workers as agents in the fight against social exclusion and the development of a model of practice that can incorporate a broader community focus as well as an individual or family approach. (NISW, 1996)

In this context, I am prompted to recall Douglas's (1993) observation, cited earlier, of the historical connection between groupwork and equality and democracy.

The challenge of social exclusion demands that we take account of what we have come to know about the systematic oppression of excluded groups, anti-discriminatory practice and empowerment (Mullender and Ward, 1991; Rees, 1991; Thompson, 1993, 2007; Adams, 2003) and, in this context, groupwork reasserts its significance. This is because, according to Butler and Wintram (1991: 77), the group can be:

- a source of immediate support, of friendship, where the knowledge that a meeting will take place regularly provides a safety net in itself
- a place to recognise shared experiences and their value
- a way of breaking down isolation and loneliness
- the source of a different perspective on personal problems
- a place to experience power over personal situations, with the capacity to change and have an effect on these.

Also, beyond these foundations, 'in groups there is a better chance of addressing the inseparability of private troubles and public issues' (Breton, 1994: 31). Even though matters may surface as private troubles, in groups these private troubles soon become shared troubles, providing the ground for the analysis of their structural sources, and action together to bring about change (Mullender and Ward, 1991).

Butler and Wintram (1991), Lee (1994) and Mullender and Ward (1991) have articulated specific models for practising anti-oppressive groupwork. What is distinctive is their insistence on taking account of an interconnectedness of values, methods and skills right through practice. Helpful guidance can be found in Brown (1992) and Preston-Shoot (2007), who provide invaluable inventories of areas for attention, but ones which – distinctive and essential to anti-oppressive groupwork – must be set within a searching exploration of underpinning values (Mullender and Ward, 1991). Both Brown and Preston-Shoot draw attention to:

- group composition
- style, format and group culture
- ground rules
- confronting racism, sexism and other forms of discrimination when they occur within the group
- co-working
- worker self-preparation
- supervision and consultation
- work within the group and its external environment.

To illustrate what is possible, I will conclude with practice examples from arguably the least promising areas of social work practice.

Butler (1994) writes about a group for women whose children were adjudged by social services to be at risk of significant harm from their parents. She explores how the 'facilitation' style of groupwork engendered an atmosphere of equality, enabling the women 'to explore the humour, sadness and strains of family life and no longer remain silent about these' (Butler, 1994: 178). Central to the group agenda emerged structural dilemmas facing members: women's sexuality and relationships with male partners, which were entangled with the processes of racism and the difficulties of bringing up mixed-parentage children. Faced with relentless hardships, the women easily identified the politics of poverty. Unpacking structural and individual issues was critical to these women's empowerment and the creation of their own solutions to the threats and dilemmas they faced (Butler, 1994: 163).

In the completely different setting of a young offenders penal institution, Badham (1989) and colleagues worked with the inmates to develop a through-care service that the young men would see as useful and relevant by enabling them to raise issues and complaints within the institution and prepare themselves for release. The workers sought to draw out of the young men, and provide opportunities for them to learn, skills and knowledge that would help them to survive 'inside' and after release. Confronting racist and sexist attitudes was part of this, and the worker team included women and black workers. The young men controlled the group's programme producing, amid wide-ranging discussions, advice booklets and arranging speakers on welfare rights, housing, parole and temporary release. For invited speakers, including the governor, the group prepared their briefs, organised invitations and devised questions so that they acquired the information they wanted. The governor acknowledged the value of the forum and saw in this different context hitherto unrecognised capacities in these inmates. One young man said on leaving the group: 'It made you feel as though you can do something with your life while you are inside' (Badham, 1989: 35).

Conclusion

This, then, is the shape of an anti-oppressive groupwork practice to tackle the processes of exclusion. Like so many other buzz words that have gone before – participation, citizenship and, sadly, empowerment – there is, of course, the ever-present danger of the 'fight against exclusion' being co-opted and watered down to become meaningless, ideological deodorant. Some insurance against this can lie in interlinking with an anti-oppressive approach grounded in the practice of 'real' groupwork. It is an opportunity to bring British social work with groups back in from the cold.

For further discussion of working with young offenders, see Chapter 23, and for communication skills, see Adams et al., 2009a, Chapter 10.

www.dmu.ac.uk/dmucsa   The Centre for Social Action, a research and consultancy unit at De Montfort University, Leicester, uses social action methods, grounded in groupwork and empowerment, to undertake project, research and training work. The website contains, and provides links to, a wide range of reports, articles and resources.

www.whitingbirch.net   Provides information on the journal *Groupwork* and an annual symposium in the UK for groupworkers, while **www.aaswg.org**, the website of US-based Association for the Advancement of Social Work with Groups, does the same for the American journal, *Social Work with Groups*, and the association's activities. Both journals are available in hard copy and online and are invaluable for access to examples of practice and the latest ideas from around the world.

Adams, R. (2003) *Social Work and Empowerment*, 3rd edn, Basingstoke, Palgrave Macmillan; Breton, M. (1994) 'On the meaning of empowerment and empowerment oriented social work practice', *Social Work with Groups*, 17(3): 23–38; Mullender, A. and Ward, D. (1991) *Self-directed Groupwork: Users Take Action for Empowerment*, London, Whiting & Birch. These three texts are most helpful in unravelling the notion of empowerment and providing practical guidelines for practising groupwork in that direction in mainstream social work settings.

Brown, A. (1992) *Groupwork*, 3rd edn, Aldershot, Ashgate; Doel, M. and Sawdon, C. (1999) *The Essential Groupworker*, London, Jessica Kingsley; Preston-Shoot, M. (2007) *Effective Groupwork*, 2nd edn, Basingstoke, Palgrave Macmillan. These books are excellent basic texts on practising groupwork and have extensive bibliographies for follow-up reading.

Community work 11

This chapter deals with community work, which may be regarded as a traditional part of social work, associated with a range of preventive, community-based approaches to meeting people's social needs. It begins by examining how community work still serves as an important approach to work with people. It explores different definitions of key concepts, briefly visits the wider historical context of community work and discusses current debates around its relevance as an approach to social work.

Chapter overview

'Community work has a long history as an aspect of social work' (Payne, 1995: 165). Essentially, community work brings a focus upon helping

> people with shared interests to come together, work out what their needs are among themselves and then jointly take action together to meet those needs, by developing projects which would enable the people concerned to gain support to meet them or by campaigning to ensure that they are met by those responsible. (Payne, 1995: 165)

Community work has generally been associated with holistic, collective, preventive and anti-discriminatory approaches to meeting social needs, based on value commitments to participation and empowerment.

Payne continues: 'As stated, this looks innocuous.' Public policy statements, both in Britain and internationally, abound with commitments to the values of participation and empowerment. In practice, however, as Payne goes on to point out, 'community work has proved controversial and problematic', having the capacity to draw 'attention to inequalities in service provision and in power which lie behind severe deprivation' and so to become part of the struggles 'between people in powerless positions against the powerful' (Payne, 1995: 165–6). This has been offered as an explanation for the British government's decision to conclude its own experiments in community development (the community development projects) in the 1970s, for example (Loney, 1983).

Why then, given its potentially controversial and problematic characteristics, has community work not merely survived from the 1970s, but taken on an apparently new lease of life from the 1990s onwards into the twenty-first century? This chapter starts by exploring some aspects of this question. Having summarised key features of the current context, the chapter will move on to provide some 'mapping', including a brief discussion of different definitions of key terms, together with a rapid summary of the recent history of debates around community work as an approach to social work.

The discussion will then focus on issues and debates in community work today. What are the main theoretical perspectives, and what are their varying implications for community work practice? At what levels, and in which types of practice setting, is community work most relevant and appropriate? What are the key areas of knowledge and skills that are required? This chapter will also consider a number of the more negative features and some of the key dilemmas of the contemporary context, in terms of both policy and practice. This will then provide the basis for concluding with an overall appraisal of community work's contribution, both actual and potential. What has community work to offer as an approach to reflective social work practice? And what changes in social policy might be required if community work's contribution were to be enhanced?

The context

The economic and social policy context within which social work and community work operate has changed significantly in recent years. These changes have been characterised in terms of 'globalisation', an expression that has become increasingly fashionable since the 1980s, 'when it began to replace words like "internationalization" to denote "the ever intensifying networks of social and economic relationships"' (Dominelli and Hoogvelt, 1996: 46). These changes have also been described in terms of a number of 'posts' – postindustrialism, post-Fordism, poststructuralism and postmodernism (Taylor-Gooby, 1994; Dominelli and Hoogvelt, 1996; Penna and O'Brien, 1996). There are key differences between these terms, as Penna and O'Brien point out, the first two referring predominantly to debates within political economy, the latter two having been more concerned with debates within cultural studies. These differences are beyond the scope of this chapter.

What these different terms share in common, however, is a common sense that the old order of 'modern' industrial society is in a state of flux and transition, on a global scale, whether in terms of economic change, or social, political and cultural change. These changes have fundamental implications for welfare states in general, and more specifically for the social policy context for social work and community work.

In summary, despite national and local differences, Dominelli and Hoogvelt (1996) argued that there are powerful global trends in the contract culture, including trends towards increasing marketisation, increasing privatisation, increasing fragmentation of services and the technocratisation of social work itself. These changes pose significant threats. They also pose new contradictions. For community work in particular, the current focus on the role of the community sector, within the mixed economy of welfare, could be seen to represent new opportunities as well as new challenges. This increased emphasis on the role of the community sector is, however, taking place within the wider context of reduced public resources, including reduced public resources for the support and development of the community sector itself. Similarly, the current focus on the promotion of self-help, diversity and choice offers new opportunities for some, against a background of reduced opportunities and choice for others. This makes it more important than ever that those engaged in community work are actively aware of these divergent tensions and critically reflective in their practice.

'Mapping' community work: definitions and recent history

This need for clarity starts with the concept of 'community' itself, a term that has over time been the subject of confusion and contestation (Crow and Allen, 1994; Mayo, 1994a; Payne, 1995). The uses of the term 'community' with greatest relevance for community work can be broadly summarised as follows:

- *community as shared locality* – a common geographical area, for example a neighbourhood, a housing estate in an urban or suburban context, or a village in a rural area
- *community as shared interests* – these might be interests based on cultures and identities, as in the case of ethnic minority communities, or common identifications of particular needs, as in the case of the parents of children with special needs, or ex-users of mental health services, for example.

The term 'community' is frequently applied to services to differentiate them from institutional forms of provision, for example community care services for the elderly in their own homes and/or in day centres in their localities, rather than in residential homes or geriatric hospitals. The term 'community' is often contrasted with 'state', as in the case of the 'community sector', which has been associated with small, relatively informal and bottom-up forms of service provision, in contrast to the larger, more bureaucratic forms of service provision typically associated with the public sector. Community-based services have been associated with the promotion of unpaid caring and self-help, often in response to widening gaps between shrinking services and increasingly unmet social needs. Also, community-based services have been associated with more participatory and more empowering approaches to social welfare provision, based on enhanced respect for the diversity of users' and carers' own perspectives.

As has already been pointed out, community work has a long history as an aspect of social work both in Britain and elsewhere, predating the current focus within the mixed economy of welfare. Broadly speaking, community work has been defined as being concerned 'with enabling people to improve the quality of their lives and gain greater influences over the processes that affect them' (AMA, 1993: 10). Twelvetrees (1991: 1) has suggested that, at its simplest, community work is 'the process of assisting ordinary people to improve their own communities by undertaking collective action'. Community work has been particularly concerned with the needs of those who have been disadvantaged or oppressed, whether through poverty or through discrimination on the basis of class, race, gender, sexuality, age or disability.

Community work developed from the late nineteenth-century settlement houses, starting with Oxford House (founded in 1883) and Toynbee Hall (founded in 1885), linked to social work as well as to community education. Through the work of the community association movement in the interwar period, and community work in the new towns after the Second World War, community work developed as a professional activity, alongside the unpaid work of volunteers and activists in community organisations and social movements. At the end of the 1960s, the government launched its own community development project as part of its efforts to combat poverty and deprivation through more holistic, preventive approaches to social welfare (Loney, 1983), approaches that were emphasised in the Seebohm Committee's conception for the future of the social services:

> directed to the wellbeing of the whole community and not only of social casualties, seeing the community as the basis of its authority, resources and effectiveness. (Seebohm Committee, 1968: 147)

Similar arguments were put forward by the Barclay Committee's (1982) report in the early 1980s.

This emphasis on the role of the community, and the need for partnerships between social service departments and the local communities they served, re-emerged, at the end of the 1980s, in the changing context for social work in the mixed economy of welfare (Bamford, 1990). In particular, the Griffiths Report (1988) on care in the community took up the theme of closer partnerships between statutory services and local communities as part of the new welfare pluralism. The NHS and Community Care Act 1990 enshrined both increasing marketisation and a potentially increasing emphasis upon community work, at least in theory if not necessarily in practice. Since the election of New Labour governments from 1997, these potentially contradictory policy directions have continued, in varying forms, combining an emphasis on marketisation and individual consumer choice with an emphasis on partnership working, including working in partnership with service users, their families and their communities. This all goes to demonstrate the significance of the challenges for community work, as well as for social work, more generally.

Community work and social work

Community work has a long history as an approach to social work. In the context of the NHS and Community Care Act 1990, there has been particular interest in community work in relation to community care, promoting care in the community, as well as enabling service users and carers to participate in planning, monitoring and evaluating community care services. Community social work has not, however, been confined to community care. Community-based social work has been and continues to be relevant across a wide range of social work practice, including preventive work with children and their families, for example, as studies by Cannan and others have demonstrated (Cannan, 1992; Smith, 1995).

While community work has a continuing role, as an approach to social work, however, community work has not been confined to social work. Community work has featured as an approach to youth work, and it has featured and continues to feature within other professional settings, including housing and planning, and more recently in relation to area regeneration and community cohesion. In addition, community work has also been carried out, and continues to be carried out, by volunteers and unpaid activists within communities.

There have been long-running debates on whether or not community work should be defined as a professional activity at all, professionalisation having been posed as potentially undermining to community activism and autonomous community movements (Banks, 1996). In summary, then, community work has had its place as an approach to social work, but community work has not been confined to the social work profession.

Alternative perspectives and implications for practice

By this time, it should have become apparent that community work can be and has been based on competing perspectives, associated with both Right and Left positions on the political spectrum. Community work has been promoted to encourage self-help and informal caring, compensate for reductions in public service provision within the context of the increasing marketisation of welfare, support strategies to combat poverty and oppression, and facilitate community participation and empowerment.

Texts such as Twelvetrees (1991) have distinguished between alternative community work perspectives, contrasting the 'professional' approach, which seeks to promote self-help and improve service delivery within the wider framework of existing social relations, with the 'radical' approach. This radical approach seeks to go further, contributing to shifting the balance of existing social relations through empowering the relatively powerless to question the causes of their deprivation and challenge the sources of their oppression, 'drawing upon insights from neo-Marxist structural analyses, together with insights from feminism and from anti-racist analyses' (Twelvetrees, 1991). This is the type of approach that supports minority ethnic communities, for example, in drawing 'attention to inequalities in service provision and in power which lie behind severe deprivation' (Payne, 1995: 166).

While these distinctions have relevance, the terms 'professional' and 'radical' have inherent problems, in the current context, as Twelvetrees has also recognised. In particular, in recent years, the term 'radical' has become even more confusing, since its adoption by the 'radical' Right. The use of the term 'professional' to describe one perspective could also be taken to imply that the alternative perspective was in some way 'non-professional' or even 'unprofessional', although this was not actually suggested by Twelvetrees. Given that professional values, knowledge and skills are essential to community work, whatever the perspective in question, it has been suggested that it would be less confusing to categorise community work perspectives in terms of a '"technicist" approach on the one hand, and a "transformational" perspective, emphasising community empowerment and social transformation, on the other hand' (Mayo,

1994b). Banks (2006) employs a similar set of distinctions, distinguishing between committed/radical, professional and technical-bureaucratic models of social work practice, more generally.

These types of categorisation have also been broken down into further subdivisions when related to the different types and levels of community work practice. Dominelli (1990), for example, has characterised the traditional, 'neutral' views of community work in ways that are comparable to the 'technicist' approach (see Table 11.1). She defines these views in terms of their assumptions that 'the system' is basically sound, although individual and community pathologies need to be ironed out through the community work process; she quotes Biddle and Biddle's comment that 'the poor and the alienated must overcome their inner handicap practically through the cultivation of their own initiatives' as a classic text to illustrate this approach (Dominelli, 1990: 8).

Table 11.1 Two perspectives on community work

Perspective	Goals/assumptions
Professional/traditional/neutral/technicist	To promote community initiatives, including self-help, and improve service delivery, within the framework of existing social relations
Radical/transformational	To promote community initiatives, improve service delivery and to do so in ways that empower communities to challenge the root causes of deprivation and discrimination, and to develop strategies and build alliances for social change, as part of wider strategies to transform oppressive, discriminatory, exploitative social relations

Dominelli goes on to characterise three models of community work – community care, community organisation and community development – in terms that can be related to this broad type of traditional/neutral/technicist approach (see Table 11.2). Community care schemes based on the use of unpaid and typically white, middle-class women volunteers to cover gaps in statutory provision would fit into this neutral approach, for example, although the effects may be far from neutral, in terms of reinforcing inequalities of race, gender and class, in service provision. Similarly, Dominelli places community organisation – or community work that focuses on improving the coordination between various welfare agencies – as typically forming a tool of corporate management rather than a tool for more fundamentally challenging the inequalities in resource allocation – including the specific inequalities experienced by women and black people. The term 'community organising' has been used somewhat differently in North America, generally being associated with community mobilisation/community. Dominelli then considers the community development model, which focuses on the promotion of self-help skills, and fits it into this broad type of approach; this is especially the case, it is suggested, when leadership in community development programmes is provided by outside professional experts brought into so-called 'problem areas' to tackle social problems as defined by the state. However, Dominelli also points out that, where community development involves collective struggles to achieve groups' demands, this community development model may turn into 'community action'.

In contrast, Dominelli considers three models that would be more consistent with the transformational approach, as outlined above – class-based community action, feminist community action and community action from a black perspective (Table 11.2). These models are all, in their different ways, about more fundamental social change, including a change in the consciousness of those affected, whether focusing on addressing inequalities of class, gender and/or race. Dominelli (1990: 11) describes class-based community action in terms of bringing people lacking power together 'to reduce their powerlessness and increase their effectiveness', typically using conflict, direct action and confrontation as well as negotiation to achieve their ends. Feminist community action has:

transcended the boundaries of traditional community work by challenging fundamentally the nature of capitalist patriarchal social relations between men and women, women and the state and adults and children. (Dominelli, 1990: 11)

Community action from a black perspective has made the struggle for racial equality central to their work, while anti-racist feminist community work has been committed to eliminating both racial and gender inequality.

Table 11.2 A continuum of community work models

Model/level of work	Perspective typically associated with model
Community care Community organisation Community development	Professional Traditional Neutral Technicist
Class-based community action Feminist community action Community action from a black perspective	Radical Transformational

As Dominelli and others have also recognised, however, there is, in practice, a degree of overlap between these different models, 'particularly in the areas of techniques and skills adopted' (Dominelli, 1990: 7), and there have been continuing debates, including debates about differences within both feminist and anti-racist approaches, which are beyond the scope of this particular chapter. (For a guide to these debates, see, for example, Williams, 1989.)

As has already been suggested, in the context of the particular pressures and tensions of the mixed economy of welfare, this makes it all the more important that community workers are critically aware of the potential implications of different models and are reflective in their practice. More specifically, this context requires increasing knowledge and skills, as community workers have to operate within the more complex, fragmented environment of the mixed economy of social welfare provision. Whatever the history of community organisation, in terms of whether or not this model has necessarily implied a more traditional, less structurally challenging/transformational perspective in the past, in the current context, community workers neglect community organisation work at their peril – not to mention the potential peril of the communities they work with professionally. The local authority, although a key player with overall responsibility, can no longer be expected to be the key provider of relevant services. Communities may need to negotiate with a wider range of agencies, public sector agencies, quangos, private sector agencies, voluntary, not-for-profit and other community sector organisations. In the current policy context, considerable emphasis is being placed on 'partnership working', as in the case of the 2004 Children Act, for example. Partnership working is far from unproblematic, however, and partnership structures can be experienced by the less powerful professions, groups and communities as being effectively excluding and disempowering (Balloch and Taylor, 2001). Community workers have a potentially more vital role than ever in empowering communities to address these situations effectively. Community workers need to be effective, then, at the levels of interagency work, local and regional planning, and grassroots neighbourhood work.

Similarly, I would argue that, in the current context of the mixed economy of welfare, a considerable proportion of community workers will need to address community care issues, whatever their own perspectives. Models of community work practice, which place community care at one end of the spectrum, through to community action and feminist, black and anti-racist community work at the other end, need to be reconsidered in the light of these changing conditions (Popple, 1995).

Community care can be approached from different perspectives:

- *traditional perspectives* that focus on the promotion of self-help and volunteering in ways which substitute for rather than enrich public service provision
- *more transformational perspectives* that address issues of immediate needs within the context of wider strategies for community empowerment, supported by anti-discriminatory, anti-oppressive community work practice.

The latter approach has been set out, for example, by Shaw (1996) when he addresses the possibilities as well as the problems for community care, drawing upon the Scottish experience. The point to emphasise here is that whether community workers are focusing on community care issues and/or tackling interagency community organisation issues, they need to reflect on their practice critically. Is their practice informed by relatively traditional, technicist perspectives on community work, which focus upon managing social problems and containing social needs? Or, is their practice informed by more transformational perspectives, geared not only towards meeting social needs, but also towards addressing the causes of oppression and discrimination and promoting community empowerment (Table 11.3)?

Table 11.3 Beyond a continuum: alternative perspectives on community care, community organisation and community development

	Models	Alternative perspectives and practice
	Traditional/technicist	Radical/transformational
Community care	Promote volunteering	Empower users and carers
Community organisation	Promote interagency coordination	Negotiate/campaign for organisational change to improve services/support for the community sector
Community development	Promote self-help to tackle concentrations of deprivation	Empower communities to develop strategies to tackle deprivation and disadvantage

Whatever their underlying perspective, however, community workers need an increasingly sophisticated core of background knowledge, techniques and professional skills (see Beresford and Trevillion, 1995). Broadly speaking, as a starting point, community workers need to be confident of their skills in the following areas:

- engagement and partnership working – with a range of individuals, groups and organisations
- assessment – including needs assessment, via area profiles
- research – including participatory action research with communities
- groupwork
- negotiating – including working constructively in situations of conflict
- communication across a wide range of contexts
- counselling
- the management of resources – including time management of self
- resourcing – including grant applications
- recording and report-writing for a wide range of purposes
- monitoring and evaluation.

These are, of course, typically skills that are widely transferable. In addition, community workers need a sound background knowledge of social policy and welfare rights, together with a specific knowledge of the fields in which they predominantly operate, such as health and welfare policies and practice in relation to community care, child protection legislation for those concerned with children and families in the community, and housing and planning legislation for community workers involved in housing, planning and urban or rural regeneration programmes. In addition, as argued by Mayo (1994b: 74):

> community workers need to have knowledge and understanding of the socioeconomic and political backgrounds of the areas in which they are to work, including knowledge and understanding of political structures, and of relevant organisations and resources in the statutory, voluntary and community sectors. And they need to have knowledge and understanding of equal opportunities policies and practice, so that they can apply these effectively in every aspect of their work.

Some current issues and dilemmas

In recent years, community work has had to respond to the criticism that it is an area of practice that is 'both imprecise and unclear' (Popple, 1995: 1), leading to publications such as *The Community Development Challenge* (DCLG, 2006), which set out the case for more systematic definitions and approaches, if community work is to be taken more seriously in the current policy context, recognising that government agendas for user and community involvement and empowerment need community development support.

In a period of increasing pressure to target scarce resources more precisely, with clearer performance indicators, there has been decreasing scope for generalist, preventive community work, the type of work with children and families in deprived areas that Holman (1983), for example, has carried out and analysed so effectively and with such inspiration. Crisis management in child protection, for example, has tended to divert resources from community-based approaches to the support of children and families in need, for example through community-based family centres and particular initiatives such as childcare projects and credit unions.

More specifically, community work has tended to be promoted within particular, short-term initiatives, such as projects to promote community participation in government-initiated regeneration schemes, in time-limited strategies to tackle social exclusion, including the effective exclusion of young people not in employment, education or training, and in programmes for children and families such as Sure Start, subsequently mainstreamed, but with some loss of community involvement in the process, it has been argued (Stepney, 2006). By their very structure, these initiatives have had a focus on short-term outcomes and specific performance indicators. The point to emphasise here is absolutely not that there is a case for exempting community work from the fullest public accountability. However, the contemporary emphasis on short-term interventions, evaluated by overly narrow performance indicators, has risked being ultimately self-defeating, marginalising the more holistic, preventive, longer term approaches to community work – the type of community work pioneered by Holman (1983) and developed in the more community-based family centres (Cannan, 1992; Smith, 1995; Durrant, 1997). While there are some encouraging signs of increasing recognition of the need for longer term strategies to promote neighbourhood renewal, there is still some way to go in terms of more holistic approaches to evaluation.

Area-specific programmes can be potentially divisive in communities, too, where community groups find themselves competing against each other for limited resources. The point to emphasise here is that, even if particular groups and individuals take a more positive view of programme outcomes, communities overall could be left even more fragmented and alienated following community regeneration interventions. Community workers need to be critically aware of this potential for negative as well as for positive outcomes. This is a key point and one that relates to a long history of debates over how far community work, like other approaches to social work, can be controlling rather than caring and enabling. There are parallels here with debates around contemporary notions of communitarianism, including debates about how far this actually focuses on responsibilities rather than rights, on communities policing themselves and/or competing with neighbouring communities for limited resources, eked out via self-help, rather than working together to challenge the policies in question.

Conclusion

In the contemporary context of the mixed economy of welfare, community work has a potentially more vital contribution than ever to make. Community workers can support service users in coming together to work out their needs, and then take action together to meet those needs. Also they can work in ways that empower users and communities to develop strategies to challenge the inequalities in service provision and indeed to begin to challenge the underlying causes of discrimination and deprivation, working in partnership with the relevant agencies, organisations and social movements. Community workers can facilitate the promotion of social solidarity, combating the current tensions within and between established and more recently arrived communities, in the context of contemporary preoccupations with community cohesion and the so-called 'war on terror'.

Conversely, however, this contemporary context is also more problematic than ever, with the risk of further fragmentation and increasing intra- and intercommunity conflicts. This means that community workers need greater professional expertise than ever. Most particularly, their practice needs to be informed by critical theory if they are to address these challenges as reflective practitioners.

Community social work has been advocated precisely because of its potential for 'working with local groups to achieve change', addressing 'structural issues of poverty, exclusion, racism and disadvantage and how these feed into local problems of inadequate facilities, crime, ill health, isolation, breakdown in relationships and so on' (Stepney, 2006: 1300). Without significant changes in the wider context, including significant changes in the social policy context, however, community work risks remaining severely constrained as an approach to social work. It will continue to be hampered by the short-termism that has reduced rather than increased support for the community sector and focused on crisis management, to the detriment of longer term, more holistic strategies of meeting social needs in preventive and anti-discriminatory ways, ways which are both participatory and empowering.

For further discussion of working with community groups, see Adams et al., 2009a, Chapter 24, and for relevant aspects of empowerment, see Chapter 16.

Balloch, S. and Taylor, M. (2001) *Partnership Working: Policy and Practice*, Bristol, Policy Press. Explores aspects of partnership working.

Beresford, P. and Croft, S. (1993) *Citizen Involvement: A Practical Guide for Change*, Basingstoke, Macmillan – now Palgrave Macmillan. Provides a discussion of user involvement.

Bulmer, M. (1987) *The Social Basis of Community Care*, London, George Allen & Unwin. Analyses the background to sociological and social policy debates.

Butcher, H., Banks, S., Henderson, P. with Robertson, J. (2007) *Critical Community Practice*, Bristol, Policy Press. Discusses community work in relation to related areas of professional practice.

Cannan, C. and Warren, C. (eds) (1997) *Social Action with Children and Families*, London, Routledge. Readings in community social work with children and families.

Dominelli, L. (1990) *Women and Community Action*, Birmingham, Venture Press. Discusses issues of gender, race and class in community work.

Ledwith, M. (2005) *Community Development*, 2nd edn, Bristol, BASW/Policy Press. Provides the theoretical frameworks for community development.

Popple, K. (1995) *Analysing Community Work*, Buckingham, Open University Press. A textbook on community work.

Taylor, M. (2003) *Public Policy in the Community*, Basingstoke, Palgrave Macmillan. Analyses community development in the wider policy context.

Twelvetrees, A. (2008) *Community Work*, 4th edn, Basingstoke, Palgrave – now Palgrave Macmillan. An important textbook on community work.

Psychosocial work: an attachment perspective

12

Intrinsic to children's development is a tendency towards inter-action with the world around them and attachment to those people, notably adults, who are closest to them and therefore best placed to protect them. Good social work needs to appre-ciate how the psychological and social interact, through people and their environments. This chapter offers an attachment perspective on psychosocial practice.

Chapter overview

It would be possible to argue that, in essence, social work is psychosocial work if by 'psychosocial' we mean that area of human experience which is created by the inter-play between the individual's psychological condition and the social environment. Psychosocial matters define most that is of interest to social work, particularly people who are having problems with others – parents, partners, children, peers and profes-sionals – or other people who are having a problem with them. There is a simultaneous interest in the individual and the qualities of their social environment.

For example, a woman neglected as a child may have low self-esteem, feel anxious and agitated in close relationships, becoming depressed when she feels unable to control what is happening to her. She needs to be loved and valued but can never take other people for granted or trust them. Her partner comes from a similarly adverse 'socio-emotional' background. Their relationship is characterised by mutual anxiety as each fears that the other may abandon them, and mutual anger as each believes that the other is capable of causing them hurt. The result is that their relationship is full of conflict and turbulence, anxiety and depression. The emotional needs of both people are so great that any children of their union are, in their turn, likely to experience a disturbed upbringing.

The basic dynamic between psychology and setting can be used to explore all aspects of people's psychosocial functioning. The developmental frameworks that help to analyse social behaviour and the quality of people's past and present relationships provide social workers with a powerful theory to guide all aspects of practice, includ-ing observation, assessment, evaluation of risk, decision-making, the choice of methods of help and treatment, worker reflectivity and models of practitioner supervision.

One of the first accounts of a psychosocial approach was given by Florence Hollis (1972). In this work, she defines the essential elements of a psychosocial approach. She argues that clients and the contexts in which they find themselves have to be thought about and handled simultaneously. Using the knowledge bases of her time, Hollis was inclined to use Freudian psychology to inform the 'psycho' element of the approach, and social systems theory to develop the 'social' component of the practice. Her aim was to help people who were having problems in their interpersonal relationships.

The socialness of self

Although the idea that we are 'social selves', whose being and personality form within social relationships, is not new, there has been a resurgence of interest in the 'socialness of self' in the social sciences (see, for example, Bakhurst and Sypnowich, 1995). The self and personality form as the developing mind relates with and tries to make sense of the world in which it finds itself. As it does this, it takes on many of the properties of the environment that it seeks to understand and negotiate. How we understand, think, feel, see and conceptualise, although heavily influenced by inherited temperamental and biological dispositions, is also shaped by our social, cultural and linguistic experiences. Individuality is socially based, and personality forms as social understanding develops (Burkitt, 1991: 2).

Children are born with an instinct to relate and interact with other people, particularly at the emotional, psychological and social level. Infants also arrive with a biological need to feel understood. Exquisite confirmation of these ideas has been given by recent developments in the brain sciences. The baby's brain is a self-organising developmental structure programmed at birth to make sense of experience, particularly social and interpersonal experience. However, it needs exposure to emotional, psychological, social and cultural experiences in order to make sense of them, neurologically as well as psychologically.

Thus, as children interact with those around them, their minds form. Schore (2001) a neuroscientist, says that 'young minds form in the context of close relationships'. It is not possible to understand children's psychological development without taking into account their social environment. We are fundamentally psychosocial beings. If social work practice is to be effective as well as sensitive, it has to understand the interplay between the psychological and the social, and how people and their environments interact. This is the essence of the psychosocial approach.

The developmental implications of this perspective are that the quality of relationships with other people during childhood has a direct bearing on the development of personality and the emotional make-up of the individual. The poorer the quality of people's relationship history and social environment, the less robust their psychological make-up and ability to deal with other people, social situations and emotional demands. Therefore, the way in which different personalities handle and develop their current social environment is in large measure a product of their past relationship experiences.

Internal working models

Different types of personality indicate the different ways in which people attempt to make sense of and adjust to their relationship environment. Adverse environments that lack love, mutuality and empathy are less conducive to the formation of secure, organised and confident personalities. The coherence of people's psychological organisation reveals the type of psychological adjustments they have had to make in order to cope with their social environment. The individual's personality is judged by the characteristic ways in which they make sense of and handle social relationships and experiences. In our development, what is on the social outside therefore establishes itself on the psychological inside. In this sense, external relationships become mentally internalised (Howe, 1995: 24).

Everyday life is a matter of understanding and negotiating the world of other people. The more children and adults are able to make sense of their social world and understand their own place within it, the more adept, skilled and relaxed they can be in social relationships. In turn, this improves their chances of enjoying good mental health, developing mutually rewarding friendships, entering reciprocally based intimate relationships, becoming caring parents and emerging as socially competent beings.

Frith (1989: 169) reminds us that 'the ability to make sense of other people is also the ability to make sense of one's self'. Children learn about their own psychological states within relationships. The more sensitive, emotionally attuned, empathic and reciprocal the communication within relationships, the more fully children learn to understand the nature and effect of their own mental states on themselves and those around them. The more they can understand the basis of their own thoughts and feelings, the more skilled they will become at understanding and interacting with other people. Imbalances, insensitivities and inconsistencies in the carer–child relationship mean that the infant's attempts to model interpersonal experience are more difficult to achieve. Not being able to make sense of experience is confusing, stressful and anxiety provoking. When other people are unpredictable and not susceptible to influence or control, children are less able to learn how to conduct themselves socially. The argument is that, if human beings are social beings, the ways in which we develop social understanding and become socially competent are of great relevance to those who work with both children and adults.

Attachment and relationship-based theories are good examples of how a psychosocial perspective can help us to understand and assess the quality of people's social relationships. The success with which people relate with others is a measure of their emotional intelligence and 'social competence' (Howe, 2008). Modern attachment theory provides us with a coherent, well-researched and elegantly argued set of ideas about the feelings, behaviours, defences and psychological strategies we all use in our dealings with others, including parents and children, partners and professional practitioners (see Bowlby, 1979, 1988).

Parents are the people most likely to provide children with their early, close relationship experiences. Attachment theory explores how the quality of children's relationships with their carers affect their socio-emotional development, which then influences the way in which they relate to and deal with other people. Therefore, if we are to understand the quality of children's social environments, we also have to understand the parents, their personalities and the kinds of relationships they generate with each other and their children. If the social outside influences the child's psychological inside, we need to pay careful attention to the quality of the relationship between the two.

Attachment behaviour

Attachment behaviour is a biologically adaptive response designed to ensure that highly vulnerable, dependent babies get into close, protective relationships. They need to get into such relationships at times of anxiety, distress and danger. They also need to be in close relationships with their primary carers in order to develop social understanding, interpersonal competence and language. By the time they are one year old, most children have established strong selective attachments to one or more adults or older children typically within their own family.

Attachment behaviours are triggered when children experience stress or anxiety. At such times, children seek out one of their attachment figures. This person is experienced as a 'safe haven' – a place of safety and comfort at times of need. When children are not anxious or in need of comfort, they are free to play and learn about their environment, particularly their social environment. Here the attachment figure acts as a 'secure base' from which the child can explore. It follows that children who experience a lot of anxiety have less time and emotional energy to explore and learn how to become socially adept.

One of the key tasks of attachment figures is to help children to understand and regulate their emotions. This is achieved in a variety of ways that involve the body, the senses and the mind. As adult minds interact with infant minds in a process known as 'intersubjectivity', children slowly develop a sense of self, the ability to regulate their own arousal, and the ability to make sense of other people as emotional and psychological beings, known as 'social cognition'.

Four types of relationship experience and their impact on psychosocial development and competence

Researchers and clinicians who have studied interactions between parents and their children have observed that the type of relationships they form depend on the parent's physical and emotional availability, emotional sensitivity, reliability, predictability, responsiveness, level of interest and level of concern. Children who experience their attachment figures as usually available and responsive feel secure. Those who do not experience their attachment figures as reliably available and responsive feel varying degrees of insecurity and anxiety.

Although there are now many refinements, we might recognise four basic types of attachment experience (Ainsworth et al., 1978). Each type represents a certain kind of emotional relationship within which a child has to make particular kinds of psychological adjustments if they are to cope and survive in the social world. We have already said that aspects of the child's personality and ability to develop social understanding form within these important relationships. Natural temperaments, genetic character, degrees of resilience and cultural contexts certainly have a strong part to play, but the classification remains extremely useful in helping social workers to understand children's emotional experiences and psychosocial functioning. The theory insists that many features of our personality and emotional life form within the history of our relationships with others. Therefore, the different patterns of attachment lead to particular personality and relationship styles during childhood and beyond into adulthood. Indeed, there is now a considerable body of research and clinical literature devoted to adult attachments, including much that is relevant to mental health, couple relationships and psychopathology (for example Rholes and Simpson, 2004).

The four types of attachment are:

1   secure attachments
2   insecure, ambivalent attachments
3   insecure, avoidant attachments
4   disorganised and controlling attachments.

A basic understanding of these four relationship environments helps practitioners to make sense of the way in which children and adults react to and deal with the social and emotional demands of others and the stresses of everyday life (for a more in-depth discussion, see Howe et al., 1999).

Secure attachments

In secure parent–child relationships, care is loving, emotionally attuned, responsive, predictable and consistent. There is a sensitivity to children's needs, thoughts and feelings. Parents tend to have children who are secure in their attachments, if they:

- are good at reading their children's minds and meeting their emotional needs
- treat their children as burgeoning psychological beings in their own right
- are good at making their children feel emotionally safe and contained
- are skilled at finding effective ways to comfort their children.

Over time, secure children get distressed less frequently, and when they do find themselves upset, they are more quickly calmed and settled.

Communication between carers and children is busy and two-way. There is mutual interest and concern in the thoughts and feelings of the other. Within such relationships, children begin to understand and handle themselves and their social relationships with increasing skill. They feel valued, socially competent and interpersonally effective. Other people are seen as trustworthy and available. These children are usually sociable and well liked by peers. They cope reasonably well with the conflicts, upsets and frustrations of everyday life. As they mature into adulthood, they continue to feel good about themselves. Such people are only likely to come the social worker's way at times of great environmental stress, such as hospitalisation, a disaster, the physical demands of a disability or old age, or in the guise of a resource – foster carer, adopter or volunteer.

Insecure, ambivalent attachments

When parental care is inconsistent and unpredictable, children begin to experience increasing levels of anxiety. The problem is one of neglect and insensitivity rather than hostility. Parents often fail to empathise with their children's moods, needs and feelings. Parents are caught up with their own needs and anxieties. The child is never quite sure where they are within the parent–child relationship. The child becomes increasingly confused and frustrated. Distress and anxiety lead to a clingy dependence. To this extent, children feel that the world of other people is hard to fathom and impervious to their influence and control. Love comes and goes in what seems an entirely arbitrary way. This generates a fretful, constant anxiety. Children become demanding and attention-seeking, provocative and needful. They create drama and trouble in an attempt to keep other people involved and interested. Feelings are acted out.

Insensitive and inconsistent care is interpreted by children and adults who have experienced such care to mean that they are ineffective in securing love and sustaining comforting relationships. Their conclusion might be that they are not only unworthy of love, but also might be unlovable. This is deeply painful. It undermines self-esteem as well as self-confidence. Thus, there is a need for closeness but a constant anxiety that the relationship might not last: 'I need you, but I am not sure I can trust you. You may leave me and cause me pain, so I feel anger as well as fear.' Such thoughts provoke feelings of insecurity, jealousy, conflict and possessiveness in relationships. There is a reluctance to let go of others, yet a resentment and fear that they may be lost at any time. The result is that people cling to relationships – including those with social workers – yet conduct them with a high level of tension and conflict. Lives, therefore, are full of drama, chaos and crisis, many of which will land on the social worker's doorstep.

Insecure, avoidant attachments

Children who develop avoidant patterns of attachment have parents who are either indifferent, rigid or rejecting. Although these parents may respond reasonably well when their child appears content, they withdraw when faced with distress and the need for comfort and attention. The clinging, complaining behaviour of children in ambivalent attachment relationships serves no purpose in these cooler styles of parenting. Attempts at intimacy only seem to bring distance, even rebuff. Carers encourage independence and de-emphasise dependency. When separated from their parents, these children show few signs of distress. It seems better to become emotionally self-reliant. Negative feelings are contained and rarely expressed.

Lack of emotional involvement and mutuality mean that both children and avoidant adults find it hard to understand and deal with their own feelings. They may find it difficult to form intimate, emotionally reciprocal relationships. Getting too close brings the fear of rejection and pain. So although there is a desire for intimacy, close relationships can cause anxiety. This might be dealt with defensively by seeking emotional distance or emotional anaesthesia through the use of alcohol or drugs.

Disorganised and controlling attachments

This type of attachment is observed most often in cases where children suffer abuse, neglect and trauma in relationship with their attachment figures (Howe, 2005). It must be noted that even in these cases of hostile (abusive) and helpless (neglectful) parenting, the primary carer is still the child's attachment figure. Therein lies the child's dilemma. The cause of the child's distress, the thing that triggers their attachment behaviour is the hostile or helpless behaviour of the attachment figure herself or himself. As the goal of attachment behaviour is proximity with the attachment figure at times of need, perversely the child experiences an increase in arousal and distress as they approach the primary carer, the very opposite of what happens in the case of secure children. In cases of abuse and neglect, children experience the simultaneous activation of fear – in which they try to escape from the parent as the source of danger – and attachment – when arousal compels them to approach their attachment figure as the supposed source of safety. When these two incompatible behavioural responses are activated by the same person – the abusive or neglectful parent – it is not possible to organise an attachment strategy that increases feelings of safety and comfort, hence the description 'disorganised' attachment.

With maturation, disorganised children do manage to develop fragile and more coherent representations of themselves as less helpless and at the mercy of others. With carers who are helpless, unavailable, frightening or out of control, children begin to take control of their own safety and needs. This results in the development of various controlling behaviours and strategies. Controlling strategies represent desperate attempts by abused and neglected children to take charge of their own safety, wellbeing and regulation. They display a range of behaviours that suggest that psychologically they are in frightened 'survival mode' for much of the time. In environments in which children suffer 'relational trauma', emotions go unregulated, minds lack integration, and brain development is compromised.

Children and adults whose attachments are classified as disorganised/controlling are at significantly increased risk of a range of behavioural and mental health problems including depression, anxiety disorders, personality disorders, and post-traumatic stress disorder.

Assessments

Using a psychosocial approach places a great deal of emphasis on making thorough, carefully observed, theoretically informed assessments of people, their relationships and their sociocultural environment. We need to know how people act and relate with each other, how they behave with their children, neighbours and officials, how children respond to parents, peers and teachers, and how they play and react to demands and difficulties. How people react to 'outer world' events tells us about their 'inner world'. Indeed, among the 'people professions', social work remains peculiarly well placed to appreciate how people bring feelings to situations and how situations provoke feelings in people (Winnicott, 1964; Schofield, 1996).

There is a need to identify the stresses in people's lives. Do they have unsupportive partners, live in poverty or experience isolation? What children and adults say and do, then, needs to be interpreted within the logic of a psychosocial framework.

Although working within a psychosocial perspective does not require social workers actively to inquire about people's past experiences, large amounts of information will in practice be acquired about their childhoods, relationships with others, including sexual partners, encounters with authority, material problems and interpersonal ups and downs. This information can be fed into the assessment to help the social worker to understand the way people are psychologically relating to their social and material environment.

Practice

A detailed psychosocial assessment allows social workers to begin to make sense of what people say and do. It sees links between past and present relationship experiences. Connections can be made between the emotional and behavioural impact of people on each other. The ability of people to feel in control of their own mental, social and economic state is recognised as fundamental to their general wellbeing. When control is absent, anxiety rises. And when anxiety mounts, a variety of feelings and behaviours may be triggered, including anger, despair, worthlessness, aggression, denial and avoidance, which brings them to the attention of social agents.

Using a psychosocial approach allows social workers to understand and 'stay with' the apparent confusion and complexity that seems to characterise the lives of so many clients. The ability to make sense of what is going on allows practitioners to respond with calm compassion. In this way, they are able to contain difficult emotional situations and continue to be available to people who feel frightened and confused, angry and impotent. Using their knowledge of self and others, social workers are able to maintain high levels of interest in and understanding of the emotional and psychological experience of the other. They show emotional intelligence (Howe, 2008). Service users who feel understood at the psychological and emotional level are more likely to engage with the social worker. Within the context of a secure, psychologically attuned relationship, clients and service users begin to feel safe and supported as they begin to explore their situation, practically as well as psychosocially. Such client–worker relationships provide the opportunity for reflection, emotional growth, rational planning and decision-making.

Working within a psychosocial perspective defines two major areas of interest for the practitioner. The first concerns the notion of risk factors – what elements of the individual's psychosocial environment place their development, emotional wellbeing and social competence at risk. Social workers and clients need to identify such risks so that they may be avoided, decreased, changed or removed. Risks range from the obvious, for example physical and sexual abuse, to the more subtle, for example marital discord, the absence of emotional support, neglect, social isolation and financial worries.

The second requires the social worker to identify the protective factors in an individual's psychosocial environment – what elements are promoting their wellbeing, sound socio-emotional development and social competence. Social workers and clients seek to increase, introduce and improve factors that strengthen and protect psychosocial functioning. Emotional, social and economic support are among the most effective protective measures we can receive. Such support may be introduced in a variety of ways. Conflict may be reduced between parents. Depressed mothers may be encouraged to meet other women at a family centre. Social workers may provide frequent, low-intensity visits (Jones, 1985). Attempts may be made to increase social security benefits. In extreme cases, in order to reduce risks to psychosocial functioning, clients may need to be removed to new social environments, as happens in the case of the adoption of older children or the transfer of an old person into a residential home.

Conclusion

At a deep level, a psychosocial approach taps into important contemporary debates about the development of behaviour and personality, and the social nature of being human. Increasingly, social scientists are recognising that our natures and development are the exclusive result of neither genes nor experience. Rather, there is a complex interaction between the two, in which the way our inheritance expresses itself and develops depends on the physical and social environment in which we find ourselves, and the ways in which our environment is shaped and reacts depends on our individual characteristics (see, for example, Rutter, 2006). These insights provide the basic intellectual outlook of a psychosocial approach.

Not surprisingly, psychosocial theory has been seen to have greatest relevance in childcare and family work. However, the perspective is being increasingly used in work with other client groups. The quality of the social environment appears to be an important factor in understanding the onset and experience of those at biological risk from either schizophrenia or depression. Social developmental models might help us to understand a range of mental health problems, and the various kinds of relationships that develop between dependent elderly parents and their adult children.

Always at the heart of practice, psychosocial theories are being revitalised in social work as other disciplines, particularly in the psychological and neurological sciences, explore how people develop (or fail to develop) social understanding and interpersonal competence. If social work is about people's emotional wellbeing, personal development and social behaviour, a psychosocial approach provides theories that help to explain personal experience in a social context and guide practice.

For further discussion of the life course in childhood, see Adams et al., 2009a, Chapter 10, and for aspects of risk and safeguarding children, see Adams et al., 2009c, Chapter 4.

Dunn, J. (1993) *Young Children's Close Relationships: Beyond Attachment*, Newbury Park, CA, Sage. Written by a leading developmentalist, a stimulating read that takes a well-rounded look at young children's development in the ever-changing context of family, peer and cultural relationships.

Goldstein, E.G. (2002) *Object Relations Theory and Self-psychology in Social Work*, New York, Free Press. Excellent overview of current psychodynamic thinking as it applies to social work.

Howe, D. (2008) *The Emotionally Intelligent Social Worker*, Basingstoke, Palgrave Macmillan. Introduction to the emotions and why an understanding of the part they play in social work underpins so much of professional practice.

Howe, D., Brandon, M., Hinings, D. and Schofield, G. (1999) *Attachment Theory, Maltreatment and Family Support: A Practice and Assessment Model*, Basingstoke, Macmillan – now Palgrave Macmillan. Broad outline of the main features of attachment theory, backed by a comprehensive review of the research literature, plus an application of developmental attachment theory to child abuse and neglect.

Mattinson, J. and Sinclair, I. (1979) *Mate and Stalemate*, London, Institute of Marital Studies. First-hand account, backed by analytic and attachment-oriented theories, of working with marital problems in a social services department, packed with case examples.

Rutter, M. and Rutter, M. (1993) *Developing Minds: Challenge and Continuity across the Life Span*, Harmondsworth, Penguin. Examination and review of the research literature that looks at human development over the lifetime, paying particular attention to the continuities and discontinuities in the psychological growth process.

Cross-cultural and black perspectives through the life course

13

This chapter argues that many well-known psychological theories are developed by white people based on their observations of white people and assume that largely European cultural norms and practices are universal. These theories have not had sufficient explanatory power to account for the behaviour of black people. This is not to say that there are only 'white' psychologies and 'black' psychologies, but that the different accounts need to be handled with greater sensitivity when considering the diversity of human experience.

Chapter overview

Life course studies may draw on different theoretical perspectives – sociological, economic, political, biological, anthropological and psychological. Social work has turned to the social sciences, particularly psychology, for accounts of human behaviour that can be applied in practice. This chapter will focus mainly on the psychological perspective. It argues that traditional psychological theories have not had sufficient explanatory power to account for the behaviour of black people. The term 'black' in this chapter has been used to describe people from Asian and African-Caribbean backgrounds.

The issues discussed in this chapter are offered as the initial steps towards an understanding of some concepts covered in the literature on the life course from a cross-cultural and black perspective: attachment theory, black identity development, the family and older people. These perspectives have been widely researched and developed in the US (Cross, 1971, 1980; Greenfield and Cocking, 1994; Crittenden and Claussen, 2000; Cross and Vandiver, 2001).

During the late 1980s, social work education 'became increasingly aware of the impact of oppression and discrimination on clients and communities' (Thompson, 1993: 1). For example, the Central Council for Education and Training in Social Work (CCETSW), which at that time approved qualifying social work programmes, attached a high priority to an anti-discriminatory approach in college and placement teaching and assessment (see CCETSW Paper 30, 1991). The guidance notes for the teaching of childcare on qualifying programmes stressed that:

> all social work students should have a sound knowledge of human growth and development, [and] the significance of race, culture and language in development must be understood. (CCETSW, 1991: 14)

While CCETSW has now been replaced by the UK care councils, these policies have had immense influence on the direction and content of UK social work education.

The Children Act 1989 states that the race, culture, language and religion of children and young people must be addressed in the provision of services. In order to meet the needs and help the development of any child, black or white, it is essential that social workers operate with adequate knowledge, understanding and sensitivity.

As Western society has become more heterogeneous, cross-cultural effectiveness has emerged as an essential skill for all social workers who work with children and young people. Over the past two decades, social scientists (mainly in the US) have become increasingly aware of the contributions that cross-cultural research findings can make to our understanding of human development (for example Segall et al., 1998). Little of the current social work literature in the UK has addressed the issue of cross-cultural development.

Inadequacies of Western psychology

The conventionally accepted paradigms and discoveries of much Western psychology do not provide an understanding of black children, adolescents and older people. Even a casual observation of the history of psychology will demonstrate that psychological literature from the past 100 years has been based on observations primarily on Europeans, predominantly male and overwhelmingly middle class. A model of white middle-class personality has been 'utilized as a measuring stick against which all other psychological development is assessed' (Sinha, 1983: 7), 'the standard against which others must measure up' (Segall et al., 1990: 93).

The formulations of notable thinkers who have shaped the thought of Eurocentric psychology, such as Sigmund Freud ([1913]1950) and Carl Jung (1950), have all directly or indirectly asserted the superiority of European races over non-European races. Despite the diversity of the various schools of Western psychology, they seem to merge unequivocally in their assumption of the Eurocentric point of view and the superiority of people of European descent. It is not surprising, therefore, that the conclusions reached from the application of their concepts and methods are invariably of the inferiority of non-European peoples (Robinson, 1995, 2008; White, 2004).

A main feature of Eurocentric psychology is the assumption among psychologists that people are alike in all important respects. In order to explain 'universal human phenomena', white psychologists established a normative standard against which all other cultural groups were to be measured. What appeared as normal or abnormal was always in comparison to how closely a specific thought or behaviour corresponded to that of white people. Hence, normality is established on a model of the middle-class,

Caucasian male of European descent. The more one approximates this model in appearance, values and behaviour, the more 'normal' one is considered to be. The obvious advantage for Europeans (whites) is that such norms confirm *their* reality as *the* reality and flaunt statements of their supremacy as scientifically based 'fact'. The major problem with such normative assumptions for non-European people is the inevitable conclusion of deviance on the part of anyone unlike this model. In fact, the more distinct you are from this model, the more pathological you are considered to be (Robinson, 1995, 2008; White, 2004).

Social workers in Britain and the US have been influenced greatly by the psychoanalytic approach in psychology. This approach is based on Sigmund Freud's work but has been developed by neo-Freudians, for example Erikson, Melanie Klein and Jung. In contrast to the critiques of Freud for sexism (Mitchell, 1974; Frosh, 1987), the racism of the psychoanalytic approach is relatively unknown. Mama (1995: 127) criticises Freudian psychoanalysis for:

> its universalism and ethnocentrism … A theory which takes sexual repression and taboo as the bedrock of 'civilisation' is also highly culture-bound.

Fernando (1991, 2002) notes that Freud (1930) envisaged the development of civilisation being dependent on suppressing instinctual behaviour under the guidance of the superego, elaborated into a 'cultural superego'; it was natural for him that the 'leadership of the human species' should be taken up by 'white nations' (Freud, 1915, 1930) and that 'primitives have a lower form of culture' (Fernando, 1991: 41). In his book *Totem and Taboo*, Freud ([1913]1950) refers to the practices and behaviours of African peoples as 'savage' or 'primitive'. However, 'although Freud adhered to racist thinking, it was Jung who integrated racist ideas more fully into psychological theories' (Fernando, 1991: 42).

Carl Jung, at one time Freud's star pupil, has been referred to as the father of 'transpersonal psychology'. He believed that certain psychological disorders found among US Americans were due to the presence of black people in America. Jung (1950: 29) noted that:

> The causes for the American energetic sexual repression can be found in the specific American complex, namely to living together with 'lower races, especially with Negroes'.

Jung identified the modern African as 'primitive' in every sense of the word. Dalal (1988) maintains that Jung considered black people to be inferior rather than just different.

Erikson's (1968) psychoanalytical theory focuses on one distinctive feature of adolescence: the development of a sense of identity. He proposed a process whereby adolescents begin with an unclear sense of their identity, experience a 'crisis' and achieve a clear sense of their identity. He felt that 'identity crisis' was normative to adolescence and young adulthood. Erikson (1964) spoke of ethnic self-doubt and a pathological denial of one's roots as being seminal to Negro identity. He could not conceive that, for some individuals, their colour might actually be a source of pride. In an article 'Memorandum on identity and Negro youth', Erikson (1964: 41) states:

A lack of familiarity with the problem of Negro youth and with the actions by which Negro youth hopes to solve these [identity] problems is a marked deficiency in my life and work which cannot be accounted for by theoretical speculation.

Towards a black perspective in psychology

There is a consensus among most black psychologists and professionals that explanations of black behaviour that are alternative to white European perspectives must be developed. A black perspective in psychology is concerned with combating (negative) racist and stereotypic, weakness-dominated and inferiority-oriented conclusions about black people. This perspective is interested in the psychological wellbeing of black people and is critical of research paradigms and theoretical formulations that have a potentially oppressive effect on black people. Black psychologists (mainly in the US) have presented alternative perspectives on black child development. However, the research of black scholars, who have unique insights into the problems of minority children and adolescents, has largely been neglected by mainstream developmental psychology (Spencer, 1988; Jones, 2004).

Cross-cultural considerations

How can a cross-cultural perspective contribute to our understanding of human development? Gardiner (1994) has pointed to a number of important benefits:

- Looking at behaviour from this perspective compels researchers to reflect seriously on the variety of ways in which their cultural beliefs and values affect the development of their theories and research designs.
- Increased awareness of cross-cultural findings provides an opportunity to extend or restrict the implications of research conducted in a single cultural group, most notably the US and similar Western societies.
- This perspective reduces ethnocentrism – by looking at behaviours as they occur in another culture.

Although it is essential for social workers to have a basic understanding of black people's cultural values, there is the ever-present danger of overgeneralising and stereotyping. Information about Asian and African-Caribbean cultural values should act as guidelines rather than absolutes. Members of every group are shaped by culture, but also by acculturation, gender, roles, age, income, education and so on. Recognising intra-group differences is critical and helps to avoid stereotyping (Robinson, 2007). Race, gender and class inequalities all play a part in shaping dominant and minority groups' cultures, defining opportunities and moulding traditions (Mirza, 1992).

Attachment

An example of a developmental theory criticised for its assumptions of universality is attachment theory, originally described by Bowlby (1969). As we saw in the last chapter, this concept refers to the special bond which develops between the infant and the carer and which provides the child with emotional security. Once attachment is established, babies are distressed by separation from their mothers (called separation distress or anxiety). Ainsworth et al. (1978) delineated four different styles of attachment: secure, avoidant (children who shun their mothers or carers), ambivalent (children who are uncertain in their response to their mothers or carers) and disorganised and controlling. One of the assumptions about the nature of attachment in the US and Britain is that secure attachment is the ideal. Cultures differ, however, on their notion of 'ideal' attachment. For example, German mothers value and promote early independence and regard avoidant attachment as the ideal, seeing the 'securely' attached child as 'spoiled' (Grossman et al., 1985; Crittenden, 2000).

Some cross-cultural studies also challenge the notion that closeness to the mother is necessary for secure and healthy attachment (for example Tronick et al., 1992). Indeed, this notion is prevalent in traditional theories of attachment based on research in the US. Tronick et al. (1992) found the children in their study to be emotionally healthy despite having multiple carers.

Theories of attachment appear to be central to social work practice with children and families. However, most of the social work literature on attachment is Eurocentric and does not address issues of working with black children and families (Robinson, 2007). Howe's *Attachment Theory for Social Work Practice* (1995: 78) refers briefly to 'cultural variations in the distribution of the different types of attachment patterns' but takes no account of Britain's black population. In a later publication, Howe et al. (1999: 33) note that:

> cross-cultural and intercountry comparisons of attachment patterns confirm that the modal type is that of the secure attachment, typically around 55–60 per cent infant–mother dyads showing the pattern.

Gambe et al. (1992: 30) argue that:

> the processes of colonization, migration, refuge-seeking and the effect of immigration controls have led to black families developing the capacity to maintain relationships and attachments over vast distances and time.

Attachment theory fails to take into account such issues and fails to appreciate the strengths of black families. Thus, the Eurocentric bias of attachment theory 'can contribute to inappropriate and racist assessments, [and] inappropriate interventions' (Gambe et al., 1992: 30).

There is still much to be done to understand the attachment patterns in other cultures. The studies that do exist, however, are clear in suggesting that we cannot assume that what is seen most in Euro-American culture is best or most descriptive for all. Notions concerning the quality of attachment and the processes by which it occurs are qualitative judgements made from the perspective of each culture. Each culture has values different from but not necessarily better than those of others.

Black identity development

This section argues that the model of psychological 'nigrescence' (Latin for the 'process of becoming black') is more relevant to the psychological life experiences of black adolescents in Britain than the more traditional psychological theories. It will enable us to gain a better understanding of the difficulties experienced by black adolescents in Britain.

Black identity has been discussed extensively in the social science literature using various terms and measures. According to Looney (1988: 41): 'Black identity deals specifically with an individual's awareness, values, attitudes, and beliefs about being Black.' It can also be viewed as 'an active developmental process which is exposed to various influences within and without, and can be selective and/or adaptive' (Maxime, 1986: 101). These definitions will be used as the 'operating definition' in the discussion of black identity development.

A perspective that has largely been ignored by traditional Eurocentric psychology is the research on the psychology of nigrescence. Nigrescence models tend to have four or five stages, the common point of departure being not the change process per se but an analysis of the identity to be changed. These models are useful as they enable us to understand the problems of black identity confusion and to examine, at a detailed level, what happens to a person during identity change. Perhaps the best known and most widely researched model of black identity development is Cross's model of the conversion from 'Negro' to 'black'.

Cross (1971, 1980, 1991) suggests that the development of a black person's racial identity is often characterised by their movement through a five-stage process, the transformation from pre-encounter to internalisation–commitment. Briefly, the five stages are:

1   *Pre-encounter:* In this stage, the individual's racial identity attitudes are primarily pro-white and anti-black, that is, the individual devalues their ascribed racial group in favour of Euro-American culture.
2   *Encounter:* Encounter attitudes describe the awakening process experienced by black people. This awakening is often the result of a critical incident in one's life that leads one to reconceptualise issues of race in society and reorganise racial feelings in one's personal feelings. For example, a white individual with racist attitudes and practices may act as a catalyst to racial identity attitude change.
3   *Immersion–emersion:* This stage involves learning and experiencing the meaning and value of one's racial group and unique culture. Immersion attitudes are pro-black.
4   *Internalisation:* This is the stage of racial identity in which the individual achieves pride in their racial group and identity.
5   *Internalisation–commitment:* In this stage, the person finds activities and commitments to express their new identity.

The internalisation and internalisation–commitment stages are characterised by positive self-esteem, ideological flexibility and openness about one's blackness.

There is an extensive empirical literature that confirms Cross's model of black identity development (see Cross, 1971, 1991, 2001). Although Cross's identity development model has been developed with African-American samples in the US, it is argued by various authors (for example Maxime, 1986; Sue and Sue, 1990) that other minority groups share similar processes of development. In Britain, Maxime (1986) has used Cross's model in the understanding of identity confusion in black adolescents.

Parham has expanded Cross's nigrescence model and considers that:

> The process of psychological Nigrescence ... is a lifelong process, which begins with the late-adolescence/early-adulthood period in an individual's life. (Parham, 1989: 194–5)

More recent developments in nigrescence theory and research have added to the expansion of specific stages (see Cross et al., 1998 for a detailed description) and opened the model up to renewed criticisms (Constantine et al., 1998). Emphasis on stage theories for capturing racial/ethnic identity formation has fallen under heavy criticism by some researchers as being too linear and not recognising the multidimensional nature of ethnic identity (Phinney, 1990; Yeh and Huang, 1996). Work continues on advancing the nigrescence construct (Cross et al., 1998; Cross, 2001; Marks et al., 2004).

An understanding of Cross's model should sensitise social workers to the role that oppression plays in a black individual's development. Maxime (1993) has used Cross's model in the understanding of identity confusion in black children and adolescents in residential, transracially fostered and adoptive care settings. It was clearly apparent from Robinson's study of racial identity development and self-esteem among African-Caribbean adolescents in residential care in a city in the West Midlands that residential care staff found Cross's model extremely useful in therapeutic work with African-Caribbean youngsters (Robinson, 2000).

Cross's model serves as a useful assessment tool for social workers to gain a greater understanding of black youth. Pre-encounter attitudes have been linked to high levels of anxiety, psychological dysfunction and depression (Parham and Helms, 1985; Carter, 1991; Cross et al., 2004), and low self-regard and self-esteem (Parham and Helms, 1985). Young people's perceptions of the social worker are likely to be influenced by their racial identity development. Thus, young people at the pre-encounter stage are more likely to show a preference for a white social worker over a black worker.

Finally, social workers need to be aware that raising children in a white-dominated society places special pressures on the black parent. Although the basic mechanisms for socialisation are the same for black and white children – reinforcement, modelling, identification and so on – the transmittal sources and content may exhibit some subtle and obvious differences for black children. The need for adaptive responses to social, economic and political barriers helps to shape the socialisation of black children (Harrison et al., 1990; Stevenson and Davis, 2004). Peters (1985) indicated that many black parents focused on racial barrier messages and emphasised learning to cope with and survive prejudice in a white-dominated society. Hill (1999: 102) noted that racial socialisation was nearly universal among black parents, 'who can scarcely escape talking about racism and racial pride and who engage in myriad subtle strategies to challenge the denigration of blackness'.

Social work with black families

This section will focus on the dominance of pathology models of black family functioning – with reference to models of African-Caribbean and Asian family structures in social science and social work literature and practice.

Many social work texts paint crude cultural stereotypes of black families. The 'norm' against which black families are, implicitly or explicitly, judged is white. The norm presents a myth of the normal family as nuclear, middle class and heterosexual. Black families are seen as strange, different and inferior. The pathological approach to black family life is evident in the British research on black people. It is also evident in social workers' perceptions of black families. Barn (1993: 120) notes that social workers' 'negative perceptions of black families led them to develop a "rescue mentality" which came into force very quickly when dealing with these families'. Various studies (for example Barn, 1993, 2002) have indicated the high presence of black children in the care system. Social workers tend to rely on Eurocentric theory and practice that devalues the strength of black families (Ahmad, 1990; Graham, 2007). For example, Stubbs (1988: 103) observed:

> the ease with which negative models of Afro-Caribbean culture and family functioning, already prevalent within the social work literature ... fit into the frameworks of knowledge held by social workers to be relevant to their task.

Asian families have also been described in terms of cultural stereotypes (Ghuman, 2003). Parmar (1981: 21) notes that:

> the traditional Asian household organised through the extended family kinship systems is held out to be responsible for a number of problems that Asians face in the context of British society.

Parmar (1981: 21) argues that the 'rebellion' that

> Asian parents face from sons and daughters is ... to be expected and deserved particularly if they [Asian parents] insist on practising such 'uncivilised' and 'backward' customs as arranged marriages.

Young people, particularly young women, are said to be torn between two cultures (Anwar, 1976, 1998), unable to tolerate strict rules, particularly arranged marriages, and ill-equipped to integrate into British society. Complex family situations tend to be reduced to simplistic, catch-all explanations such as 'endemic culture conflict', which offer no real understanding and fail to give any positive regard to the client's cultural roots (Ahmed, 1986). Implicit in the idea of 'culture conflict' is the assumption that the values of the British family are modern and superior while Asian culture is in some way backward and inferior.

White social workers are more likely to tolerate intergenerational conflict between parents and adolescents in white homes than in black homes. However, the little research that exists suggests that young Asians are no more alienated from their parents than any other group of young people (Westwood and Bhachu, 1988).

Dwivedi (1996, 2002) argues that if social work perceptions and practice are largely Eurocentric, the Children Act 1989 can easily work against the best interest and protection of the black child. Thus:

> The instrument of 'race, culture, religion and language' can be easily abused to perpetuate the dominance of professional control as a manifestation of their perception of ethnic minority families as culturally deficient, dysfunctional or pathological from whom the children need to be rescued on the one hand, to a justification of non-intervention even when a child desperately needs intervention and protection, so that the professional could appear to be culturally sensitive in case abuse is culturally acceptable! (Dwivedi, 1996: 9)

According to O'Hagan (2001: 116), social work has 'no roots in cultural sensitivity or cultural competence'. He argues that 'even today its literature adopts a distinctly anti-cultural stance, compatible with its monocultural theories and practices'.

Social work with older black people

Older people, both black and white, face discrimination on the grounds of age or 'ageism'. Fennell et al. (1988: 97) define ageism as: 'ageism means unwarranted application of negative stereotypes to older people'. Unlike other older people, black elders face additional problems arising from racial, cultural and economic differences and disadvantages.

The comparative literature on black and white elders is dominated by the theme of 'double jeopardy'. This concept, first popularised in the US (National Urban League, 1964), asserts that the adverse living conditions of black older people in America is compounded by the social fact of their overall treatment as minority group members (Jackson et al., 1982). In Britain, the term has been applied to 'emphasise the double disadvantage of being poor (in income, housing, health, status and role) and a member of a minority group which suffers racial discrimination' (Patel, 1990: 5). In addition to 'race' and age, gender and social class are also important dimensions to inequality (Patel, 1990, 2003). Thus, older black people could face triple jeopardy, which is defined as the combined impact of race, age and social class on the lives of people in disadvantaged minorities (see Jackson et al., 1982).

British research has suggested that the service needs of older people from black groups may be considerable as a result of low incomes, poor housing, isolation and comparatively poor health (Askham et al., 1993; Dominelli, 2002c). However, older black people 'have been virtually neglected by statutory bodies and have seldom found provisions addressing their specific needs' (Dominelli, 1988: 117). In a recent study of the housing and care needs of black elders in Tower Hamlets, London, Bowes (1998: 41) concludes that 'existing provision ... is not appropriate and is not meeting their needs', and that despite earlier research studies, the housing and care needs of black elders remain unmet.

Dominelli (1988: 117) notes that myths about the support of the extended family in caring for its older members have been used by white social workers and their institutions to deny the need for making appropriate provisions available. This approach ignores the fact that 'immigration controls since 1962 have made it virtually impossible for black family units to exist in their totality in Britain' (Dominelli, 1988: 96). Therefore, not all older Asians live with family members and, even when they do, they may still have problems of isolation and lack of daytime support. The strains on the extended Asian families, partly as a consequence of cramped accommodation, have been mentioned in many of the reports presenting the need for Asian day centres (for example Rochdale County Council, 1986). Older black people, especially older Asians, are ill-informed about their welfare rights and the social services. Positive action is, therefore, required by social services departments and other organisations to increase awareness (Askham et al., 1993; Butt, 2006). However, social work practice in this area is largely ethnocentric, if not colour blind.

The dominant psychological theories on ageing do not provide an adequate understanding of older black people. For example, disengagement theory (see Cumming and Henry, 1961) claims to be universal, but the theory is based on a model of middle-class, white, older people living in the US mid-west (Hochschild, 1975; White, 2004). Blakemore and Boneham (1994: 138) suggest that:

> ethnicity and race do make a difference to the experience of ageing, whether this is in connection with ... roles in the family ... culture-specific needs for care by voluntary and statutory services, or problems of racism and stereotyping.

Thus, the main theories on ageing 'need to be reconsidered with ethnic and racial diversity in mind' (Blakemore and Boneham, 1994: 137).

Conclusion

The issues discussed in this chapter indicate that black and white people have different experiences at different stages of the life course. Social work training and practice must question whether theories that have originated in Euro-American settings have relevance in working with black clients in Britain. A Eurocentric perspective in psychology has meant certain theoretical deficits when social workers attempt to apply it in practice. Traditional psychology perpetuates a notion of deviance with respect to black people. Social workers need an understanding of the black perspective in psychology and social work theory in order to be able to deliver effective services to black clients and communities.

Research that focuses on attachment theory, identity development, the black family and older black people from a black and cross-cultural perspective will enable social workers to gain a better understanding of the difficulties experienced by black children, teenagers and adults in Britain.

For further discussion of perspectives on later life, see Adams et al., 2009a, Chapter 11, and for issues arising in work with asylum seekers and refugees, see Adams et al., 2009c, Chapter 9. For a discussion of the social and political dimensions of anti-oppressive social work, see Adams et al., 2009a, Chapter 5.

Cross, W.E. (2001) 'Encountering nigrescence', in J.M. Casas, L.A. Suzuki and C.M. Alexander (eds) *Handbook of Multicultural Counseling*, 2nd edn, Berkeley, CA, Cobb & Henry. Provides a discussion of racial identity development models.

Cross, W.E., Parham, T. and Helms, J.E. (2004) 'The stages of black identity development: nigrescence models', in R.L. Jones (ed.) *Black Psychology*, 4th edn, Berkeley, CA, Cobb & Henry. Provides a detailed discussion of nigrescence models and directions of future theorising and research.

Dwivedi, K.N. and Varma, V.P. (eds) (2002) *Meeting the Needs of Ethnic Minority Children, including Refugee, Black and Mixed Parentage Children: A Handbook for Professionals*, 2nd edn, London, Jessica Kingsley. Provides social workers with theoretical and practical information on the health, education and social care of black children.

McAdoo, H.P. (ed.) (2002) *Black Children*, 2nd edn, Thousand Oaks, CA, Sage. This comprehensive book discusses black children's development.

Patel, N. (2003) (ed.) *Minority Elderly Care in Europe: Country Profiles*, Leeds, PRAIE. Provides social workers with information about minority elderly care in Europe.

Robinson, L. (2008) *Psychology for Social Workers: Black Perspectives*, 2nd edn, London, Routledge. Essential introductory text for all social workers in training and practice.

Robinson, L. (2007) *Cross-cultural Child Development for Social Workers: An Introduction*, Basingstoke, Palgrave Macmillan. This unique text offers an introduction to cross-cultural perspectives on child development for social workers.

fuRtHer
ReadinG

14 Cognitive-behavioural practice

Chapter overview

A wide variety of health and social care practitioners undergo training in cognitive-behavioural therapy (CBT). They use it because of its proven effectiveness. By providing an outline of learning theories, with live practice examples, this chapter aims to encourage social workers to integrate CBT into their work.

Rapid expansion of theoretical and empirical research in applications of learning theory (see British Association for Behavioural and Cognitive Psychotherapies, www.babcp.com) has not been matched by growing awareness and interest of social work practitioners. Fischer's (1974) 'quiet revolution' – the gradual integration of learning theory processes into social work – has gained some ground in the British context but, well over three decades later, not as much as expected. Later in this chapter, we shall consider some of the reasons for this.

During this same period, terminology changed, reflecting shifts in emphasis. For example, Payne, writing in 1991 about theories in social work, divided the cognitive (thought processes) from the behavioural (the 'doing') and discussed their theoretical bases in separate chapters. The journal *Behavioural Psychotherapy* changed its name to *Behavioural and Cognitive Psychotherapy* in 1993, in line with its parent association. Sheldon revised his 1982 text *Behaviour Modification*, publishing it in 1995 as *Cognitive-behavioural Therapy*. The hyphen denotes a linking of cognition and behaviour: a deliberate indication of how the one informs the other and how both elements are important for therapeutic practice. Sutton (2000a) gives an excellent account of the development of CBT.

Careful examination of the role cognition plays in deciding whether a behaviour will be repeated or not, or how it helps, either in learning behaviours or in eliminating unwanted behaviours is a particular contribution that social workers can make to the literature and to practice skills (although, of course, not uniquely; see, for example, the earlier work of Herbert, 1987a, 1987b; Falloon et al., 1993; Webster-Stratton and Herbert, 1994). Social workers' broad remit, attention to the immediate and the wider environment and their tradition of intervention in the service user's own home setting put them in an ideal position for developing applications of CBT to the real and often untidy, oppressive world of users of social welfare in local authority and other non-clinical settings. This chapter will concern itself with such applications.

The policy context of social work

Superficially, the recent and present political and social policy climate would seem favourable to the advancement of the principles of cognitive-behavioural practice. Pragmatic concentration on presenting situations and problems, planned, focused work, contracts, the attention to goals, outcomes and evidence for 'what works': all these fit into Best Value and performance indicators of effectiveness. Furthermore, current legislation and procedures, while rarely acknowledging the influence of learning theory and competency-based approaches, have nevertheless absorbed several of their essential principles. Examples are:

- the Children Act 1989 and its guidance (DfES, 2006), with the emphasis on working in partnership with professionals, parents and children, clear assessments, written, negotiated plans and systematic reviewing
- the frameworks for quality services and assessment (DH, 2000a; DH/DfEE/Home Office, 2000; DH, 2001b).

Meanwhile, a backlash against such approaches within the broader agenda of 'what works' and evidence-based practice is popular in social work (for example Gorman, 2001; Bilson, 2006).

First, many misconceptions prevail about learning theory approaches: they are mechanistic; they are about punishment; they are concerned with institutions and token economies. Such uninformed views ignore the many research-based British texts published over the past two decades (for example Hudson and Macdonald, 1986; Falloon et al., 1993; Sutton, 1994, 1999, 2000b; Iwaniec, 1995; Scott et al., 1995; Cigno and Bourn, 1998; Herbert and Harper-Dorton, 2002), as well as the number of case studies written by social workers from the position of mainstream social work and social services (Iwaniec et al., 1985a, 1985b; Bunyan, 1987; Bourn, 1993; Cigno, 1993; Matthews, Harvey and Trevithick, 2003). However, this convincing body of research, and its availability, is not commensurate with practitioner readiness to use it or social work educators to teach it (Sheldon and Chilvers, 2000; Payne, 2005), largely in contrast with healthcare professionals.

This leads to the second point: keeping up with research on the effectiveness of different social work approaches is hard work, although there are some reviews available to make the task easier (for example Macdonald et al., 1992; Macdonald, 1994; Sheldon, 1994; the Cochrane database). It requires considerable commitment to seek after truth and carry out our ethical duty of using only those approaches where there is evidence that they work in that situation, with this family or person, with those problems (Cigno and Wilson, 1994), rather than following our own predilections. In 1991,

Payne noted that social workers use psychoanalytic theory and do not find CBT attractive: this is still true today. Decisions to use one approach rather than another are not based on evidence of 'what works' (Newman et al., 1996; Davies et al., 2000).

The third reason is that some North American research is based on clinical studies of what hard-pressed local authority social workers would rightly regard as esoteric problems unlikely to come their way in their work with the disadvantaged, poor, oppressed, multi-problem section of the population in crowded inner cities or isolated, amenity-deprived rural areas. This, of course, ignores the important and ground-breaking studies by social work academics such as Thomas (1974), Fischer (1978) and Gambrill (1983, 1997). A recent US American text, although directed at social workers in clinical settings, contains material useful to all (Ronen and Freeman, 2007).

To sum up, many practitioners are reluctant to use CBT because they object 'on vague philosophical grounds … they just don't like the look and sound of anything "behavioural"' (Sheldon, 1995: 31). Hollin et al. (1995) point out that service user resistance is much less than that of practitioners.

We now go on to consider more precisely what we mean by cognitive-behavioural practice, its underpinning theories and how an understanding can help us to identify people's problem behaviours as well as work out programmes with them to improve significant aspects of their lives.

Cognitive-behavioural practice

Before describing procedures and giving examples of their relevance to social work, I shall briefly attempt to define and discuss what is meant by learning theory (or, more properly, theories) on which cognitive-behavioural intervention is based.

Behaviour is, largely, a result of prior learning, and what we learn is acquired in different ways. Sometimes we learn inadvertently or without deliberate intention. This kind of learning by association is known as 'classical conditioning': Pavlov's dogs produced saliva at the sound of a bell or approaching footsteps, which they had learned to associate with the bringing of food; a child's fear of the dentist who has drilled into a tooth after an unpleasant injection may spread to fear of anyone in clinical settings.

We also learn through others' reactions to our behaviour or through environmental consequences: our behaviour is established and maintained by reinforcement, commonly called a 'reward', although it may not necessarily look 'rewarding'. Volunteers may work in an Oxfam shop because they find it a pleasant environment in which to meet people and also because they feel good to be doing something worthwhile, but many of us would not work unless we got paid. This kind of learning is known as 'operant conditioning'. Here we can see how our thoughts, or 'cognitions', have a role to play in deciding whether a behaviour will be repeated or not, as well as whether it is reinforced.

Many behaviours, such as the way we talk (regional accent), walk (swagger or glide), cook or drive a car, are acquired by watching or listening to someone we like or respect doing it. This is called 'modelling' or 'vicarious learning'. We may think about others' performances and talk it over with ourselves – What effect will we have? Will we be able to imitate the behaviour successfully? – before we repeat the action. Sutton (1994) uses the term 'social learning theory', which encompasses a good deal of what we have briefly outlined above. She describes it thus:

> Social learning theory comprises a large body of concepts which, happily, are recognised by researchers in the disciplines of both psychology and sociology. It concerns how children and adults learn patterns of behaviour, as a result of social interactions, or simply through coping with the environment … it suggests how to focus upon the practical rather than the pathological, upon people's strengths and potentials rather than upon their weaknesses or shortcomings, and upon how to empower those with whom we work. (Sutton, 1994: 5–6)

Clearly, the effects of what we do are going to determine which behaviours will be repeated and in which circumstances. It is this knowledge of how and why we learn that enables the cognitive-behavioural practitioner to make a thorough assessment of a 'problem' behaviour, which, according to its possessor or one or more significant others, needs changing. It may be that more of the behaviour is desired, as in cases of non-school attendance, or less, as in cases of adults who have difficulty in controlling their anger. Much family social work focuses on controlling parental anger, which can lead to the potential or actual abuse of children, and where techniques include relaxation, role-rehearsal and self-talk (Scott, 1989; Leadbetter, 2002). Getting a child back to school often entails changing the parent's or the teacher's behaviour, often the reason for the child's absence in the first place. Fear of maths or sports, worsened by a teacher's sarcasm or shouting, may be the antecedent to sickness or truanting.

Fundamental to CBT is the observation that being aware of our thinking does not necessarily alter behaviour. Understanding, achieving 'insight' into why we do what we do, by no means inevitably leads to behaviour change. We may think 'This is bad for my teeth' as we reach for another chocolate, or 'These harm my health' and 'I must give this up' as we light a cigarette, or 'This never really works and I shouldn't do it' as we raise a hand to smack a child. We listen to the sound of our voice as we quarrel with our loved ones and think 'This is awful; I'm making things worse.'

Anxious thoughts, maladaptive interpretations of self, unrealistic expectations of others and disturbing ruminations affect behaviour in many, often serious, ways. Awareness of these processes is a start, but a consideration of our professional and private experiences tells us that this alone does not lead to desired behaviour change. Crucially, strategies are also required. Cognitive restructuring – challenging, for example, negative thoughts about ourselves ('I'm no good') and teaching others to do so – has been described and applied by social workers, such as Scott et al. (1995); much cognitive-based work derives from the seminal studies of Beck (1976) and Beck and Emery (1985). There is still much work being done in this area, but most practitioners would agree that a mainly cognitive approach needs to be evaluated by indicators of behavioural and environmental change. One has only to think of the implications of a service user with a serious addiction or a parent whose child has been identified as being at risk of overchastisement telling the worker, 'I think things are better now', and the practitioner going away satisfied that the intervention has been a success on this evidence alone. A careful combination of cognitive and behavioural techniques can be useful and appropriate, provided that clearly defined behavioural goals are identified to ensure that an evaluation of practice as 'a success' is soundly based.

Areas of practice and links with effectiveness

There are, then, many areas where research and experience indicate that CBT helps with behaviour problems in home and community settings. Herbert (1987b), in his preface to a book on helping children and their parents with problem behaviours, describes his conversion to a behavioural approach. When he was practising as a child psychologist, a despairing mother told him that she wanted to know what to *do* when her child screamed and cried. People want strategies to help them cope.

One area where families of children with learning difficulties do not get sufficient help is behaviour problems (Burke and Cigno, 1996, 2000). Sinclair et al. (1995) report that 30 per cent of children in the care system are referred because of problematic behaviour. Research shows that helping carers to learn different responses to a child's behaviour and teaching them parenting skills can help to prevent abuse or stop it escalating (see Chapillon, 1996, for a student social worker's account of a parenting skills group).

Social skills training (SST) has been used effectively with different service user groups:

- people with various degrees of learning difficulty (for example McBrian and Felce, 1992; Cullen et al., 1995)
- adults in different situations and with diverse problems (Hollin and Trower, 1986)
- people with mental health problems (Hudson, 1982; Oliver et al., 1989; Oliver and Hudson, 1998)
- young people leaving care (Biehal et al., 1992)
- young offenders and alcohol-related crime (McMurran and Hollin, 1993; Long et al., 1998).

SST combines well with other CBT approaches. It is not to be confused with punitive 'boot camp training' (Gendreau and Ross, 1987; Gendreau and Andrews, 1990). After such treatment, young offenders become leaner, fitter criminals. The authors conclude that cognitive-behavioural intervention, rather than short, sharp shocks, works. Different levels of CBT with homeless men with histories of violence and substance misuse are having some success (Maguire, 2006). Older people are not often thought of as having goals or as being suitable for the attention of social work intervention (Lymbery, 2005). Gambrill (1986), however, reports a successful, step-by-step approach to helping older people in the community express what they would like to achieve. They can be assisted to improve the quality of their lives by, for example, making telephone calls to friends and organisations to increase social contacts. The behaviour is rehearsed then reinforced by encouraging comments; successful calls become self-reinforcing. Cigno

(1993, 1998) describes a behavioural programme carried out in residential care with a 70-year-old woman to decrease unwanted aggressive behaviour and increase helpful acts and contacts in the wider community (see below).

Motivational interviewing (see Rollnick and Miller, 1995) developed from learning theory principles such as the use of positive modelling, cognitions and selective reinforcement of self-statements to change the behaviour of adults, including young offenders, with addictions (Tober, 1998). Indeed, motivational interviewing, because of its promising results, is now used in other fields too (de Jonge and Berg, 2007).

In the area of child welfare, what is familiarly known as the 'Dartington research' has drawn attention to key criteria for assessing outcomes with young people (Bullock et al., 1993, 1999; DH, 1995a). In order to evaluate outcomes, it is not only important to take into account factors such as maturation and other variables that operate externally to the intervention, but also to draw up a baseline on features of wellbeing such as health, educational achievement, level of social skills and troubled behaviour of the person concerned prior to intervention and service provision. It is possible, for example, to assess outcomes for children and young people according to how far they conform to accepted social norms of behaviour.

Consumer research, from the early British study of Mayer and Timms (1970) to the many studies now available, confirms that service users of all ages value attributes such as reliability, openness, honesty and clarity in their social worker, quite apart from any particular approach adopted. Happily, these qualities are the basis for the service user–worker relationship in CBT. Freeman et al. (1996) report the feelings of young people on being let down by social workers over such matters as cancelled visits and postponed meetings. Many missed visits are due to poor planning and lack of consideration of the meaning of such disappointments for vulnerable, powerless service users. Similar findings of appreciated practitioner attributes are found in a study by Cigno (1988) of the views of mothers attending a family centre.

Evocative accounts of users on the receiving end are important feedback as long as other, more objective, outcome criteria are employed alongside. Technical skills are to no avail if the practitioner lets the service user down as described above. It is crucial that students learn this during their practice placements, for one of the ways we learn is by modelling ourselves on others' behaviour. 'Show me' is a reasonable position for a student to take towards practice teachers. It is common often not to connect one's own behaviour with those to whom we are close and over whom we have influence. As a parent once said apologetically of her child: 'I don't know why he **** swears like that. I'm always telling the little **** not to **** well do it.'

Assessment and intervention

The key to good practice is thorough, detailed assessment. Apart from adhering to the basic social work values mentioned above, social workers need to practise from within a relationship of warmth, genuineness and empathy. Assessments may vary, but a good starting point for many situations where the aim is behaviour change is an ABC (antecedents, behaviour, consequences) analysis. It has the advantage of being easy to remember and is an excellent guide to the questions to be asked. In brief, these are as follows:

- *Antecedents:* What are the circumstances in which the behaviour takes place? What happens just before the behaviour in question? It is often useful to obtain information about more distant antecedents, too.
- *Behaviour:* How can the actual behaviour be described? What does the person do?
- *Consequences:* What happens immediately after the behaviour?

Worker and service user together discuss the relationship between the three. Many of our service users, living in poor housing, jobless, ill-educated and often suffering from health problems, exhibit what Seligman (1975) has called 'learned helplessness'. They do not think or feel that they can make any impact on their situation; it is their destiny to suffer the 'slings and arrows of outrageous fortune'. In some areas of their life this may be true; however, if they can learn to take action in one small part of their life, the results can be greatly reinforcing, can increase self-esteem and encourage the service user to take small steps to improve other aspects of living.

CASE EXAMPLE

Ms A's three children were on the child protection register because of her ex-partner's abuse and her own lack of parenting skills. The children, aged three, five and seven, were, according to their mother, 'out of control' and 'did what they liked'. She attended a parenting skills course where she constantly said 'Things are no better'. Gentle exploration of this statement by the worker revealed that she was now managing to get the children to school and that she was thinking of taking a course at the local college, 'but I'm thick'. She was surprised when the worker praised her efforts and discussed how she might go about getting information about courses. A home visit indicated that Ms A was now talking to the children and had some control over them. She subsequently went to the library to obtain leaflets about part-time courses. Giving her credit for the changes she was making to her behaviour and the benefits to her made her smile. She was further encouraged by the other parents in the group 'evaluating' her progress by telling her 'You should have seen how you were a month ago.'

Pointing out that Ms A's negative self-statements were not true was a start. Tracing her attempts to improve her management of the children, praising her and observing how they responded encouraged her to continue these new behaviours. She began to see that she could take steps to change elements in her environment and was not forever destined to be a 'bad mother' and 'thick'. (For a discussion of these issues from a user self-help perspective, see Adams, 1996.)

This is an example of challenging the learned helplessness of a mother where there was risk of neglect and abuse to children, and of shaping coping behaviour mainly through cognitive restructuring and positive reinforcement. The next example is of a case where careful observation of a person's environment, behaviour and its consequences led to an ABC assessment, hypotheses, intervention plan, review and evaluation. It is based on Sutton and Herbert's ASPIRE assessment framework (Sutton, 1994), where AS is assessment, P – planning, I – intervention, R – review and E – evaluation. (An example of the use of ASPIRE in work with a child with learning disabilities can be found in Burke and Cigno, 2000.)

◇◇◇ **case example** ◇◇◇◇◇◇◇◇◇◇◇◇◇◇◇◇◇◇◇◇◇◇◇◇◇◇◇◇◇◇◇◇◇◇◇◇◇◇

The problem concerned a young man, Colin, who attended a centre for adults with learning disabilities. Various activities took place, and, as well as participating in these, service users were encouraged to take responsibility for other tasks. Colin was often asked to take messages from one member of staff to another. He was willing and pleased to do this but usually returned after a long while with the message undelivered. Staff could not understand why this was so and renewed their attempts to impress upon him where he had to go. One worker volunteered to study the problem, observing Colin over the space of two weeks. Her analysis was as follows:

- *Antecedents:* An activity room, often the education room (because one of Colin's goals is to improve his literacy skills). Colin is asked to take a message to someone in another part of the building.
- *Behaviour:* Colin sets off. Talks to the manager on the way. Walks round the building, sometimes stopping at different rooms. Returns to where he started, message undelivered.
- *Consequences:* Staff express disappointment. Colin misses much of the teaching/activity session. Colin cannot tell why he has not delivered the message. Colin's learning goals are not achieved.

One hypothesis is that Colin enjoys wandering about rather than participating in an activity. If so, it is good that he is having a pleasant time but less good that he is not achieving his own learning objectives. The second is that he fails to understand the instructions given or understands but forgets. Further observation showed that both hypotheses are partly right. Colin likes being entrusted with a message but also enjoys chatting to the manager and walking about. Nevertheless, he is not happy when he realises that he has failed to carry out the task, nor when he misses an activity.

The volunteer observer discovered that the instructions given to Colin did not follow the same pattern. This is related to the second hypothesis. Here are some of the instructions he was given over the observation period:

- Take this to Mr Jones
- Take this to Mr Jones' room
- Tell Mr Jones the forms are here
- Take this to the craft room, and so on, with the substitution of another name or room.

So he is sometimes directed to a person and sometimes to a room or activity in a fairly random way. After a while, and particularly after a chat with the manager, Colin would either have forgotten where he was going or would not remember the name of the person to whom he had to give the message. Writing the name down for others to read would reduce Colin's responsibility. This longstanding problem was solved by giving Colin, along with the message, something to remind him of his destination: a piece of wood, a cotton reel, a tube of paint, a book and so on. The manager was also asked to prompt him by asking to see the object he was carrying. This programme worked: messages were delivered, Colin's pride in his achievement and competence increased and he spent more time on improving his literacy and other skills.

Putting this plan into operation required working together as a staff team in order to achieve a coherent response. Otherwise, Colin's wandering behaviour and failure to complete a given task would have been intermittently reinforced, perpetuating his confusion over what was expected of him.

The next situation also demonstrates how important it is to try to make sure that anyone involved in a behavioural programme is aware of how essential it is not to respond in different ways to a behaviour targeted for elimination or increasing. Parents will be well aware that the child refused sweets, staying up late, going out to play and so on by one parent may achieve success by making the same request to another parent or a grandparent.

Professionals often do not consider that older people have goals, but rather as recipients of resources, important though the latter may be. Yet, in both field and residential settings, the quality of life of older people and their family or co-residents can be improved.

CASE EXAMPLE

Miss B is a resident in a home for elderly people. Miss B's problems were that she shouted, upsetting and frightening other residents as well as exasperating staff. Sometimes she would throw things on the floor during mealtimes. This got her attention from staff, while at other times, when she was calm or helpful, she tended to be ignored. The places where these behaviours took place could be almost anywhere and could be triggered by a look perceived as hostile (antecedents). Miss B would then shout, swear, insult someone or argue (behaviour), resulting in complaints from residents and scolding from staff, sometimes ending in a shouting match (consequences). Further consequences were exclusion from a social event because of fears that she would make a scene.

Miss B was helped, by the use of a chart, to record periods free from outbursts and, by rewards that she selected, to reduce her aggressive behaviour and increase her social skills. Gradually, the charts were withdrawn as the changes in Miss B's behaviour began to alter the way in which residents and staff reacted to her. In other words, enough reinforcements were present in the natural environment to render the use of a chart redundant. (A detailed account of the case of Miss B is found in Cigno 1993, 1998.)

Devices such as charts and other symbolic rewards and monitoring systems are useful for clarifying and establishing desired behaviours – a diary is often a good way of recording and reviewing progress – but these should be withdrawn once the behaviour has been firmly established or eliminated. Tangible rewards, such as special outings, comfort food and so on, should always be accompanied by social rewards such as smiles and praise.

Conclusion

CBT has a place in mainstream social work. There is a case for thoughtful, systematic intervention as part of a 'package of care' to be carried out by the practitioner and not referred to other professionals (Sinclair et al., 1995). Once the therapeutic component of social work is lost through privatisation or loss of competence, it is doubtful whether it will ever be regained.

Although social work and social care will continue to go through many stress-provoking changes, social workers should make sure that their work is as competent as it can be in the light of current knowledge of what works. Learning about cognitive-behavioural intervention is part of this preparation. To do this, we need the best prepared people to practise social work: to paraphrase Pearson (1983), if this is elitist, so should we all aspire to be.

For further discussion of theoretical associations and practice applications, see Chapter 9, and Adams et al., 2009c, Chapter 5.

www.babcp.org.uk   British Association for Behavioural and Cognitive Psychotherapies, good for information and links.

www.livinglifetothefull.com   Life skills courses for adults, carers and professionals.

www.nice.org.uk   National Institute for Clinical Excellence.

Cigno, K. and Bourn, D. (eds) (1998) *Cognitive-behavioural Social Work in Practice*, Aldershot, Ashgate. Contains case studies and practice examples by distinguished contributors to cognitive-behavioural theory and practice. Includes interventions in childcare, probation, youth offending, mental health, addictions, disability and older people.

Keenan, M. and Dillenburger, K. (2000) *Behavior Analysis: A Primer*, a multimedia tutorial (computer software), New York, Insight Media. Lively, visual demonstration of theory and applications by UK-based authors versed in social work and psychology.

Task-centred work   15

This chapter explains a method of social work practice that helps people to reach agreed goals using carefully negotiated tasks. It sets this method in a wider context, including its contribution to the personalisation of services, emancipatory practice and the development of social work as a discipline.

Chapter overview

Introduction

One of the biggest challenges facing the social work profession is how to square professional practice with the 'circle' of organisational constraints. The break-up of social work into its constituent tasks and the increasingly proceduralised nature of the work of agency practitioners are two factors that lead back to Brewer and Lait's (1980) question, *Can Social Work Survive?*

This chapter will present task-centred social work not as *the* answer to the question of survival, but as one of the best available. It will also seek to clarify what task-centred social work is, in the light of misconceptions deriving from its name.

Task-centred social work has its roots in North American casework practice. It is widely known that J. and Shyne's (1969) research project, *Brief and Extended Casework*, looked at the effectiveness of short-term casework, but perhaps fewer understand that what they experimented with was a curtailed form of long-term work, cut short after a number of sessions. They found that the interventions that were allowed to run their full course were no more and no less effective than those which were foreshortened. It was Reid and Epstein (1972) who made a virtue of the short interventions by developing a short-term therapy, making positive use of a time limit to achieve a 'goal gradient effect'; in other words, the closer we approach a deadline, the more motivated we are to take action.

From these beginnings in the mainstream of social casework, the model has grown and been adapted to a wide variety of contexts. It has been tried and tested in work with children, families and older people; in large public welfare agencies, small voluntary agencies, probation, school and hospital settings; and in fieldwork, day, domiciliary and residential work. It is used by students, experienced practitioners and managers; with individuals, groups and communities; with a wide range of difficulties and problems; and with people from diverse cultures and backgrounds (see Doel and Marsh, 1992: 118–22 for a comprehensive guide to the task-centred literature). In short, task-centred social work is a generic practice method whose effectiveness has been subject to more evaluation and scrutiny than any other social work practice method.

In the process, task-centred casework has become task-centred practice, an indication of its development from individualised, therapeutic beginnings to a broader stage; a move away from relatively conservative practices into more radical territory, embracing notions of partnership, empowerment and anti-oppressive practice, and signalling practical ways of realising these ideas.

Task-centred work and other social work ideas

The influences on task-centred social work have been broad and various. From its inception in the psychosocial tradition, it soon became embroiled in the heat of the inquisition over behaviourism – just how behaviourist was task-centred work? In a debate that now seems unfashionable, task-centred work was seen as merely 'soft' – as opposed to the 'hard' behaviourism of those whom traditionalists considered beyond the professional pale. What these questions served to show was the growing influence of learning theory as a way of understanding why people behave as they do. This in turn led to consideration of alternative patterns of behaviour and an increasing focus on outcomes and the ways in which these can be defined and measured (Jehu, 1967). All this was consistent with the developing technology of task-centred practice, with its aim for a more precise statement of problems and goals, and a philosophy of 'small successes rather than large failures'.

As the behaviourist controversy faded, systems theory became the latest fashion statement, its essential design being detailed by Pincus and Minahan (1973). The systems approach in general, and the task-centred one in particular, contributed much to providing a unified appeal to social work practice. Tolson et al. (1994) made a strong case for task-centred as a generalist practice, using concepts from systems theory to demonstrate how task-centred practitioners can move within and between systems at different levels. This approach places the problem centre stage, so that it is the problem rather than the person that is 'the client'.

Task-centred practice is a member of the family of problem-solving models. In addition to developing its own techniques, such as the task planning and implementation sequence (Tolson et al., 1994: 73), it borrows from many others, such as 'positive reframing' from family therapy. The vogue for social skills training in the late 1970s and early 1980s made its mark on the task-centred methodology – for example in the use of techniques such as 5W+H, what? when? who? where? why? and how? – when investigating the specific nature of the problem, and coaching and rehearsal methods to help people to achieve success with tasks (Priestley et al., 1978).

In the 1980s, task-centred practice was well placed to give voice to the clients' rights/consumer choice movement (BASW, 1979). With its emphasis on working with people around issues that they considered prime, it provides a strong counter to paternalistic professional practice. Its links with open and shared recording (Doel and Lawson, 1986) and the requirement for explicitness about the purposes of the work gave task-centred practice an ambiguous attraction to both radical and managerial elements in social work. This tension continued into the 1990s and beyond to the present day; task-centred practice provides a visible means of shaping the good intentions of partnership and the concrete expression of anti-oppressive principles, while also attracting interest from agency managers keen to have measurable outcomes and explicit systems of accountability.

Task-centred practice is primarily about learning. Indeed, the task-centred encounter between social workers and service users can be likened more to a teaching session than, say, a medical consultation, an administrative interview, a gatekeeper's assessment, a salesperson's pitch or a therapy session. The task-centred encounter should have the feel of a highly participative workshop.

The essence of task-centred work

A brief description of the components of the task-centred model will help to place in context the themes and issues raised in this chapter. For a detailed exposition of the British variant of the task-centred model, see Doel and Marsh (1992) and Marsh and Doel (2006). In addition, a briefer summary is available in Doel (1994).

Task-centred casework was first described as a method to help people with 'problems of living' (Reid and Epstein, 1972). It is a systematic model of social work with a coherent and explicit value base. It has a 'practice technology' that has developed out of a body of research to examine what works well and what works less well. There is, therefore, a 'how to' aspect of the model, in addition to a clearly expressed 'why'. Its value base is anti-oppressive, in that it addresses issues of power and oppression, both in the immediate encounter between worker and service user and in the broader social context.

There are three phases in task-centred social work, plus the 'book ends' of entry and exit.

Entry

The point of entry for a social worker is often muddy. The purposes of any contact may initially be unclear and ambiguous for the worker, the service user or both. Conversely, the participants may have clear but contrary purposes. Unlike most other services, the social work service might be unwelcome.

It is essential that practitioners use a method of work that accommodates these complex factors. It should not enforce consensus where none exists, but should ease the process of reaching agreement where one is possible. Above all, it should be sensitive to the service user's 'world' – the context in which the work occurs and the relative power of the participants.

There is, rightly, a debate about the extent to which partnership is really possible.

Dominelli (1996: 157) writes that 'the real extent to which "clients" gain control through task-centred approaches remains a matter of controversy'. She sees financial constraints, policy imperatives and the practitioner's value base as setting boundaries which pre-empt the possibility of real power-sharing. Of course, these are factors common to all social work interventions, whichever method is used. However, the task-centred model ensures that discussion of power is part of the work itself.

Phase 1: exploring problems

There is no neat cut-off point between the entry period and the first phase of exploring problems. In many instances, the early parts of the investigation of problems will confirm or challenge the mandate for further work. The worker may have spent much time helping the person to 'engage with the problem'; de Shazer (1988) uses the term 'visitors' for those people who think that the problem is someone else's.

The encounter between the task-centred worker and the service user is a systematic approach that links areas of concern to desired changes, which are achievable through a relatively brief and intensive plan of action. As well as an outcome, there is an explicit attempt to learn from this particular experience of problem-solving, in order to generalise to other circumstances. The learning is mutual; the service user learns to generalise to problem-solving with other life difficulties, and the practitioner evaluates this example in the light of other task-centred encounters in order to learn what tends to work and what tends not to work.

This first phase is composed of a number of smaller stages:

- Problem-scanning, which involves a wide review of problematic areas (the 'headlines') and a deliberate avoidance of explanations and solutions.
- Additional problems, consisting of problem areas evident to the practitioner but not mentioned by the service user.
- Detailing each of the identified problems, with an investigation that focuses on the problem as a way of gaining a better understanding of it, rather than to provide causal explanations or fodder for a social diagnosis. Questions such as 'What will be the first sign that you are overcoming the problem?' and 'What are you doing that stops things from being worse?' help the person to colour in the details (George et al., 1990: 10).
- Selecting a problem (or, to use the jargon, 'targeting'), in which the service user makes a choice about the problem area they want to work on, based on their informed judgement and having considered factors such as the feasibility of working on the various problems. There may also be 'mandated' problems, which the worker is sanctioned to work on, even though they are not recognised as a problem or a priority by the client.

Phase 2: agreeing a goal – the written agreement

Having focused on difficulties, problems and concerns, the work now turns to what it is the person wants. Goals may already have been mentioned, and they can often be confused with problems – 'I need to get out of this house' sounds like a problem but is in fact a goal, and it may not be the best way to address the problems it is intended to resolve. All involved in the work need to be aware of how the agreed goal(s) will resolve or alleviate the selected problem(s). The goal must be one that is within clients' control to achieve, one they are well motivated to work towards and which workers consider ethically desirable, in other words, they can lend their support to it.

A significant factor in the success of the goal is to decide a time limit by which the goal will be achieved, an agreed pattern for contact between worker and client, and concrete indicators of how success will be recognised. The time limit sets the work in a framework, and the indicators for success allow all involved to pace their progress and gauge the distance to achievement.

Together, the selected problem(s), the agreed goal(s), the time limit and frequency of contact make up the agreement. This should be recorded, usually written, with copies for all involved, but other formats should be considered in work with people with a visual impairment or difficulties with literacy.

Phase 3: planning and implementing tasks

Once the written agreement is in place, the rest of the task-centred work follows a recognisable pattern from one session to another, in which past tasks are reviewed and evaluated, and future tasks are developed and implemented.

The 'task' is a central construct of task-centred social work, yet there is much confusion over this notion. The everyday English use of the word carries misleading implications, for example that tasks are always 'physical doings', when, in task-centred practice, they can be cognitive reflections, mental lists, a log of feelings and so on. Everyday tasks are usually free-standing ('My task today is to get the ironing done'), which is why many practitioners consider that they are working in a task-centred way when all they are doing is performing tasks. In task-centred work, tasks are carefully negotiated steps along the path from the present problem to the future goal. They build in a coherent fashion, sometimes completed in the session itself, sometimes completed between sessions, some for the user and some for the worker, some repeated, others unique (see Doel and Marsh, 1992: 60–79, for a full account of the significance of task development and review).

The importance of task development to the service user's success in achieving their goal has led to a five-stage task planning and implementation sequence (Tolson et al., 1994). This is based on research into what promotes task achievement. Reid (2000) provides a comprehensive guide to possible task 'menus' in a wide range of circumstances.

Exit

The end of task-centred work has been planned from the beginning; indeed, the built-in time limit is a powerful motivator for success, whether the intervention is a short, intensive burst over a few days or a number of sessions spread over several months. The length of work is a judgement based on how long it is likely to take to achieve the goal. Any change should be negotiated explicitly rather than allowing a sense of drift.

In situations where there is long-term contact between the service user and the agency, for example in residential care, task-centred agreements can be renegotiated periodically.

Issues

A systematic practice method

It is evident from the preceding description that task-centred work is a systematic method of practice. One way of illustrating what is meant by 'systematic' is to consider one task-centred practitioner acting as 'a fly on the wall' watching the work of another. Although the observer has not been involved in the work and knows none of the background or context, they will recognise the practice as task-centred, identify the particular phase of the work and any specific technique being used, and predict the shape of the next sequence of work. For example, the observer might state:

> This is the middle phase of the work. They have been reviewing the work on the tasks agreed at their previous session, using the scoring method to help the service users make a judgement about their success. They are now developing new tasks. The practitioner is helping them to generate these by using the headlines technique, usually associated with the earlier problem exploration stage. The practitioner might provide some coaching later, depending on the nature of the tasks, and the tasks will certainly be recorded so that they all have a copy. They will agree a time by which the tasks should be completed and the practitioner will probably refer back to the original agreement, so they are all clear about why these tasks are relevant and when the work will end.

The observer will even be able to make some comments and judgements about how well the work was progressing and how skilled the observed practitioner was:

> I've never seen the headlines technique used at this stage – that was very imaginative and I'm going to try it myself. I liked the way the practitioner asked 'What changes have happened since I last saw you?' rather than 'Have any changes happened since I last saw you?' I think the worker should have been clearer about the reasoning behind the scoring – even when a task has not been completed, there are things to be learned from that failure and the practitioner came over as half-hearted at that stage ... and so on.

Although each task-centred encounter is recognisable as such, it is not a question of 'painting by numbers'. The mood and feelings of the service users, their particular circumstances and the context of the work all guide the practitioner, so that each encounter is unique. It has been likened elsewhere to a tidal progress, often slow and with one pace back for each two forward, but overall there is movement (Doel, 1994: 23).

Who is task-centred work for?

Earlier, we explored how task-centred practice has been influenced by psychosocial, behavioural, systems and problem-solving theories, in addition to broad movements such as clients' rights and anti-oppressive practice. Is the task-centred model, therefore, a coat of many colours?

There is certainly anecdotal evidence that many practitioners subscribe to task-centred practice. Payne (1995: 119) suggests that it is 'a popular model of social work, widely used in the UK'. In an unpublished survey of 25 student placement reports, 17 mentioned that task-centred practice had been used, while counselling was second, mentioned in 7 reports. However, there is a suspicion that if social workers wish to convey a sense that their work is purposeful and active, they label it 'a task-centred approach'.

Task-centred practice has perhaps become the new eclecticism, popular but undifferentiated. In the audit of practice undertaken in the 'social work in partnership' action research, which employed a task-centred model of practice, Marsh and Fisher (1992: 41) found that the initial response from participants was 'We do all that already.' It is an irony that its apparent simplicity makes task-centred practice a victim of its own success, yet the explicitness and clarity of the process of task-centred work should not be mistaken for easiness.

If social work is appropriate and possible, task-centred work is appropriate and possible. Social workers find themselves in situations where they are not practising 'social work', for example when they are policing or administering, and task-centred work will not be appropriate in these circumstances. Similarly, if the service user's capacity for rational thought is severely limited, the use of the method will be similarly limited, as will other methods of social work practice. However, Marsh and Doel (2006) record the use of task-centred practice in some remarkably challenging situations, including with a severely disabled person with very limited communication.

Task-centred work and empowerment

In using a problem-solving approach, task-centred practice links us all, users of social work or not. The task-centred philosophy does not pathologise service users but sees them as fellow citizens who are encountering difficulties. These difficulties are often more severe and more enduring than those which non-service users experience, but the problem-solving techniques used in task-centred practice are universal, even if the specific application in task-centred work is unusually systematic. In effect, the service user undergoes a training course in problem-solving techniques, and – with appropriate coaching from the worker – can use this method independently when the work ends.

Although the focus of task-centred work is primarily with individuals, families or groups, the method recognises the significance of context on individuals' problems (Tolson et al., 1994: 395). In other words, there is often a dissonance between the level at which analysis takes place (structural) and the level at which effective action can be taken (local). The reasons that a person is without a job might be analysed at a macroeconomic level, but the possibility of doing something about it remains at the micro-level. Task-centred work helps to expose the subtle relationships between these different systems.

Conclusion

Professional practice in an organisational context
Task-centred social work helps the practitioner and the service user by providing a framework to consider whether there is just cause for the work to begin. Whatever methods practitioners use for the ensuing encounter with the person, the idea of developing a mandate for the work is one of the most valuable contributions the task-centred model has made to social work practice. Social workers practise in diverse fields, with a broad range of systems and in uncertain circumstances, and task-centred practice offers a unifying model of practice for social work in all these circumstances.

Practitioners must behave professionally. This means an ability to handle uncertainty, use discretionary power and responsibilities, and subscribe to a code of ethics drawn from outside any particular employer. Practitioners are under equal pressure to behave bureaucratically, by following procedures established in large organisations, driven increasingly by administrative and financial considerations. In these circumstances, it is necessary to establish ways of working that allow professional practice to engage with agency realities. Task-centred work can provide the cog that gears profession to organisation.

Task-centred work lends itself to professional practice because of the skills needed to negotiate with the service user in ways that are truly empowering and anti-discriminatory. The explicit focus on power and discrimination, and the emphasis on qualitative outcomes, means that it is significantly more than a systematic procedure. It can help to promote the 'personalisation' of services that is central to current policy in social care (HM Government, 2008).

There are also aspects of task-centred work that could fall foul of professional practice, if not properly exercised. For example, it could be seen as routinised practice, in which the instruments of the model are used mainly to exercise social control; and tasks (or failure to complete tasks) become sticks with which to beat the service user or provide evidence of their incompetence or lack of motivation.

There are aspects of task-centred work that fit well with agency imperatives, such as the accountability of an explicit approach, the potential to quantify outcomes and the potential economy of time-limited interventions. However, the emphasis on negotiation can be problematic for agencies, since it implies a willingness to work on issues that might not, at first sight, be defined as the kinds of problems with which the agency deals. Moreover, the need for relatively 'short, fat' interventions in task-centred working, rather than 'long, thin' ones, needs to be accommodated by the agency.

The task-centred model has proved itself to be an effective method that is popular with practitioners and service users. It has the potential to maintain professional practice while satisfying agency requirements. However, this degree of accommodation can appear ambiguous and perhaps explains why the task-centred method is described, on the one hand, as 'supporting managerialist objectives' (Dominelli, 1996: 156) and on the other as 'offering much potential for empowering clients' (Ahmad, 1990: 51).

A systematic strategy of training in the task-centred method, from pre-qualifying to post-qualifying levels, is the best way to retain a clear understanding of what it means to undertake work that can be called 'task-centred'. Only when there is confidence that task-centred work *is* task-centred work can agencies, practitioners and service users benefit from experiences that are commonly understood and which accumulate into a better knowledge of how and when task-centred social work performs best.

For further discussion of intervention, see Adams et al., 2009a, Chapter 18, and for legal and regulatory frameworks for practice, see Adams et al., 2009a, Chapter 8.

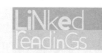

Doel, M. and Marsh, P. (1992) *Task-centred Social Work*, Aldershot, Ashgate. Offers a detailed account of the task-centred model in contemporary British practice.

Marsh, P. and Doel, M. (2006) *The Task-Centred Book*, London, Routledge/Community Care. Task-centred practice told via the recorded stories of practitioners' actual task-centred work with service users in a wide range of circumstances. Also considers teaching, learning, supporting and supervising task-centred work.

Reid, W.J. (2000) *The Task Planner*, New York, Columbia University Press; Tolson, E.R., Reid, W. and Garvin, C.D. (1994) *Generalist Practice: A Task Centered Approach*, New York, Columbia University Press. Both books provide interesting accounts of developments in the task-centred model, especially with regard to its position as a generalist practice method, and task-centred techniques.

Reid, W.J. and Epstein, L. (1972) *Task-centred Casework*, New York, Columbia University Press. Allows you to understand the origins of the model by returning to the first text.

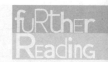

16 Advocacy and empowerment

Chapter overview

This chapter deals with two quite distinct, but neighbouring ideas – advocacy and empowerment – which both have applications in social work. Advocacy and empowerment are multifaceted notions, each with a historical legacy, the imprint of which is visible in contemporary practice. Although both are mainstream, and even quite traditional in one way, there is a sense in which each, by its nature, contributes to critical practice.

Advocacy and empowerment are concepts whose origins can be traced back several centuries, both of which, however, share certain features and make an important contribution to contemporary social work. Each is a multifaceted concept, the practice of which has developed in relation to social work practice in the UK largely since 1990. This chapter considers their main common and separate features and some of the key practice issues associated with them.

Shared contexts of advocacy and empowerment

The historical and conceptual roots of advocacy and empowerment are to an extent common to them both, although when we consider them separately below, we shall see that the authenticity of each derives from its unique heritage. Empowerment and advocacy are heirs to radical and critical traditions, which we could argue are, after the Act of Union 1707 between England and Scotland, specifically 'British' or, after the Act of Union 1800 between Britain and Ireland, 'UK-wide', concerned with social change and community action, and, at the same time, with 'conservative' aspects of individual and collective self-help and mutual aid by people who use services. To take these conservative aspects first, any party political association is incidental, since they relate to institutions and processes that are fundamental to the conservation of many societies. The activity of mutual aid, in particular, is as old as many communities. From the eighteenth century onwards, friendly societies were founded in England, Ireland, Wales and Scotland, encouraged by the Friendly Societies Act 1793; they were the forerunners of later mutual insurance companies. By the end of the nineteenth century, there may have been as many as 30,000 friendly societies. Many poorer people saved small weekly or monthly amounts from their wages in a friendly society, perhaps 1p a week to pay for their funeral. 'Mutuals' are fundamentally different from limited companies, since the mutual is co-owned by its members, whereas independent shareholders invest in the company and take profit shares in the form of dividends. Thus the purpose of the 'mutual' is to benefit its members, while the limited company exists primarily to enable its shareholders and directors to draw off profits. A modern form of the friendly society is the credit union, a collective method by which people of limited means can save and borrow through a not-for-profit society, offering an alternative to emergency loans from loan sharks at high interest rates.

These associations are not entirely straightforward. Mutual aid is a close neighbour to the idea of self-help, which since the Victorian era has expressed individualist rather than collectivist attitudes to society and social policy. 'Individualism' is a set of beliefs that puts the achievement of individual goals before social goals, promotes the interests of the individual over those of society and values independence, self-reliance and the freedom to achieve one's personal goals. 'Collectivism' relates to beliefs in prioritising social rather than individual goals, valuing public, that is, state, control of the production and distribution of services, and cooperation and mutual dependence between people.

So, we can see that empowerment and advocacy share an ambiguity in their basic concept, between their individualist – self-serving – and collectivist – community and society-serving – purposes. In their application to practice, they share another ambiguity. This can be expressed in terms of the tension between the idea of self-advocacy or self-empowerment and the actuality of receiving a service from a professional. It concerns the extent to which people's capacity to self-advocate and self-empower is mediated or intervened in by professionals. There is a sense in which professional intervention undermines or even contradicts the basic principles of empowerment and self-advocacy. Both of these are ideas about people helping themselves, which were given enormous impetus in Victorian England by the publication by Samuel Smiles of *Thrift* in 1875 and *Self-help* in 1890. These reflected Victorian values of the same name, which, along with the other Victorian values of respectability and hard work, combined to create the unique mix of radicalism and conservatism that permeates the concepts of advocacy and empowerment in the twenty-first century.

We have spent a little time teasing out those elements shared by advocacy and empowerment. We turn now to their distinctive features.

The concept of advocacy

Advocacy is a concept that originates largely in the individually based 'casework' of professions such as the law which represent people's interests, although, as we recognised above, this is reflected in the power of the judicial system and professions and in the informal interactions between people supporting each other as they live in communities (Bateman, 2000). These twin origins mean that advocacy takes place in the somewhat contested space between professional help and support and informal/amateur self-representation. The word 'advocate' is most commonly used in the various judicial settings, including civil, criminal and family courts, where barristers and solicitors practise. In this connection, advocacy means arguing or presenting a case on behalf of somebody. The implication is that the professional possesses the specialist knowledge and expertise and therefore the power to act, while the 'client' waits on the sidelines. In social work, the idea of advocacy not only refers to the work a professional does on behalf of service users but also refers to the work service users do on their own behalf. Advocacy may include the work of particular professionals on behalf of people as well as the work of a group of service users campaigning for their own rights. The Mental Capacity Act 2005, which became law in 2007, introduces the idea of advocates for people whose mental capacity requires advocacy, while ensuring that legal safeguards are in place to protect their interests (see Chapter 7). This illustrates the tension encountered in some social work settings between advocating for people and enabling them to advocate for themselves.

The reality is that advocacy varies according to fitness for purpose in particular circumstances. According to Johnstone (2001: 77), there are five forms of advocacy: self-advocacy, individual advocacy, citizen advocacy, legal advocacy and group advocacy. Brandon (1995) also writes of advocacy by families, peer advocacy and collective advocacy, which corresponds to Johnstone's group advocacy. Most of these labels are self-explanatory, except citizen advocacy, which is a specific form of long-term partnership between a person and a lay advocate who receives basic training to advocate for them on a long-term basis. It is clear that the concept of advocacy covers a range of areas, from individual advocacy to group-based advocacy. Brandon (1995) identifies only three basic forms of advocacy: paid/professional advocacy, unpaid/amateur advocacy and self-advocacy. According to Brandon (1995: 1), advocacy:

> involves a person(s), either an individual or group with disabilities or their representative, pressing their case with influential others, about situations which either affect them directly or, and more usually, trying to prevent proposed changes which will leave them worse off.

Professional advocates include a variety of practitioners, from legal advocates to social workers acting on behalf of people. Unpaid advocacy includes a range of peer and family advocates as well as schemes such as citizen advocacy. Self-advocacy includes the tasks people take on for themselves and this can take place individually or in groups. Service user groups or advocacy groups may act to safeguard vulnerable or disabled people. Not every person prefers another person advocating for them. For example, in cases of abuse, advocates may insist that all cases of substantiated abuse should be treated as criminal matters by the police. However, carers and disabled people may not wish to pursue this option, on the grounds that the associated investigation and judicial process are too stressful.

One function of advocacy is that it enables people's rights to be upheld. The concept of rights is central to advocacy. Moreover, according to Brandon, advocacy plays a crucial part in enabling us to appreciate that the roots of people's suffering lie in social rather than individual causes:

> " Advocacy has an important role in the overall movement to identify the major causes of unnecessary suffering as external to the individual. It promotes an increased awareness of rights and participation – rejects paternalism and moves towards greater political involvement. This leads directly to a struggle with the various professionals, often seen as oppressors; increasing demands for anti-discrimination legislation; and for greater involvement in both the planning and running of services. (Brandon, 1995: 5) "

A particular tension in the practice of advocacy is highlighted by Shakespeare (2006) in the field of disability. In response to the argument that disabled people do not benefit from advocacy, he argues that it is too simplistic to claim that advocates for disabled people invariably heighten their stigmatisation and exclusion. He points out that the reality for many disabled people is complex. He does not deny the credibility of the social model of disability, but notes that it may tend to underplay the reality of physical or mental impairments that affect some people. Their disability undoubtedly is made more pronounced by social factors, but there are often important physical impairments that they have to cope with at the same time. These may come about through a combination of hereditary and current medical conditions. For example, a person's disability may be a consequence of the mistakes made by medical professionals, perhaps during pregnancy or birth. In such circumstances, the advocate may play a role in obtaining adequate compensation and services.

This brings us finally to the question as to where advocates are located in relation to other services. While this may seen relatively straightforward, it remains the case that advocacy can be a somewhat contested, or even precarious, activity. This is because of the range of roles that advocates are likely to carry out in working with people. Advocacy can act to reinforce traditional practice and sustain rather unhelpful stereotypes by helping people who use services and disempowering them in the process. On the other hand, advocates can act supportively and may even play a part in corroborating the views of people who use services, enabling them to be transmitted to those who need to hear them. Southgate (1990) identifies five main roles: nurturing, witnessing, protesting, translating, and supporting. Among these, protest is likely to be one of the most problematic and conflict-ridden roles, perhaps involving the advocate in empowering people – whistle-blowing or safeguarding the interests of individuals and groups who represent minorities, excluded groups or people who are seldom heard. This reference to empowerment is the appropriate point for us to turn to consider it in more detail.

The concept of empowerment

As indicated at the start of the chapter, empowerment is a multifaceted idea that can mean different things to different people. It can be quite a radical concept, linked with consciousness-raising and collective, community or social action. On the other hand, it may be used in a diluted sense almost as a synonym for enablement. Between these limits, empowerment remains an imperfectly theorised idea, somewhat patchily related to the main social work approaches to working with people. Undeniably, empowerment is a somewhat problematic concept to apply in social work, in that 'it does not correspond with a single, existing method, although it can be shown to have links with all of them' (Adams, 2008: 4). Empowerment has been defined as:

> the capacity of individuals, groups and/or communities to take control of their circumstances, exercise power and achieve their own goals, and the process by which, individually and collectively, they are able to help themselves and others to maximise the quality of their lives. (Adams, 2008: 17)

Empowerment has quite commonly been linked with participation by people, on a ladder ranging from a significant degree of disempowerment to an empowered status.

It is more creative not to take a hierarchical view of empowerment at different levels, but to regard it as taking place in a number of different but linked and sometimes overlapping domains, ranging from self-empowerment, through empowering other people individually and in groups, to empowerment in organisations, communities and political systems. In many situations, a practitioner will engage with a person in more than one domain simultaneously. Often a degree of self-empowerment enables a person to develop the knowledge, skills and confidence to help others. Croft and Beresford (2000: 116) have linked empowerment with moves to democratise health and social services through enhancing public and service user participation. They claim that 'for service users, empowerment means challenging their disempowerment, having more control over their lives, being able to influence others and bring about change'. Thus, self-empowerment is linked with empowering other people and the political goal of achieving greater collective power.

We need to distinguish between the focus of the considerable, and growing, literature on participation by individual citizens in aspects of their own health and social care and social work services and the much broader concept of empowerment, which has collective as well as individual dimensions. Social work empowerment in the UK has been influenced strongly by the civil rights movement and campaigns for black power in the US, as well as by the theory and practice of personal and political consciousness-raising in South America. The former is well expressed in the writing of Solomon (1976: 21), who perceives empowerment as an appropriate means of social intervention with an individual, group or community experiencing a 'present and pervasive condition of systematic institutionalized discrimination'. Freire's work (1972) was rooted in his experiences of poverty in the Great Depression of the 1930s in his home country of Brazil. He advocated democratic and reciprocal approaches to educating people, which did not just assume that the professional was filling the 'empty' person with enlightenment. Instead, he developed the concept of *conscientizacao*, which, translated from the Portuguese, means the growth of critical consciousness or consciousness-raising, and links individual and collective empowerment.

In Western Europe, the theory and practice of empowerment were enriched from the 1970s by feminist critiques and movements to liberate psychiatric patients. Women's therapy took many forms, such as the sharing of common experiences and taking control of their own health by the Women in Mind (1986). Liberation from the stigma of being labelled a user of mental health services was a theme of the organisation Survivors Speak Out, founded in 1988.

Empowerment as an emancipatory approach spread from developed to developing countries and has become a prominent feature of initiatives and projects engaging poor and excluded groups and communities. Participatory approaches to social development and collaborative research have converged in the publications of the Intermediate Technology Centre.

The domains of advocacy and empowerment

Empowering work with people crosses back and forth between work in different domains – from self-empowerment to empowering work with individuals, groups, organisations, communities and political systems.

It is apparent that whereas empowerment can take place in these different domains, individual aspects of advocacy are more widespread than its social applications. We shall conclude this chapter by considering these briefly in turn.

Self-advocacy and self-empowerment

The most apparent overlap between the concepts and practice of advocacy and empowerment occurs in the areas of self-advocacy and self-empowerment. We can make two points about this:

1 Self-empowerment is similar to the notion of self-advocacy, which concerns being empowered to represent our own interests.
2 Empowerment and advocacy in practice are not restricted to the individual and cannot be considered in isolation from issues of taking power and exercising political (with a small 'p') expertise to bring about change.

The main stages of self-development involved in self-empowerment and the development of self-advocacy are similar, and are shown in Table 16.1.

Table 16.1 Main stages of self-empowerment

Assessment and planning
Finding a starting point
Focusing on areas for self-development
Identifying relevant skills
Clarifying learning styles and profiles
Formulating a self-empowerment plan
Action
Carrying out the self-empowerment plan
Tackling the barriers to self-empowerment
Tackling aspects of inequality
Using assertiveness, self-actualisation and personal growth
Reflection
Using reflection and reflexivity
Using perspective transformation

Source: Adapted from Adams, 2008: 86

Engaging individuals in advocacy and empowerment

The range of people's circumstances makes it necessary for the practitioner to adopt different approaches with different individuals and groups. In some situations, an authoritative, interventionist approach is required, whereas other people need support and counselling. There is also a fine balance to be struck between empowerment and disempowerment. The service user may have been treated as the victim, or simply as the consumer of services, and it may require work to enable movement towards the position of empowered contributor to service development (see Figure 16.1).

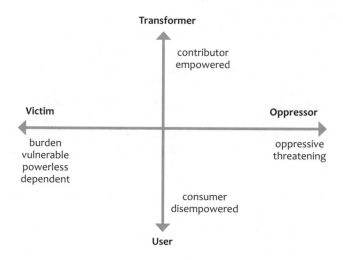

Figure 16.1 Tensions of empowering roles in work with individuals

CaSE EXaMPLE

Mary is working with 65-year-old physically disabled Malik and his 61-year-old partner Thelma who has cared for him for years, but who was recently blinded in an accident, and now is dependent on Malik for some care. In different ways each of them is dependent on the other. Mary discusses with Malik and Thelma the ways in which the principles of empowerment and advocacy can help them to retain their autonomy. Mary distinguishes between self-sufficiency and autonomy. There are aspects of professional services that will enable Thelma to learn to use Braille and have a guide dog. A guide dog will enable Thelma to retain her independence. Braille will enable her to continue reading the books and other material she loves. Mary suggests to Malik and Thelma that there are supports from which she can ensure they benefit: self-advocacy, professional advocacy and self-empowerment.

Thelma finds it a struggle to accept her new circumstances. She wants to continue to care for Malik as she did formerly, recognises that she needs services in view of her recent impairment, but is angry and upset about the ways in which blind people experience discrimination and social exclusion. On the other hand, Malik is managing the tension between being cared for and being the newly empowered carer for Thelma, as she learns to cope with being blind.

Mary has to give sufficient support, resources and advocacy to enable Malik and Thelma to empower themselves, but not so much that their dependence is emphasised and they are disempowered.

Empowering groups

Any group may be empowering or disempowering, although groups that are led by users are more likely to be set up with empowerment of members in mind. User-led groups are similar to self-help groups, defined by Katz and Bender (1976: 9) as:

> voluntary, small group structures for mutual aid in the accomplishment of a specific purpose. They are usually formed by peers who have come together for mutual assistance in satisfying a common need, overcoming a common handicap or life-disrupting problem, and bringing about a desired social and/or personal change.

EXAMPLE

A self-advocacy group with physically disabled people carried out an evaluation with the social worker who referred disabled people to them after facilitating their setting up of the group. They all contributed to the evaluation alongside the social worker, who arranged for the evaluation report to be printed and distributed. The report concluded that:

- members gained in the sense of empowerment
- members of the group shifted from reliance on the social worker to self-reliance
- the role of the social worker changed from facilitator to consultant, who only continued to participate on occasions, when invited by group members.

Empowering organisations

We need to acknowledge that many people who use services are not empowered by the organisations to which they relate. Carr (2004) has drawn authoritative conclusions from six related research studies, summarising the barriers that hindered service users from taking part in an empowered way in organisations that deliver social care services. The main barriers encountered by people include:

- a lack of policy and practice in the organisation, which is rooted in its culture and infrastructure
- resistance by different staff in the organisation, including professionals
- issues concerning the exercise of power by those representing entrenched interests in the organisation, to the detriment of people who use services.

Research has been carried out with a view to identifying a preferred strategy for developing an empowering and participative organisation (Kirby et al., 2003a, 2003b). This entails:

- building the appropriate *infrastructure:* the systems, procedures and processes that support the work of staff
- achieving *culture change* in the five components of the culture of the organisation: values, organisational systems, norms, methods of peer support, and the organisational climate
- creating three kinds of *motors for change* for the organisation in doing this:
  - its policy drivers
  - creating incentives for staff
  - taking all possible measures to increase the motivation and capacity of people who use services to become positive participants.

Kirby et al. (2003a) identify three types of organisational culture likely to be empowering, to which we have added the fourth, shown in Table 16.2.

Table 16.2 Four types of organisational culture

Type of culture	Characteristics
Consultation focused	Taking advice from people
Participation focused	Decisions on basis of ongoing participation by people. Staff determine focus of participation
People focused	Based on experiences and perceptions of service users. Some of the organisation's work changed as a result
Change focused	Much of the organisation's work changed as a result of the influence of service users

Source: Adapted from Adams, 2006: 149, Table 7.5

The end point of the process of empowering people is to enable them to advocate successfully to bring about significant change in the organisation.

Empowering communities and political systems

Personal advocacy and individual empowerment could be said to be the key to social transformation. The tasks of empowering individuals and communities are two halves of the same coin, in the sense that Freire (1972) identifies the need for social change to be rooted in consciousness-raising of the individual. Sometimes this is identified as social and political education, meaning that the practitioners 'set out to empower the communities they work with to question dominant assumptions – in Freire's terms to 'get the oppressors out of their own heads' (Mayo, 2000: 6). Corrigan and Leonard (1978) emphasise that the assessment of the needs of individuals should make links with the social problems that beset their environment. Burns et al. (2004: 131–47) illustrate at some length how community empowerment offers mainstream benefits, rather than just enabling individuals to help themselves.

We can be optimistic and assert that community empowerment plays an increasing part in urban and rural regeneration, in Western and developing countries alike. Increasingly, with the benefit of participatory approaches, community initiatives may progress to appraisal and evaluation (McTaggart, 1999).

One stage beyond empowering the community lies in targeting the political system. We shall end this chapter by assessing the viability of using practice at the individual level to exercise direct influence on the political system. Corrigan and Leonard (1978) use examples from practice to make the simple point that work with the individual needs to develop alongside an analysis of the social problems that form the context for that individual's difficulties. For example, social work with a lone parent experiencing financial hardship takes place in the context of government policies aiming to reduce family and child poverty. In developing countries, Mayoux (2000) has researched the increasing practice of using micro-finance as a strategy to fight poverty and enable people to achieve sustainability. She concludes that women and children benefit from micro-credit, but in order for social and community empowerment to result, wider changes need to follow, feeding women's savings into wider planned economic and social development. Without this, micro-finance 'is unlikely to make more than a limited contribution to empowerment' (Mayoux, 2000: 4).

Conclusion

We have seen how the overlapping but distinctly different concepts of advocacy and empowerment can be used in social work to enhance practice. However, there are some awkward junctions between these ideas and professional practice, partly because self-advocacy and self-empowerment in particular run counter to the traditional notion of services provided 'for' people rather than in collaboration with them. A further tension arises where empowered people self-advocate in ways that cast a critical light on existing services. It takes strong and secure practitioners to accept criticism from service users and admit that good practice benefits from acknowledging its frailty.

For further discussion of work with service users and carers, see Adams et al., 2009a, Chapter 15, and for tensions between intervention and empowerment, see Adams et al., 2009a, Chapter 19.

Adams, R. (2008) *Empowerment, Participation and Social Work*, 4th edn, Basingstoke, Palgrave Macmillan. Examination of the somewhat overlapping territories of empowerment and participation, illustrating social work applications in the different domains of self-empowerment, individual, group, organisation, community and political systems empowerment and empowering evaluation.

Bateman, N. (2000) *Advocacy Skills for Health and Social Care Professionals*, 3rd edn, Basingstoke, Palgrave – now Palgrave Macmillan. Useful examination of the use of advocacy in health and social care practice.

Brandon, D. (1995) *Advocacy: Power to People with Disabilities*, Birmingham, Venture Press. Somewhat polemical and critical exploration of advocacy in theory and practice.

Rees, S. (1991) *Achieving Power: Practice and Policy in Social Welfare*, London, Allen & Unwin. Meaty discussion of different perspectives, theories and approaches to empowerment.

From radical to critical social work
Progressive transformation or mainstream incorporation?

17

This chapter traces the transformation of radical social work into critical social work in light of the author's own involvement in these movements since the 1970s. It examines the diversity of approaches to critical social work and responses to the postmodern critique. The chapter concludes by outlining the key challenges to critical social work in the current context.

Chapter overview

Introduction

All writings on radical and critical social work to some extent reflect the personal and situational aspects of the writer. As a middle-aged white heterosexual male academic from a working-class background in Australia, I invariably bring some aspects of my context and personal biography into the foreground of my theorising. Just as the theoretical debates about radical social work have changed over the past 30 years, so have my own conceptual frameworks as I have responded to the changing sociopolitical landscape of social work education and practice.

I was a participant in the early radical social work movement in Australia. I studied social work in the 1970s when the debates about radical social work were emerging from the UK (Bailey and Brake, 1975) and the US (Galper, 1975). As in other countries, the early Australian radical social work literature reflected first a Marxist analysis (Skenridge and Lennie, 1978) and later incorporated feminist (Marchant and Wearing, 1986) and anti-racist approaches (Lynn and Pye, 1990).

After some years of practice in community-based services and community development projects, I moved into social work academia in the 1980s. In my teaching, I felt a need for my theorising of radical social work to be grounded in the practice reality of social workers. Thus I undertook an MA into the attempts by radical social work practitioners to construct progressive practices in their work (Pease, 1987, 1990). To further this project, in 1991 I undertook a PhD to study the subjectivities and practices of pro-feminist men in the human services who were challenging patriarchal gender relations (Pease, 1996, 2000). I began to read about the intersections of feminism, masculinity studies, postmodernism and critical theory and I started to consider the implications these developments had for changing men and masculinities in the context of a critical social work practice.

In 1997, Jan Fook and I formed a reading group on the intersections of critical theory and postmodernism and their implications for social work practice. That reading group would provide the impetus for us to edit one of the first books on the links between postmodernism and critical social work (Pease and Fook, 1999). Since then, I have co-edited a second book on critical social work (Allan et al., 2003), as well as developing further my ideas about pro-feminist approaches to working with men (Pease and Camilleri, 2001; Pease, 2002). I have also been exploring cross-cultural and global approaches to this work (Pease and Pringle, 2001; Flood et al., 2007).

Currently, I teach in a social work course in Australia that espouses a critical approach to social work theory and practice. Our mission statement emphasises the importance of critical race and gender issues, equity, power and diversity issues and anti-oppressive and empowerment approaches to social work. I would therefore seem to be in a relatively good position to review the developments in theory from radical to critical social work over the years. However, in many ways, I find it a daunting task. One of the complexities is that there are multiple theoretical perspectives on radical and critical approaches and the issue is complicated further by the different meanings given to radical, critical, structural and anti-oppressive practice in different countries.

I am also conscious of writing outside the UK context of social work. Although Australia is geographically part of the global South, we are also part of the hegemonic North, along with Britain, Canada and the US. Connell (2006) has talked about 'Northern theory' as a means of explicitly naming the way in which most social theory is produced in the global North. The 'northern-ness' of social theory is reflected in the claim to universal relevance, a tendency to 'read from the centre' and an exclusion of texts from the non-metropolitan world. So I am aware of the geopolitical limitations of the review that I am about to conduct and encourage readers to look to Latin America and Asia to globalise these debates.

The transformation of radical social work

As there are published accounts of the history of radical social work in the US (Reisch and Andrews, 2001), Britain (Langan, 2002) and Australia (Martin, 2003), I will not review these historical developments again here. Suffice to say that the early accounts credit Bailey and Brake (1975) in the UK, Galper (1975) in the US and Throssell (1975) in Australia as initiating the debate about radical social work in those three countries. It has often been noted that the overemphasis on class was regarded as a limiting factor in the early development of radical social work (Healy, 2005) and that radical social work failed to engage with the diversity of oppressions (Langan, 2002). Feminist and anti-racist approaches, along with later links to disability politics and gay sexual politics, would attempt to address this gap.

Reisch and Andrews (2001) note that by mid-1980s in the US, radical social work was replaced by what was perceived as a less threatening and more inclusive term, 'progressive social work'. This was also associated with moving beyond class analysis to consider the issues of gender, race, ethnicity and sexuality. Langan (2002) has similarly explored the legacy of radical social work in the UK, concluding that by the late 1970s, the spirit of this tradition had disappeared. Anti-discriminatory (Thompson, 1993) and anti-oppressive (Dalyrmple and Burke, 1995) social work was later developed in the UK in response to the perceived weaknesses of radical social work.

In the early 1980s, when I was reviewing the curriculum of the social work course in which I taught in Australia, I approached my head of school with a proposal to teach a new subject titled 'radical social work'. I was told in no uncertain terms that I couldn't use the language of 'radical' and that I had to find an alternative title. So 'critical social work' was born. This was over 10 years before Ife (1997) introduced the term in the published literature in Australia. I tell this story not to claim any form of ownership of the term, but rather to note how language often shifts in response to particular socio-political circumstances. I remember Maurice Moreau, in a personal conversation, describing a similar set of circumstances to account for the language of 'structural social work' that emerged in Canada in the 1970s (Moreau, 1979). Even the language of 'radical social work' was framed to avoid mentioning socialist or Marxist approaches to social work too explicitly.

The emergence of critical social work

It almost goes without saying that there is a diversity of critical perspectives in social work and a variety of conceptions of what critical social work involves. Some see it as simply another way of naming what we used to call 'radical social work' (Hick and Pozzuto, 2005), while others chart a significant departure from the radical tradition (Ferguson, I., 2008).

Critical theory was originally associated with the Frankfurt School of Marxism. However, it has now expanded to include any theories concerned with transformation and social change. Gray and Webb (2008a) argue that critical social work is moving further away from the Frankfurt School. However, I'm not sure that it ever defined its critical theory base solely within those parameters. It does mean, though, that critical social work has come to take on an almost exhaustive set of meanings.

One area of confusion is that critical social work is used in both a broad and a narrow way. In the broad sense, it is an umbrella term that encompasses a range of theoretical approaches including Marxist, radical, feminist, anti-racist, anti-oppressive, anti-discriminatory, postcolonial, critical constructivist and structural perspectives. In the narrow sense, some writers have used it to define their particular model of practice (Healy, 2000; Fook, 2002; Allan et al., 2003). Clearly there is a tension between the idea of critical social work as a coherent conceptual framework and the existence of a diversity of theoretical approaches within it.

One of the meanings of critical social work practice in the UK is in relation to critical thinking and critical reflection (Payne, 2005). This approach to critical social work is the notion of 'being critical' in the sense of developing a disposition that challenges existing ideas and practices. Such an approach, however, does not necessarily involve a structural analysis of oppression. Humphries (2005) appropriately differentiates between the use of 'critical' in critical questioning of all received ideas and the use of 'critical' to describe knowledge that challenges oppressive social relations.

A new conception of critical social work that has emerged in the UK in recent years is 'transformational practice'. Adams et al. (2005a: xx–xxi) describe it as 'reflexive and critical practice with individuals, communities, families and groups to achieve social changes that enhance social solidarity and reduce or remove inequalities in societies'. This seems an ambitious project. However, the focus seems to be more on improvement in social functioning as it emphasises that 'skills and self-confidence learnt in the process is transformational' (Adams et al., 2005a: xxi). Transformational social work is focused on developing the capacity of individuals to initiate change in their lives to enhance their social relationships and realise their potential (Adams et al., 2005b). Adams et al. (2005b) make the point that transformational social work is not synonymous with radicalism because it is concerned with continuity as well as social change. So this conception of critical social work does seem to depart more significantly from the earlier radical tradition.

A number of writers in the UK have particularly noted the contribution to critical social work emerging in Australia (Payne, 2005; McBeath and Webb, 2005; Dalyrmple and Burke, 2006; Ferguson, I., 2008). Most of these commentators associate the development of critical social work in Australia with the influence of postmodern and poststructural ideas.

Postmodernism and critical social work

Iain Ferguson (2008) says that the main distinction between critical social work and radical social work is the incorporation of postmodern theories as opposed to Marxist approaches. Payne (2005) similarly argues that critical social work departed significantly from radical social work because of its association with constructionist and postmodern theories. Dalyrmple and Burke (2006), however, are more accurate when they observe that critical social work has been influenced by both postmodern and modernist approaches and that many of us have argued that practitioners should maintain the tension between them (Allan et al., 2003).

From the beginning, postmodern ideas were controversial in relation to critical social work. It was noted by many writers that postmodern theories could be used to support conservative policies and practices. Some critical theorists are concerned that postmodern perspectives can obscure the material reality of oppression (Mullaly, 2007). Others are concerned that the commitment to social justice and human rights may be undermined by the postmodern rejection of the meta-narrative (Ife, 1997). I. Ferguson (2008) criticises postmodernism for its anti-realism and its moral relativism and Lundy (2004) similarly comments that if all accounts are equal, as postmodernists suggest, then reactionary theories and views would also have to be validated. Many critical social work theorists, however, have argued that it is possible to develop a 'critical postmodernism' (Fook, 2002; Healy, 2005) that avoids the critique of relativism. Leonard (1997) has always maintained that postmodernism has no intellectual base on its own and that it has to be linked to Marxism and feminism to be able to offer anything to an emancipatory project.

Ferguson and Lavalette (1999), however, have challenged the view that postmodern themes can be incorporated with Marxist perspectives to develop an emancipatory social work. In their view, postmodernism, in any of its forms, has nothing to offer a critical social work practice. They argue that because of its rejection of meta-narratives and materialism, there is a shift away from structurally produced oppressions towards freely chosen identities. McBeath and Webb (2005) also maintain that postmodern ideas in critical social work do not live up to their claimed radical potential and that critical social work has been weakened by its engagement with Foucault and postmodern ideas. The key issue is whether postmodernism is subordinated under critical theory or vice versa. My own view is the former and hence I have previously articulated a postmodern critical theory (Pease, 2002) as distinct from the critical postmodernism advocated by Healy (2000) and Fook (2002).

Facing the challenges in critical social work

If any form of radical or critical social work is to survive in the current context, it will need to address a series of critiques and challenges from a variety of quarters. Perhaps we should be concerned less with language categories and postmodern/modernist debates and more concerned with the substantive issues underlying the critiques. Here I engage with what I see as some of the key challenges and explore their implications for the future of critical forms of social work.

Mainstream social work

It has been noted that many aspects of radical social work, including the emphasis on empowerment, human rights and social justice, have become integrated into mainstream social work (Langan, 2002). In the Australian context, ecological systems theory and the 'multidimensional approach', which claim to acknowledge the 'bio-psychosocial-spiritual' dimensions of a person's life (Harms, 2007), have become the dominant conceptual frameworks for social work. Within these frameworks, strength perspectives, empowerment approaches, narrative therapy and solution-focused practices are all presented as progressive. Wood and Tully (2006) regard these approaches as being consistent with their structural approach and H. Ferguson (2008) sees them as consistent with his notion of critical best practice.

However, radical critiques of these approaches have not been adequately addressed by writers who promote their progressive use. Baines (2007), for example, in discussing empowerment, says that this form of social justice-oriented social work was appropriated and reshaped as individual self-promotion and advancement. Margolin (1997) argues that while social work espouses an understanding of the structural causes of social problems, it continues to focus on intervention with individuals. Consequently, discourses of empowerment and social justice serve to legitimise social work. I am reminded of Simpkin's (1983) concern expressed many years ago that bringing critical approaches into the mainstream can dilute and fragment their radical potential.

Direct practice in social work

A number of social work writers have raised concerns about the applicability of social change theories and strategies in critical social work for direct practice (Payne, 2005; Hick and Pozzuto, 2005; Healy, 2005). H. Ferguson (2008) has introduced the notion of 'critical best practice' because in his view critical social work did not move beyond the level of critique. This idea that radical social work was weak in terms of practice guidelines has, however, been challenged by those who remind critics that radical social work was enacted and informed by practitioners (Langan, 2002). Langan and Lee (1989), for example, argue that radical social work was grounded in practice and always acknowledged the importance of small progressive changes in daily practice. The challenge remains, however, about how to develop social change strategies that can be pursued at the micro-level of day-to-day practice.

The state and social work

Increased managerial control over social work practice has major implications for critical social work. We must remember that social work is mediated by the state. Ferguson and Lavalette (1999) observe that the institutions of the state are deproblematised in most contemporary social work writings. Dalyrmple and Burke (2006) also note that the anti-oppressive dimensions of critical social work are in tension with the elements of social control that are part of social workers' jobs. McDonald (2006) has further raised the question about whether critical social work can function at all within the institutional context of the contemporary state.

The debate in the 1980s about the limitations and potential to work within and against the state (London to Edinburgh Weekend Return Group, 1980) has been neglected in recent years. There was general agreement among radical social workers that the state was a source of oppression but disagreement about the potential to develop radical practices within it. One of the important legacies of the Marxist approach was the capacity to think dialectically and to develop practices that worked with the contradictions within both the state and social work itself (Corrigan and Leonard, 1978). These understandings need to be adapted to the changing context of the state.

Neoliberalism and the implications for social work

One of the major challenges facing social work is the rise of neoliberalism around the world. Neoliberalism, with its emphasis on free-market economics, the privatisation of government services, free trade and user pays services, has had a significant impact on human service provision. Welfare state provisions are cut back to allow for greater privatisation of human services with an emphasis on freedom of choice, small government, market values and individualism. Davies et al. (2006) have pointed out that one of the ways that neoliberalism works is that it encourages people to believe that they have no choices at the systemic level and they need to make choices within the system. To develop a critical practice, social workers will need to engage in a systematic struggle against neoliberalism. To begin, we need to become more aware of how our conceptions of practice are shaped by this discourse.

Evidence-based practice and social work

While the socially constructed nature of knowledge has been articulated in the social sciences and social work education and many of us have moved away from positivism, science and rationality, some forms of social work practice have moved in the opposite direction to embrace scientific and evidence-based practice (Trinder, 2000). The debates over what constitutes evidence are located in the wider divisions between objectivists and subjectivists about the nature of social reality. Social constructivists and postmodernists have emphasised the importance of seeing science and knowledge as being socially constructed. However, from a critical social work perspective, if there is no objective reality, how can we develop the foundations for emancipatory projects?

Evidence-based practice has been subjected to significant criticisms by critical social work writers. However, such critics either fail to develop alternatives or they place the emphasis on qualitative and critical reflective approaches as the way forward. Critical social work is based on an alternative research paradigm that challenges both the epistemological assumptions of positivism and the relativist underpinnings of the interpretative approach. I have suggested that critical realism seems to offer a reconciliatory position between positivism and social constructionism (Pease, 2007). I have thus proposed that critical social workers develop the foundation for 'critical knowledge-informed practice' to encompass critical social theory, quantitative and qualitative research, tacit knowledge, critical reflective practice, social justice values and consumer-based knowledge. Only a valuing of knowledge from diverse sources that is driven by a commitment to social transformation will enable social work to fulfil its emancipatory objectives (Pease, 2007).

Social work and professionalism

In their account of the history of radical social work in the US, Reisch and Andrews (2001) raise the question of whether social work has ever or could ever be a radical profession. Many of the critics of radical social work in the 1970s argued that political action has no place in professional social work practice (Specht, 1972). Others have argued that social workers have an ethical imperative to be politically active (Reisch and Andrews,

2001). Among those who advocate a radical position, there are also debates between those who regard the organisational and professional basis of social work as a limitation on radical practice (Margolin, 1997) and those who believe that social work can become a radical profession (Reisch and Andrews, 2001). If radical and critical forms of social work are in conflict with professionalism, then they can only be fully realised outside the traditional professional roles. Thus, we need to revisit some form of critical engagement with the limitations and potential of professionalism in relation to social transformation.

The individual in social work

Numerous writers have claimed that the relationship between the individual and society is both the rationale for social work practice and the primary focus for intervention. However, linking structural and sociocultural analyses to the lived experiences of individuals has been a historical tension that has plagued social work since its inception. Critical social work thus needs to address the psyche and subjectivity. Leonard (1984) made a valuable contribution to understanding the individual within radical social work in his book *Personality and Ideology*. He saw the disjuncture between our understandings of the social order and the individual as one of the major barriers to a critical social work practice with individuals and families. Thirteen years later, he argued that a critical social work practice had to be informed by a critical psychology that had not yet been developed (Leonard, 1997). I have built on Leonard's work and explored attempts within the critical tradition to theorise the relationship between self and society with a particular emphasis on challenging oppression and domination (Pease, 2003).

Oppression and social work

Intersectional approaches to oppression that have characterised critical social work have been a source of concern for many critics. In challenging the notion of a hierarchy of oppressions, specific groups are concerned that their experiences and analyses of oppression will not be adequately recognised. Ferguson and Lavalette (1999), for example, take issue with the analysis that locates class as being no more significant than other forms of oppression and they challenge the view that all oppressions are equal. In their view, the power within capitalist societies is distinctly different from that behind working-class men who abuse women or able-bodied people who abuse disabled people. The key issue here, though, is whether analyses of gender, race, sexuality and disability should be subsumed under class analysis, as the Marxists have argued.

One of the debates is about the extent to which oppression is systematic and structural as opposed to primarily interpersonal. Ferguson and Lavalette (1999) maintain that the implication that we all oppress each other in different ways ignores oppressive structures and the state as sources of oppression. We must recognise that some forms of oppression are likely to be more significant for some groups at particular times and in particular circumstances (Barnoff and Moffatt, 2007). While many advocates of intersectional analyses argue that we should not give primacy to any one system of domination, the reality is that some systems of domination are more socially significant than others at particular times. It seems to me that Perry's (2001) analysis of how the interlocking systems of domination interact within specific contexts provides the most useful insight on the impact of different forms of domination and oppression.

Privilege and social work

More attention is given in critical social work to the processes that reproduce oppression than the processes that perpetuate dominance. The struggle for social justice is thus usually conceived of in terms of empowering clients who may be oppressed by class, race, gender and sexuality. Little attention is given to the ways in which the positioning of the professional worker may embody class, race, gender and sexual privilege. Social workers need to be aware of how their own power and privilege are maintained or challenged in their encounters with both clients and other staff (Rossiter, 2000).

A number of writers have drawn attention to the need for critical social work to address privilege as the other side of oppression (Carniol, 2005; Pease, 2006; Barnoff and Moffatt, 2007). Carniol (2005) discusses the importance of analysing our own social location as a precursor to analysing the social location of others. He emphasises the importance of using our critical consciousness to deepen our awareness of our privilege as well as our oppressive circumstances. Such an awareness is an important first step if we are to become involved in undoing those privileges.

Conclusion

All books on radical and critical social work conclude with some statements of optimism and hopefulness in sociopolitical contexts that do not inspire such optimism. While we must avoid the paralysis by analysis that understandings of globalisation, international capitalism and neoliberalism sometimes invoke, we must also be careful not to promise too much by articulating models of critical practice that fail to acknowledge let alone address these obstacles to social transformation.

I remember the discomfort I felt when I first read Margolin's (1997) claim that social workers convince ourselves and others that we have changed, to enable us to stay the same. This, Margolin argues, involves us in a process of deception about our social control functions and leads us to mystify the role of social work as a profession. How do we explore and affirm the progressive potential of critical social work without deluding ourselves? Matahaere-Atariki et al. (2001), writing in the colonial context of New Zealand, argue that critical social workers must acknowledge their failures and the contradictions of their practice. This means staying in touch with our experience of discomfort and it is with that discomfort that I conclude this chapter.

For further discussion of postmodernist ideas, see Chapter 20, and for alternatives to Western practice frameworks, see Adams et al., 2009a, Chapter 21.

www.criticalsocialwork.com *Critical Social Work* is an online journal based at the University of Windsor in Canada that encourages dialogue about social justice and critical social work.

Allan, J., Pease, B. and Briskman, L. (eds) (2003) *Critical Social Work: An Introduction to Theories and Practice*, Sydney, Allen & Unwin. Edited collection that explores the tensions between modernist and postmodern versions of critical theory and their application to critical social work practices.

Ferguson, I. (2008) *Reclaiming Social Work: Challenging Neoliberalism and Promoting Social Justice*, London, Sage. Marxist critique of the postmodern turn in critical social work that argues for a return to a structural analysis of oppression.

Fook, J. (2002) *Social Work: Critical Theory and Practice*, London, Sage. Introduction to the possibilities of a critical social work practice informed by postmodern ideas associated with discourse, power, agency, identity and difference.

Mullaly, B. (2007) *The New Structural Social Work*, 3rd edn, Don Mills, Ontario, Oxford University Press. Popular Canadian text incorporating feminist, anti-racist and postmodern critiques into a reconstructed theory of structural social work.

White, V. (2006) *The State of Feminist Social Work*, London, Routledge. Reappraisal of feminist approaches to social work in the context of changes to managerial regimes within the state in the UK.

Feminist social work 18

Chapter overview

This chapter emphasises that feminist social work is not a separate way of intervening and is not for women only. Among other things, feminist analysis has contributed to the research base of social work, to mainstream practice and to discussions about the value base of social work.

The relationship between social work and feminism is interestingly complex. Both originate from a focus on women. This focus has led to political projects in both that have sought to bring the conditions of women to the fore in the policy and practice agenda. Over the past three decades, both have been informed by theoretical debates that have led to more complex understandings of the experiences of women, which inevitably include relationships with men.

Social work has been informed by feminism in a number of ways. Initially, feminist activists highlighted the particular experiences of women, and the absence of specific attention to these by social work. There was an emphasis specifically on practice with, and for, women. The suggestion was that feminist social work constituted a separate way of intervening in the lives of women users of welfare services.

Over the years, feminist approaches have influenced practice in a number of ways. Specific experiences such as domestic violence have been recognised and responded to. Different approaches to, for example, counselling, groupwork and management have been developed. Increasingly, the research base for practice has drawn on feminist analysis and utilised feminist methodologies. In attending to knowledge, theory and practice, feminist social work has also contributed to discussions about the value base of social work.

During the same period, feminist theories have been refined, reviewed and revised in a dynamic dialogue with practice, drawing on the experiences of women and men. Such developments have provided challenges to the suggestion that there is a separate way of intervening that is 'feminist social work', which is for women only. This chapter will plot how social work has responded to these challenges in ways that have reinforced the contribution that feminism has made to social work.

Context

Attention to the condition of being a woman and the conditions that women experience has been a feature of feminist analyses of social work since the 1970s. Initially associated with the radical critique (Statham, 1978; Wilson, 1980), a shared concern of feminist thought and women in social work was the family and women's role. An early contention of feminists was that most social work was undertaken by women and with women, either as clients in their own right or as part of an infrastructure on which agencies depend to support services (Hanmer and Statham, 1988). Women are either direct recipients of services and/or are users of services in their role as carers of children, older people, those who are sick, disabled or experience mental health problems. In the criminal justice system, women are sometimes the focus of intervention not only because of their own delinquency but also because they are partners of delinquent males.

However, feminism as a movement was critical of women social workers, questioning whether it was possible for them to work in women-centred ways. It was argued that, at best, social work, and therefore women who worked as social workers, reinforced women's roles as carers based on gendered stereotypes. At worst, women who were in touch with social work agencies were pathologised, that is, seen to be problematic, and held responsible for their own problems and the problems of those for whom they had responsibility (Dale and Foster, 1986). There was also ambivalence within social work about whether there needed to be a specific synthesis of feminist theory. Early commentators such as Brook and Davis (1985) were concerned that this would both institutionalise and marginalise feminist theory, thus negating its dynamism and creativity. Others (Wise, 1985; White, 1995) pointed out the dilemmas that some aspects of feminist theory created for practitioners.

The response was feminist social work, or women-centred practice (Hanmer and Statham, 1988; Dominelli and McLeod, 1989). Early social work texts described this alternatively as a movement to raise consciousness and give women control of their lives (Howe, 1987) or as an analysis of oppression and modes of empowerment – for women (Payne, 1991). There were also criticisms, the most consistent being that adopting a separatist approach detracts from the need to permeate all practice. Feminist social work was described as a form of crude reductionist sociology, with contradictory theories that create a hierarchy of oppression imposed by a form of ideological imperialism (Sibeon, 1991). In concentrating on the oppression of women, it was also accused of avoiding or negating class, race and the imperative to work with men. Finally, its influence was also seen to be limited because of a lack of clarity on how to intervene, that feminist theory did not inform social work practice (Payne, 1991).

A growing canon of feminist literature (Hanmer and Statham, 1999; Orme, 2001; Dominelli, 2002a; White, 2006), which is neither institutionalised nor marginalised, addresses the complexities of women's lives and offers guidance on the principles and practices of intervention. Also, reference to working with women and feminists' contribution to social work are now almost taken for granted in compendium texts such as this one (see also Davies and Barton, 2000; Hick et al., 2005; Gray and Webb, 2008b), and in textbooks for social work education (Trevithick, 2005; Coulshed and Orme, 2006), on management (Coulshed and Mullender, 2001) and on specific interventions such as narrative work (Milner, 2001) and groupwork (Cohen and Mullender, 2003). These texts and others also address the need to work with men (Cavanagh and Cree, 1996) and families that include men (Featherstone, 2004).

In identifying the contribution that feminist theories have made to social work practice, this chapter will draw on these and other works to address the critiques of feminist social work, arguing that it has both provided a commentary on mainstream social work and contributed to practice developments that have enhanced the profession of social work.

Feminist social work practice

A crucial factor in debates about feminist social work is the recognition that there are a number of feminist theories, or, more accurately, feminist theorising can lead to different understandings and different recommendations for practice. Feminist thought has influenced writing about social work practice in a number of ways. In the analyses of the 1980s (Dale and Foster, 1986; Wearing, 1986), there was agreement about the source of women's oppression, described alternatively as men or patriarchy. Over time, explanations of the source and process of oppression have drawn alternatively on liberal, reformist, Marxist, socialist and separatist approaches. Any form of theorising is of limited value to social work, if the understandings gained do not inform ways of intervening in the lives of service users to bring about some positive change. For feminist social work, whatever its theoretical stance, the challenge is to contribute to the transformation of social and structural relations and thus empower women through social work practice and interventions. As we shall see, the wider challenge is to understand how feminist analysis can also inform work with men. Hence an exploration of how feminism has influenced social work involves four themes: the conditions of women, women-centred practice, women's 'different' voice and working with diversity.

The conditions of women

Social work has consistently dealt with the conditions of women by ascribing female roles and defining female behaviour. In this way, social work is predicated on the expectations of women. Paradoxically, traditional theories and explanations of service users were gender neutral, they took for granted a status quo that involved women's contribution to the household, and invoked stereotypical views of women and men. At times there was a reinforcement of these roles, for example in childcare practice informed by theories of maternal deprivation.

Early feminist analyses of social work therefore argued for greater attention to the conditions that women experience. For example, over time, the economic position of women has meant that they are traditionally among the poorest in society. Although the participation of women in the paid labour force is increasing, their earnings are consistently lower than those of men. In 2007, for example, on the internationally comparable measure based on mean earnings, women's average hourly pay (excluding overtime) was 17.2 per cent less than men's pay (National Statistics, 2008).

Also, because of childcare and other responsibilities, when women are not in paid work, their entitlement to benefit or their dependence on male earners means that they constitute the poorest in society. This situation has been particularly acute for older women who are living longer but, because of employment patterns, have limited pension rights. These socioeconomic conditions often mean that women become dependent upon social services, they are caught up in the web of service provision and regulatory practices. However, social workers rarely see the focus of their work with women as the alleviation of their poverty, but focus on the attitudes, behaviour and coping strategies of individual women. Drawing on Marxist analysis, Wilson (1980) argued that the welfare state sought to keep women in the role of housewife, mother and carer, and, as employees of that welfare state, social workers themselves were purveyors of the repression of the state.

Other research highlighted how other conditions impacted on women's lives, particularly expectations of women as carers (Finch and Groves, 1983; Ungerson, 1987). Feminist social policy analysed how social workers not only negatively focused on the conditions of women but also were dependent upon them to undertake tasks to support the welfare of others. Focusing on the conditions of women meant that they were seen as both the cause of the problem and the source of the solution.

In attending to the conditions of women, and acknowledging the condition of being a woman, feminist theory therefore provided a critique, but what were the solutions? The limitations of Marxist concentration on class and the economic system were seen merely to reflect and reinforce patriarchal underpinnings. Hence some feminists established a radical perspective that identified the source of women's oppression as the social institution of gender. For social work, the recognition of sexual politics (Firestone, 1971; Millett, 1972) resonated because it emphasised the role of male power in interpersonal relationships within the family, which contributed to women's sense of personal and economic inferiority and helplessness. In practice, such analysis informed understandings of domestic violence and sexual abuse. This led to an important strand of inquiry, the exploration of the condition of being a woman. Work in the area of domestic violence (Hanmer and Maynard, 1987), child abuse (Hudson, 1992) and women offenders (Carlen and Worrall, 1987) emphasised that there were oppressions and disadvantages experienced by women by virtue of their sex. Work in the area of domestic violence has informed social work practice over time, providing a critique of the responses from various agencies (Mullender, 1996) and recognising the needs of survivors of domestic violence (Hague et al., 2003).

This condition of being a woman, with assumptions of feminine behaviour, has also led to an important critique of women and mental illness. Feminist analysis describe how mental disorder was perceived as 'a female malady' (Showalter, 1987), illustrating how women's biology was seen to be the cause of their mental instability (Ussher, 1991) and that assessing women as high risk by mental health workers was often on the basis of their transgression of gender norms (Warner and Gabe, 2008). Attention to the condition of being a woman also challenged heterosexist assumptions of state services predicated on women being in relationships with men. The contribution of feminist theory to social work was to put women, their experiences and their oppression on the agenda.

Women-centred practice

Early recognition that women had been absent from the social work discourse (Hale, 1983) led to approaches at the micro-level that sought to enhance the lives of women. Raising consciousness, changing assumptions about, and perceptions of, women while acknowledging structural oppression were themes reflected in prescriptions for women-centred practice. These included codes of practice that recognised the power of the social worker in individual interpersonal relationships (Hanmer and Statham, 1988) or those which focused on constructing an anti-sexist environment and mode of service delivery (NAPO, 1990). However, maintaining a focus on the individual sometimes led to services that reinforced women in their role as mothers and/or carers, for example mother and toddler groups or prisoners' wives groups.

There were some who argued that feminists in social work could not combat the structural imbalances of state welfare systems, which were imbued with individualised approaches that pathologised women (Wilson, 1980). Feminist social work, they argued, required women-only organisations. Indeed, a rich stream of feminist social work did emerge with the establishment of women's refuges, rape crisis lines, well women clinics and other forms of women's self-help organisations. However, others thought it imperative that feminists remained within the statutory agencies and tried to change the culture of both the organisation and the practice to reflect feminist aims (Dominelli and McLeod, 1989).

This happened more slowly than many would have wished. With the support of organisations such as CCETSW (Phillipson, 1991), feminism became a focus for study under the broad umbrella of anti-discriminatory practice, and attention to women and women's issues began to permeate the social work curriculum. Also, as has been indicated, social work texts began to reference the particular needs of women. However, official support for attention to the issues of discrimination and oppression on the basis of gender (and race) was the focus of harsh criticism (see Dominelli, 2002a for a discussion of this) and was short-lived. In the qualifying degree for social work introduced in 2003 (DH, 2003a), there is little specific attention to issues pertaining to women. As will be discussed below, the focus is on diversity.

Women-centred practice brought about other tensions. Balances of power inherent in traditional ways of working highlighted distinctions between workers and service users traditionally known as 'clients'. Feminism and social work were both accused of emanating from white, middle-class movements that ignored or denied the experiences of other women (hooks, 1984a). From the perspective of women with disabilities, Morris (1993) points out how women who were deemed to be 'clients' or users of social services became invisible. They were defined in terms of their 'condition' but were not thought to experience the oppressions and discriminations of non-disabled women (Morris, 1996). The same arguments can be made on behalf of older women (Orme, 2001). In social work practice, increasing attention to the needs of one group, women carers, further oppresses and discriminates against women who require care, who are described as a burden (Dalley, 1988). Those with needs are seen to constrain the lives of the women who provide care (Parker and Clarke, 2002).

In the first edition of *Women and Social Work,* Hanmer and Statham (1988) drew attention to these tensions by urging women workers to identify commonalities and diversities; to acknowledge the differences in experience, but recognise that women workers and service users shared some of the same oppressions. But recognising commonality and diversity is not always helpful. It may reinforce notions that women are the source of, and solution to, the problems they experience. Acknowledging diversities between women and users, and arguing that these should be transcended, denies the power relationship between these groups of women (White, 1995). Also, while recognising that commonality is a way of expressing empathy (Hanmer and Statham, 1988), requiring workers to do so raises concerns over shared information.

A further set of criticisms was that identifying women as a separate category requires workers to deny the complexity of women's responses in childcare and other situations in which social workers had to intervene (Wise, 1985). While it was important to listen to women's voices, practitioners also had to accept that women were also capable of anti-social behaviour and abuse (Crinall, 1999).

However, women-centred practice did produce some specific approaches that have informed practice, not only with women. These include approaches to management (Coulshed and Mullender, 2001) that embody different ways of negotiating workplace situations, the use of narrative approaches in counselling (Milner, 2001), and developments in groupwork with women and men informed by understandings of gender (Cohen and Mullender, 2003). These examples illustrate that practice that arose out of a specific focus on women gave a different perspective for understanding the relations between women and men.

The 'different voice' of women

A parallel development to women-centred practice was an exploration of the differences between women and men. This emerged from understandings of women's moral development explored by feminist psychologists (Gilligan, 1993). Claiming that women have developed an 'ethic of care' as opposed to the male 'ethic of justice', Gilligan argues that women therefore speak in 'a different voice'. This voice has been associated with women's facilitative nature, in which they address relational aspects of problems rather than resorting to procedures, rules and rationality. It is argued that these feminine ways have traditionally been devalued. Indeed, the very fact that social work as a profession drew on such qualities and was therefore a feminine profession had been the subject of criticism (Younghusband, 1951). The project for feminism was to valorise these qualities, and ensure that the different approaches permeated all services. For example, feminist writing has challenged the male ethos of social work management, arguing that it can be more inclusive, collaborative and egalitarian (Coulshed and Mullender, 2001). Such writings have become more significant as changes in policy have led to more 'managerial' approaches to service delivery that have implications for women's involvement in a changing organisation (Balloch, 1997) and for men (Christie, 2006).

Also, explorations of the 'ethic of care' in social work have introduced scholars and practitioners to a wealth of feminist theory to inform discussions about values. This has included reframing understandings of both care and justice (Orme, 2002) and the value base of professional practice (Parton, 2003).

The 'different voice' of women has been influential in the research base for social work. Based on assumptions that women have different ways of knowing (Hawkesworth, 1989; Belenky et al., 1997; Oakley, 1999), feminist theories have informed practice research (Green, 2003). For example, feminist writing on epistemology and methodology (see Stanley, 1990) has invoked the notion of 'praxis' – the practical application of theory (Orme, 1997). In social work, this has led to methods of inquiry that have encouraged user participation and emancipatory research, and have linked knowledge production with bringing about change (Fawcett et al., 2000). However, again there have been discussions about the dangers of adopting too simplistic an approach to the contribution of feminism to social work research. Feminist approaches can include many methods and research the experiences of women and men (Orme, 2003).

Thus privileging the 'different' voice strengthens the contribution of feminist social work to working with men. For example, early work on a feminist jurisprudence (Carlen, 1989) documents how women are adversely treated by the paternalism of the criminal justice system. In arguing for the appropriate treatment for women, Carlen recognises that dehumanising and punitive custodial sentences are not appropriate for women or men. For men to become less violent there needs to be less violent treatment within the penal system. Work with men has to acknowledge their context.

These arguments have been further developed in writings on domestic violence, where the emphasis initially and rightly was on having the problem recognised and making women safe. However, to ensure the long-term safety of all women, it is necessary to widen the project. Work has to be undertaken with men to understand and halt the violent behaviour, not by the use of punitive measures but by pro-feminist ways of working (Orme et al., 2000).

Work on domestic violence has also inevitably led to explorations of the role of men in families. The focus has been to understand abusive behaviour (Featherstone and Lancaster, 1997) in order to prevent it and to protect women. It has also recognised the need for men to be involved in family life and childcare (Featherstone, 2003). This work has led to further work by men in social work drawing on feminist theory (Scourfield, 2002).

Working with diversity

The developments in feminist social work, which acknowledge the imperative to recognise the heterogeneity of women's experiences and to address working with men, have been associated with the influence of postmodernism. The unitary category of women has been challenged by some feminist writers, who argue that the essentialist notions of femininity reflected in Gilligan's writing constrain women to subordinate functions and prevent men from undertaking caring roles. Disabled, black and lesbian women have argued that to enable them to assert their rights, there has to be recognition of diversity within the category 'women'. If this is so, the false duality of women/men also has to be challenged. If there is no single category 'woman', there can be no single category 'man' (Butler, 1990). Such an analysis has created both a crisis and a development in feminist social work. Some see postmodernism as part of a (white) male academic back- lash against feminist thought and action (Hester et al., 1996). Others see it as an opportunity for feminism to inform working with men, challenge masculinist assump- tions and recognise the oppressions of patriarchy, rather than expecting women to change their own conditions (Cavanagh and Cree, 1996). These opportunities have also enabled pro-feminist men to explore ways in which they can work to challenge the oppression of women by men (Thompson, 1995; Hearn, 1998; Christie, 2001).

Exploring gender as relational, recognising that women and men are constructed by certain aspects of their identity, challenges other dualities such as disabled/able-bodied; carer/cared for (Orme, 2001). Feminist social work therefore can work with all service users to challenge the way that their needs are constructed, interpreted and responded to.

Issues

The themes that have been identified in this account of the development of feminist social work raise a number of issues. The first is that critical debates with feminism and within feminist theory raise dilemmas about the way that the condition of being a woman is responded to. Should social workers see women as different from men, as having separate experiences, as being a special case, because of their biology, or because of the way that gender is socially constructed? If they do treat women in this way, how can they argue for equality and equal treatment?

These challenges occur daily in social work practice. In the field of childcare, issues to do with motherhood are ubiquitous. Women experience different socioeconomic condi- tions because of their capacity for childbearing, but this should not deny them equality in the workplace and in the home. Assumptions about motherhood have consequences for women and men in the way social workers intervene in families (Featherstone, 2004). Also, related to motherhood are notions of femaleness and femininity that permeate poli- cies on, and reactions to, young people's behaviour. Crimes of violence, excessive drinking and antisocial behaviour in young people have numerous gendered implications. First, there are differential expectations of young men and women, and the latter are treated more harshly when they challenge gender stereotypes. Second, simplistic analysis frequently invokes the 'failure' of one-parent families or, more accurately, lone mothers to socialise young people – the implication being that the causal factors are to do with the inadequacy of the women rather than the abdication of the men. Despite the ubiquitous nature of these dilemmas, policy continues to ignore gender (Daniel et al., 2005).

The second issue is that, acknowledging the dangers of stereotyping, feminist social work has not responded to the particular needs of women service users. To be effective, it has to recognise the contradictions of women's lives and, through a process of individualisation, accept that being a woman – be that a black or disabled woman – is part of the person-in-environment perspective that is core to all social work practice. This is not difficult because it resonates with the feminist claim that the personal is political (Collins, 1986), that the environment includes the social construction of gender, of being a woman or a man. What has to be worked with is how individual women experience their situation. To tell a woman service user that she is oppressed is no more liberating than labelling her as depressed, unless there are ways of changing the situation. Having recognised the dilemmas and clarified the accounts, it is also necessary to be open about the social control elements of the social work role. This control often emanates from the dynamic of individual relationships and the legislative framework, which reinforces gendered stereotypes or appears to circumscribe the work that has to be done (White, 2006). The challenge for feminist social work, therefore, is to acknowledge the operation of power within all relationships and influence the policy debates (Featherstone, 2005) as well as work at the level of the individual.

However, this focus on the individual and the recognition of the diversity of women's experience, and the inclusion of men within the feminist social work project, is problematic for some feminists. It is seen to lead to a deflection from focusing on the oppressions of women and to undermine research that has stressed the material realities of women's lives and men's behaviour in these (Hester et al., 1996). However, in the absence of dialogue, unless work is done with men as service users, as potential carers and as perpetrators of the abuse of women, there will be no challenge to constructions of masculine identity. Unless feminist theory and practice are used to undertake this challenge, there will be little change in the conditions and behaviours that women have had to tolerate.

What is important, therefore, is the way in which situations are worked with, the praxis that incorporates feminist analysis. It is appropriate for feminists to intervene to protect vulnerable people, whoever they may be. The notion of praxis requires feminists to be part of the debate about acceptable standards of conduct, ensuring that these are not constructed on stereotypical gendered lines and arguing for the inclusion of service users, especially women who constitute the majority of users, in the decisions. In this way feminist social work will contribute to the transformation of social and structural relations.

Conclusion

Feminist thought in social work practice has played a vital role in recognising the conditions of women and their oppression and subjugation. It has moved from a woman-centred analysis that is for women, by women and with women to a perspective that includes working with men. That is not to say that a woman-centred stance is not valid: women-only space is important, and women's thoughts and experiences should be actively heard. In working with women, feminist social work practitioners are only too aware that any one person's condition is influenced by the behaviour and expectations of others. For women service users, their lives are defined and constrained by 'malestream' thinking and organisation and male behaviour. To focus solely on women, to attempt to empower them, leads to dilemmas, conflict and frustration and can hold them responsible for change in their own circumstances and those of others. It concentrates on their feminine condition in a negative way and does not address other conditions that oppress them.

This chapter has argued for an articulation of feminist social work which draws on substantive feminist theory to provide both a critique of mainstream social work and opportunities for further theory and practice development. Feminist theories in and for social work have enhanced understanding of the experiences of women and contributed a reflexivity, a way of responding to the conditions of women. The notion of feminist social work praxis has emerged that demands attention from women and men workers, and sees as its project understanding the situations of women and men. Feminist praxis therefore recognises the diverse experience of all social work service users and seeks to challenge and transform policy, practice and the organisation of the service delivery that constrains people in gender-specific roles or oppresses them by the inappropriate exercise of power.

The themes explored in this chapter illustrate that more than most paradigms, feminist social work has been reflexive in responding to the experiences and criticisms of those whose position it seeks to explore, explain and exhibit. It has striven to ensure that women are both made visible within the organisation of service provision and empowered by individual interpersonal interventions. This emphasis on the transformational is now evident in debates within feminist social work about working with men.

For further discussion of women's reproductive rights, see Chapter 6, and for criminal violence in the home, see Adams et al., 2009c, Chapter 3.

Dominelli, L. (2002) *Feminist Social Work Theory and Practice*, Basingstoke, Palgrave – now Palgrave Macmillan. Useful overview of a range of feminist theories and the implications for social work practice, drawing on examples from global literature and practice.

Orme, J. (2001) *Gender and Community Care: Social Work and Social Care Perspectives*, Basingstoke, Palgrave – now Palgrave Macmillan. Drawing on a range of feminist theories, this text explores how these theories help us to understand how women and men service users are constructed by policy and practice.

White, V. (2006) *The State of Feminist Social Work*, London, Routledge. Gives an overview of the development of feminist theory for social work and an analysis of the viability of feminist practice in statutory organisations.

Anti-oppressive approaches

19

This chapter explores how a theorised social work practice informed by anti-oppressive principles can be sensitively and effectively used to address the inequalities and oppression that shape the life chances of service users.

Chapter overview

The complex nature of oppression is witnessed in the lives of people who are marginalised in this society. As social work practitioners, we have a moral, ethical and legal responsibility to challenge inequality and disadvantage. Historically, in attempting to understand, explain and offer solutions to the difficulties experienced by groups and individuals, the profession has drawn from, among others, the disciplines of sociology, psychology, history, philosophy and politics. This multidisciplinary theoretical framework, informed by anti-oppressive principles, provides social workers with a tool to understand and respond to the complexity of the experience of oppression.

The writings of black feminists (hooks, 1981, 1984b, 1989, 1991; Lorde, 1984; Neale-Hurston, 1986; Morrison, 1987; Jordan, 1989; Russell, 1990; James and Busia, 1993; Mirza, 1997; Hill Collins, 2000) provide a rich literature that is theoretically based and informed by the disciplines of psychology, sociology, politics, history and anthropology. It incorporates existentialist ideas, liberatory educational principles (hooks, 1994), community activism and personal experiences provided by both autobiographical and fictional accounts. It thus expands understandings of oppression and lays the foundations for the exploration of the experience of power, powerlessness and oppression.

Black feminist thought is a dynamic perspective, derived from 'diverse lived experiences', that not only provides an analysis of human interactions, based on principles of equality, but also considers the interconnections that exist between the major social divisions of class, 'race', gender, disability, sexuality and age as they impact on the individual, family and community.

Black feminist theorising has helped us to understand ourselves as black women. It has enabled us to make sense of the patterns of domination and oppression that characterise our professional and personal lives. We hold the view that personal experiences are inextricably linked to and determined by social, cultural, political and economic relationships within specific geographical and historical situations. This process of location allows us to challenge those who see only our visible differences of race and gender, failing also to take into account the invisible differences such as class and sexuality. For us, what is important are the interconnections between the range of social divisions to which we belong that ultimately defines who we are and the nature of the oppression we may experience (Lorde, 1984). In our view, developing an understanding of the concept of anti-oppressive practice is a means of working with the complexity of the impact of oppression and discrimination in practice situations.

What is anti-oppressive practice?

There are a number of definitions, ranging in complexity and length. Anti-oppressive practice has been debated by a number of writers, whose works are informed by differing perspectives (Thompson, 1993; Clifford, 1994; Braye and Preston-Shoot, 1995; Featherstone and Fawcett, 1995; Dominelli, 1996; Dalrymple and Burke, 2006). However, for the transformative potency of anti-oppressive practice to be realised, the reader needs to be critically aware that the choice of words used to define reveals not only the value and ideological base of the definer, but also the nature of the practice that will emanate from that definition.

Anti-oppressive practice is a dynamic process based on the complex changing patterns of social relations. It is, therefore, important that a definition is informed by research within academic institutions, practitioner research and the views of service users. For the purposes of this chapter, we provide a 'definition' – with all the attendant problems of defining – that incorporates points already discussed as well as providing a framework to clarify and inform practice.

Clifford (1995: 65) uses the term 'anti-oppressive':

> to indicate an explicit evaluative position that constructs social divisions (especially 'race', class, gender, disability, sexual orientation and age) as matters of broad social structure, at the same time as being personal and organisational issues. It looks at the use and abuse of power not only in relation to individual or organisational behaviour, which may be overtly, covertly or indirectly racist, classist, sexist and so on, but also in relation to broader social structures, for example the health, educational, political and economic, media and cultural systems and their routine provision of services and rewards for powerful groups at local as well as national and international levels. These factors impinge on people's life stories in unique ways that have to be understood in their socio-historical complexity.

Within this definition, there is a clear understanding of the use and abuse of power within relationships on personal, family, community, organisational and structural levels. These levels are not mutually exclusive – they are interconnected, shaping and determining social reality. Informed by the writings of black feminist and other 'non-dominant perspectives', Clifford (1995) formulated the following anti-oppressive principles, which provide the foundation for a social work assessment that is theorised and empowering:

- *Social difference:* Social differences arise because of disparities of power between the dominant and dominated social groups. The major divisions are described in terms of race, gender, class, sexual preference, disability and age. Other differences, such as those of religion, mental health and being a carer, exist and interact with the major divisions, making the understanding and experience of oppression a complex matter.
- *Linking personal and political:* Personal biographies are placed within a wider social context and the individual's life situation is viewed in relation to social systems such as the family, peer groups, organisations and communities. For example, the problems associated with ageing are not solely due to the individual but should be understood in relation to the ageist ideologies, policies and practices that exist within the social environment in which the individual is located.
- *Power:* Power is a social concept that can be used to explore the public and private spheres of life (Barker and Roberts, 1993). In practice, power can be seen to operate at the personal and structural levels. It is influenced by social, cultural, economic and psychological factors. All these factors need to be taken into account in any analysis of how individuals or groups gain differential access to resources and positions of power (Lukes, 2005).
- *Historical and geographical location:* Individual life experiences and events are placed within a specific time and place, so that these experiences are given meaning within the context of prevailing ideas, social facts and cultural differences.
- *Reflexivity/mutual involvement:* Reflexivity is the continual consideration of how values, social difference and power affect interactions between individuals. These interactions are to be understood not only in psychological terms, but also as a matter of sociology, history, ethics and politics. The reflexive practitioner will be aware, for example, of the impact of social divisions, power differences, life history and values on the developing relationship between the service user and themselves.

The above principles relate to each other, interconnecting and overlapping at all times. Working from a perspective that is informed by anti-oppressive principles provides an approach that begins to match the complex issues of power, oppression and powerlessness that determine the lives of the people who are recipients of social care services. An understanding of these principles brings with it a fundamental transformation in the relationship that exists between the assessment of a situation and the nature of the action that is required to change the existing state of affairs.

In anti-oppressive practice, the process of change is driven by the practitioner's challenge of situations of inequality and oppression, where the act of challenging will be informed by the principles of anti-oppressive practice. Challenges are not always successful and are often painful for the person or group being challenged or challenging. A challenge, at its best, involves changes at macro- and micro-levels. If anti-oppressive practice is to provide appropriate and sensitive services that are needs-led rather than resource-driven, it has to embody:

> a person centred philosophy; an egalitarian value system concerned with reducing the deleterious effects of structural inequalities upon people's lives; a methodology focusing on both process and outcome; and a way of structuring relationships between individuals that aims to empower users by reducing the negative effects of social hierarchies on their interaction and the work they do together. (Dominelli, 1994: 3)

Work in welfare organisations is constrained by financial, social, legislative and organisational policies (Healy and Meagher, 2004). Social workers operating within such an environment will inevitably face conflicting and competing demands on their personal and professional resources. The use of anti-oppressive principles offers the worker a way of responding to and managing these sometimes hostile and disempowering situations (Strier, 2007), which affect both worker and service user.

The dynamic link between theory and practice will be demonstrated through the use of a case scenario, written in autobiographical form. It is through the critical and reflexive analysis (Healy, 2005; D'Cruz et al., 2007) of practice that theories, principles and methods can come alive. By reading the following scenario, you, the reader, are directly involved in a young black woman's 'lived experiences' (Hill Collins, 2000). Through the act of reading, you become both participant and observer. You begin to start the process of critical thinking, reflection and analysis of her life, bringing with you to the interpretation of her story your values, assumptions and practice wisdom. It is important to remember, when reading Amelia's story, that it contains the stories of others – her son, the professionals involved, her community networks and her family. Within the scenario and the analysis, we have attempted to utilise the principles to explore various issues raised by the scenario, for example we make specific reference to social difference, such as gender and ethnicity, as this will have an impact on the relationship between service user and practitioner.

To set the scene: following a period of 18 months' engagement with social services, a decision was made by a social services department that changed the life of a family. A young, single, 19-year-old black woman was told that the care plan regarding her 20-month-old son was that of adoption. The decision was based on evidence from intensive social work involvement, and the influential information obtained from reports written by a white male psychologist and a white female psychiatrist.

CASE EXAMPLE

Amelia's story as told to a friend

Leaving home at 16, I spent most of my time trying to find a place to live and make ends meet. I relied on shoplifting and my friends to survive. At 17, I met a man who was 27. We lived together; when I became pregnant, things began to change. He became violent towards me. I was placed in a hostel for mothers with children, I wasn't very happy at the hostel, I disliked the racist name-calling – no one in charge did anything about it. Drugs were easily available. I tried heroin.

My baby was born three months prematurely. While he was in hospital, he nearly died, I was really frightened. I visited him every day for the two months he was in hospital. I kept asking for social work help. I needed money to travel to and from the hospital and I needed someone to talk to. The nurses asked for help for me. I never got any. I returned to the hostel with my son. Then he became ill. I took drugs to help me to stay awake so that I could look after him. Everything seemed too much. When he was in hospital, I told one of the nurses that I had 'tapped' him when he would not stop screaming. They told social services. So when I tried to leave the hospital with him, I was stopped. My son was placed in respite care for a couple of weeks. I was told that I could have him back when I felt better.

When I wanted him back, they said that they had to do an assessment to see if I was able to care for him. I began to scream and shout. I begged them to give my baby back, but they placed him with white foster carers. I did not agree, but there were no black foster carers. I saw him every day. It was decided that I needed to have a psychological and psychiatric assessment. I felt that I needed someone to talk to. I know I am not mad. The social workers spent time with me and wrote a report saying I should have my son back. My son was put on a supervision order for a year.

I moved into a new house. I told my social worker that I really did not feel ready to live on my own. The social worker arranged for a childminder two days a week and a home help. I wanted a nursery place. I was lonely in the new house. I went out a lot. I told someone I knew that six months earlier, while on drugs, I had tried to harm my son. She said we should tell the social services and they would help me to sort it all out. I agreed. They took my son into care again.

A month went by. They were trying to find a place where I could live with my son and get the help I needed. They never really told me anything. I felt very frustrated. It was hard being without my son. One day, after access, I did not return my son to the carer. I kept him overnight. They found me the next morning. They took him away. Now I can only see him for two hours a day at the foster carers, and at weekends.

I cannot think straight. I cannot be upset or depressed as this would go against me. All the time I was told that I was capable of looking after my son and that they were working on us being together. They knew I loved and wanted him very much. But now they have told me that they have plans for adoption. I am so angry and frightened, but I cannot show my anger or this would upset the workers. My son has had so many changes. I am not sure what to think or do.

Should I start thinking about when I will not have him? I know that I need someone to talk to about all the things that have happened to me. But I cannot do this without my son. Why do they need to take him away when I know I can look after him with help? I do not know how I can fight any of this.

Theory into practice

Using anti-oppressive principles, which incorporates challenging as a central process, we will analyse Amelia's story, highlighting issues and dilemmas that workers face in attempting to empower a service user.

The anti-oppressive principle of reflexivity demands that workers continually consider the ways in which their own social identity and values affect the information they gather. This includes their understanding of the social world as experienced by themselves and those with whom they work.

Involvement in Amelia's life is not a neutral event. It is determined by the interaction between the personal biographies of the worker and Amelia, and will be expressed in the power relationships that arise from their membership of differing social divisions.

For example, a white male social worker – because of the social divisions he represents – brings to the situation a dynamic that has the potential to reproduce the patterns of oppression to which black women are subjected in a racist and sexist society (Thompson, 2003). In this scenario, Amelia feels she is silenced. Her plea for 'someone to talk to', to be listened to and taken seriously, is neither understood nor acted upon. This is highlighted in the powerlessness expressed in the telling of her story.

The challenge to you, the worker, is to reflect on your social division membership, your personal and professional biography and to be aware of the impact that this will have on your involvement with Amelia. Are you the right worker for her? If the answer is no, the challenge is not only to find a more appropriate worker but to look to ways in which you may minimise the potential for oppressive practice at the point of referral. In and through this process of thinking and reflecting, which should take place in supervision, team discussions and interactions with service users, you will begin to work in an anti-oppressive way.

Society is divided along the major divisions of race, class, gender, sexual preference, disability and age. There are also other divisions that occur as a result of inequality and discrimination, such as poverty, geographical location, mental distress and employment status. The social difference principle is based on an understanding of how the divisions interconnect and shape the lives of people.

Amelia is young, black, unemployed, female, of a particular class background, living in poverty and a single parent. Yet in the scenario, she is seen merely as a young woman suffering domestic violence and in need of accommodation. Her needs as a black woman from a particular background with a specific history are not fully considered. Amelia's experience of racism in the hostel compounded her overall experience of oppression, forcing her into independence before she was ready.

The challenge for you, the worker, is to understand both the specific and the general nature of social division membership and how it may contribute to the individual's experience of oppression. As a worker, you must make a systematic analysis of the social division membership of all the individuals involved in Amelia's life and understand the relevance of this for your intervention.

It is important to locate the life experiences and events of Amelia and her son within a historical and geographical context. Those experiences need to be chronologically charted and their relevance clearly understood and applied to Amelia's story. In doing that, you, the worker, will get an accurate picture of how events within the family, community and society have influenced Amelia's current situation. Amelia's story will have been influenced by previous specific historical and geographical factors.

As the worker, you need to be aware of how prevailing ideologies have influenced legislation, agency policy, procedures and practice relating to childcare, homelessness and parenting by single mothers. The challenge is to use that analysis to inform your assessment and decision-making. You need to question the agency's policies on work with homeless young women. Amelia's needs as a homeless, black young woman were never assessed with reference to research evidence, which documents the oppression and lack of services faced by this specific user group.

The principle of historical and geographic context directs the worker to consider not only the individual worker's relationship with the service user, but also the team and agency practice. The following are some of the questions that need to be considered:

- How does a prevailing ideology of a mixed economy of care affect practice within the team?
- How does the team prioritise work with homeless young people?
- How far has the historical development of service provision in the area determined current practices?

Such questions will help workers to understand what is constraining their practice. Anti-oppressive thinking moves the worker beyond the confines of agency policy and practice and directs the challenge more appropriately.

In understanding the personal as political, the everyday life experiences of individuals need to be located within social, cultural, political and economic structures that are historically and geographically specific. This process of location ensures that, in practice, the individual is not pathologised, and weight is given to the interconnections and interactions between that individual's story and the social systems they encounter.

Amelia is defined in terms of the domestic violence she has experienced. The assessment is not placed in a wider context, failing to make sense of Amelia's whole life experience. You, the worker, need to take into account the structural factors that contribute to women's experience of violence and how, for Amelia, the dimension of race and her membership of other social divisions added other layers to her experience of oppression.

The social worker's decision to formulate a care plan that put forward adoption as a solution to Amelia's problems needs to be analysed. Their decision appears to be highly influenced by the expert evidence, which focused on Amelia's psychiatric and psychological functioning. How did these assessments inform the worker's analysis of Amelia's ability to parent adequately? Here, we see a failure to locate assessment evidence within a framework that takes into account all aspects of Amelia's existence – her gender, her race, her poverty, her single parenthood – as well as making reference to assessment evidence from other professionals.

The challenge to the worker is to examine the range of evidence used in decision-making, asking questions about why any one piece of evidence is given more weight than another. Does that weighting pathologise the individual by not taking into account the assessments made by other professionals, such as the health visitor and the foster carers? For example, was support from the extended family and other informal community support networks considered? Did particular assumptions about black families influence the workers' views about Amelia's ability to parent? By ignoring the impact of oppressive social values and policies in the decision-making process, the worker can further devalue the service user's capacity to reach their full potential. A more sophisticated and nuanced approach is necessary, which will involve:

> a paradigm shift from essentialist notions of race that view culture in rigid and inflexible ways to one in which cultural sensitivity is understood within the context of power relations. (Barn, 2007: 1432)

In addressing power and powerlessness, it is essential to understand how the differential access to power shapes and determines relationships on an individual, group, community, organisational and societal level. We get a glimpse of Amelia's feelings of powerlessness when she says, 'I do not know how I can fight any of this.' Central to her powerlessness is the lack of access to many social resources. There is evidence in Amelia's story of her being denied access to the resources she feels will help her to parent effectively.

You, as the worker, need to take into account the professional and personal power – based on your particular social division membership – you hold. As a practitioner, you need to identify and assess the power and the strengths that Amelia brings from her previous life experiences.

An anti-oppressive practitioner will consider issues of power in their assessment and intervention strategies. The worker in this situation could have advocated on behalf of Amelia, working creatively to explore other more collaborative, service user-focused options that would have supported her in her parenting. For example, the availability of culturally appropriate community resources could have been explored. It appears that the workers ignored the personal strengths of Amelia, gained from her experiences of oppression, leading to practice that compounded her feelings of powerlessness. They failed to listen and work in partnership with Amelia.

The misuse of power by the worker culminates in a situation in which decisions can be made where the outcome labels Amelia as a non-deserving case. Amelia, however, is not alone in her powerlessness. There are clear differences of the power ascribed to the opinions of one professional group over another. It appears that extended social work practice had little impact on the overall decision regarding the future of the family. Explanations of Amelia's behaviour are reduced to the opinions of one professional group who are seen as 'expert', reducing complex explanations of her behaviour to psychology and psychiatry.

Social workers are well placed to make assessments that are theoretically informed, holistic, empowering and challenging. Anti-oppressive practice does not negate the risks posed to the child. Intervention based on anti-oppressive practice incorporates a risk and needs analysis of both mother and child as well as taking into account the issue of cultural relativity (Barn, 2007).

To work effectively from an anti-oppressive perspective, it is important to:

- be open to other views, be willing to listen and be prepared to change
- include the views of oppressed individuals and groups
- be theoretically informed in a critical and reflexive way
- challenge and work to change existing ideas, policies and practice that undermine principles of justice and equality
- analyse and challenge the oppressive nature of organisational culture and its impact on practice
- have a clear framework for continuous reflection and evaluation of practice
- have a range of strategies that incorporate the concepts of networking, user involvement, partnership and participation
- have a critical understanding and analysis of the concept of power and how it is used at the personal, professional and structural levels.

Anti-oppressive practice remains the focus of numerous contentious debates regarding its utility and relevance to current practice situations (Nellis, 2000; Wilson and Beresford, 2000; O'Hagan, 2001; Mullaly, 2002: Sakamoto and Pitner, 2005; Dalrymple and Burke, 2006; Millar, 2008). Service users, practitioners, students and academics continue to try to find ways of dealing with issues of oppression in the delivery of health and social care services. This has generated a number of theoretical positions that promote particular ways of working, such as 'critical practice' (Healy, 2000), 'emancipatory social work practice' (Pease and Fook, 1999), 'culturally competent practice' (O'Hagan, 2001), 'transformational practice' (Adams et al., 2005b) and 'critical best practice' (Ferguson, 2003; Jones et al., 2008b). Common to all these positions are the principles of anti-oppressive practice.

This chapter was originally written using Amelia's story. It is to her we have returned. She has tried to make sense of the social work intervention to which she was subject and its impact on her and her child. In keeping with black, feminist and anti-oppressive principles, which advocate the use of narrative, we have updated this chapter using Amelia's reflections.

CASE EXAMPLE (cont'd)

Amelia's reflections

It is now four years since I experienced difficulties in caring for my son. Following the care plan for adoption, and the court hearing, my mother took care of my son for the next two years. I now have full care of him without a care order.

Looking back, I would say that it is really important for the worker to look at you as a whole person. Not just focus on what you did and make you feel like a bad person. I knew I had done something wrong. I always wished they could have understood me as a young person, who was very confused. I was also black, a single parent and homeless.

I felt the workers needed to listen to my views more, and work with me. They were only OK with me when I agreed with their views. I needed to understand why they made certain plans for me and my son. I wanted them to be honest with me. I feel it is important for those who want to go into social work to have had some experience of life. I realise I still have a lot to learn, but I do know some things about myself and what I need.

The strength of anti-oppressive practice is that it combines the concepts of participation, partnership and empowerment, offering the potential for the service user's voice to be heard and acted upon. The challenge for practitioners is not to act as 'mere functionaries of agencies' (O'Sullivan, 1999: 35), following practice guidelines without questioning the underpinning knowledge and value base. It requires workers to be reflexive, informed and challenging in their practice.

Amelia asks for workers to understand her needs and her child's needs by locating her individual act within a social and political context, taking account of her many differences and how they contributed to her situation. In her reflections, Amelia asks for her voice to be heard and respected, not merely when it coincides with the workers' professional views (Holland, 2000). Anti-oppressive practice extends the choices available for service users and can prepare workers and service users to deal effectively with power differences by addressing the impact of oppression at both the micro- and macro-level.

If the principles of anti-oppressive practice are to move the practitioners' thinking beyond agency policy and practice and make a difference, they need to invest time and energy in the application of those principles, enabling them to analyse situations systematically and think through the action that needs to be taken. Anti-oppressive practice then moves beyond descriptions of the nature of oppression to dynamic and creative ways of working. These ways of working, informed by a complex, critical, politicised and geopolitical view of our culturally plural society, will contribute to the development of relevant and appropriate services. The principles of reflexivity, social difference, historical and geographical location, the personal as political, and an understanding of power and powerlessness, together with the act of challenging, provide a framework that can be used to inform work with people in need.

Conclusion

Through the use of a real practice situation we have made visible some of the complexities of the broader societal patterns of discrimination and oppression that can be replicated in the micro-relationships of service user and practitioner. In our analysis of Amelia's experiences, our intention was to signal the dangers of replicating these patterns of oppression, and so challenge the individual worker to be aware and appreciate the potential impact that their gender, cultural background, sexuality, class, ability and other differences can have in shaping and determining their relationship with those who are deemed as 'other'. To practice anti-oppressively, we need to be ethnically sensitive, self-aware, reflective and reflexive if we are to develop the capacity to engage in open and honest dialogue with service users and other professionals.

For further discussion of anti-oppressive perspectives, see Adams et al., 2009a, Chapter 5, and for issues in emancipatory research, see Adams et al., 2009c, Chapter 25.

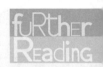

Clifford, D. (1998) *Social Assessment Theory and Practice*, Aldershot, Ashgate. Provides a theoretically informed anti-oppressive framework for undertaking assessments. Looks at the personal, structural and methodological dynamics that impinge on the assessment process and demonstrates his ideas in relation to a practice example.

Healy, K. (2005) *Social Work Theory in Context: Creating Frameworks for Practice*, Basingstoke, Palgrave Macmillan. Outlines critical theoretical perspectives and approaches including the strengths perspective and anti-oppressive practice as well as look at the links between theory, context and skills.

Humphries, B. (ed.) (1996) *Critical Perspectives on Empowerment*, Birmingham, Venture Press. Interrogates the concept of empowerment and raises questions about the political context in which debates about empowerment take place.

O'Hagan, K. (2001) *Cultural Competence in the Caring Professions*, London, Jessica Kingsley. Explores the ideas and definitions of 'culture' and 'cultural competence' and their relevance for health and social care practice.

Spencer, S. (2006) *Race and Ethnicity: Culture, Identity and Representation*, London, Routledge. Provides a range of theoretical perspectives on race and ethnicity and links the analysis of race and racism with ideas regarding the nature of identity and culture.

Walker, A. (1983) *The Color Purple*, London, Women's Press. First-person account of domination and abuse, it is also a story of recovery and the love and support that women can offer to each other.

20 Postmodern and constructionist approaches to social work

Chapter overview

This chapter explores what postmodernism means and how the ideas associated with it relate to social work. It examines some of the debates about the nature and relevance of modernist and postmodernist ideas, concluding that they cannot be dismissed as unduly negative. On the contrary, they have much in common with views of social work as inherently uncertain, characterised by a diversity of perspectives and perceptions rather than one 'truth'.

It is only in the last twenty years that postmodern and social constructionist perspectives have been drawn upon to think about, analyse and directly contribute to social work practice (see, for example, Howe, 1994; Parton, 1994; Hall, 1997; Leonard, 1997; Meinert et al., 1998; Chambon et al., 1999; Jokinen et al., 1999; Pease and Fook, 1999; Fawcett et al., 2000; Healy, 2000; Parton and O'Byrne, 2000; Taylor and White, 2000; Hall et al., 2003; Gorman et al., 2006). In many respects, the starting point was the recognition that social work had been experiencing a major period of change and uncertainty in its organisation and day-to-day practice, such that it seemed qualitatively different from what went before and so requiring new skills and new forms of knowledge in order to practise. Social work's engagement with postmodern and constructionist perspectives is a recognition that these changes and experiences are not particular to social work but reflect much wider transformations in Western societies and have been the subject of considerable and often heated debate within social theory. More particularly, the significance of postmodern perspectives is that they draw attention to a number of areas of social transformation in terms of:

- the increasing pace of change
- the emergence of new complexities and forms of fragmentation
- the growing significance of difference, plurality and various political movements and strategies, and the pervasive awareness of relativities

- the opening up of individual 'choice' and 'freedom'
- the increasing awareness of the socially constructed nature of existence.

Perhaps most centrally, such perspectives have reactivated a question that has lain dormant in social theory for many years but which touches the heart of much social work – what kinds of human beings have we become (Rose, 1996)?

At the outset, however, it is important to recognise that the term 'postmodern' has been hotly contested so that it is almost impossible to impose, by definitional fiat, an agreed set of terms for the debates (Turner, 1990). While the primary concern has been to consider how far and in what ways 'current times' are different from what has gone before, a number of commentators have argued that it is inappropriate to periodise history in this way (Heelas et al., 1996), that the changes and breaks have been exaggerated (Clark, 1996) and that, rather than characterise the present in terms of the postmodern, it is better characterised as high or late modern (Giddens, 1990, 1991). It is for this reason that I have previously consciously used parenthesis for the '(post)modern', pointing to a provisional and somewhat sceptical use of the term (Parton, 1994), and have argued that postmodern interpretations are in danger of not taking the situation of actually living human actors sufficiently seriously (Parton, 1998b). Even so, the debates provide an important vehicle for developing our insights into the nature of the contemporary complexities, uncertainties and experiences, and for opening up new and creative ways of thinking and acting.

Certainly, reference to the postmodern is much older than the recent fashion in social theory might suggest and goes back many years in art history and aesthetic theory (Featherstone, 1988). The term 'postmodernism' was first used in the 1930s but became increasingly used in the areas of literature, architecture, philosophy and the arts more generally from the 1960s onwards (Turner, 1990; Smart, 1999). The perspective came to particular prominence with the publication of Lyotard's *The Postmodern Condition* in 1984. While postmodern perspectives are united by a number of cultural projects that claim a commitment to heterogeneity, fragmentation and difference, it is perhaps their critiques of modernity that have proved most influential but contentious.

As a summary term, 'modernity' is seen to refer to the cluster of social, economic and political systems that emerged in the West with the Enlightenment in the late eighteenth century. Unlike the premodern, modernity assumed that human order is neither natural nor God-given, but is vulnerable and contingent. However, by the development and application of science, nature could be subject to human control. The distinguishing features of modernity are seen to be:

- the understanding of history as having a definite and progressive direction
- the attempt to develop universal categories of experience
- the idea that reason can provide a basis for all activities
- the idea that the nation-state could coordinate and advance such developments for the whole society.

The guiding principle of modernity is the search to establish reliable foundations for knowledge. It aims to identify central truths about the world but also assumes that truth does not reside on the surface of things but is hidden by appearances. The two crucial elements of modernity in the post-Enlightenment period were thus seen as the progressive union of scientific objectivity and politicoeconomic rationality (Parton, 1994).

In the modern 'frame', the goal is to produce knowledge about a chosen aspect of the physical or social world by which we can claim greater certainty. At that point, we can confer a sense of truth about that knowledge, and also confer on the people producing knowledge, for example scientists or professionals, the status of holder of truth and expert about that aspect of the world. In short, the modernist equation is:

> external reality – objective knowledge – certainty about that knowledge – claim to truth – expert status given to holder-of-truth/knowledge. Modernist truth is indeed bound to certainty, external reality and objective knowledge for modernism both relies on (and produces) a clear splitting of the subject who wants to know and the object which is being observed for knowledge and truth. (Flaskas, 1997: 5)

Increasingly, however, there is a recognition that we now inhabit a world that has become disorientated, disturbed and subject to doubt. The pursuit of order and control, the promotion of calculability, belief in progress, science and rationality and other features that were so intrinsic to modernity are being undermined by a simultaneous range of unsettling conditions and experiences. In part this is related to the major social, economic and cultural transformations that have characterised recent times in terms of:

- globalisation
- the increasing significance of the media and the widening networks of information technology, which transform and transmit knowledge
- the changes in modes of consumption and production
- the increased awareness of risk and uncertainty.

Social work and the postmodern

Howe (1994) has usefully outlined the possible significance of such debates for social work. His central argument is that, if social work was a child of modernity, it now finds itself in a world uncertain of whether or not there are any deep and unwavering principles that define the essence of its character and hold it together as a coherent enterprise.

He suggests that not only can the emergence of social work from the mid-nineteenth century onwards be seen as a particular manifestation of the development of the modern, but also that the three traditional cornerstones of social work – care, control and cure – can be seen as particular manifestations of modernity's three great projects. Howe (1994: 518) suggests that:

> in its own way social work has pursued the beautiful (aesthetics), the good (ethics) and the true (science) as it attempts to bring about a pleasing quality of life and a just society by using the insights of the social sciences.

Howe (1994) and Parton (1994) both suggest that the high point of modern social work in the UK came in the 1970s when major attempts were made to rationalise and reorganise social work's practices, skills and approaches. This was exemplified by the creation of unified social services departments and the generic social worker at the organisational and practice level and the search for a common base for social work (Bartlett, 1970) via the development of the systems approach (Pincus and Minahan, 1973) and integrated methods (Specht and Vickery, 1977).

However, Howe (1994) suggests that contemporary social work is, in many respects, experiencing a number of features that have been characterised as symptomatic of the postmodern condition. Modernism's promise to deliver order, certainty and security has been unfulfilled, and it is increasingly felt that there are no transcendental universal criteria of truth (science), judgement (ethics) and taste (aesthetics). The overriding belief in reason and rationality is disappearing, as there is a collapse of consensus related to the 'grand narratives' and their articulation of progress, emancipation and perfection, and what constitutes the centres of authority and truth. The rejection of the idea that any one theory or system of belief can ever reveal the truth, and the emphasis on the plurality of truth and 'the will to truth', captures some of the essential elements associated with postmodern approaches.

Truth takes the guise of 'truth' centred neither in God's word (as in the premodern) nor in human reason (as in the modern), but is decentred and localised so that many 'truths' are possible, dependent on different times and places. Notions of 'truth' are thus related to context and are culture specific so that there is a refusal to accept that some groups have a monopoly on what constitutes truth, beauty and the good. Relativities, uncertainties and contingencies are no longer seen as marginal and problems to be overcome as yet beyond the reach of reason, but as central and pervasive. In fact, the modern approach, rather than being humanitarian, progressive and emancipatory, is seen as invariably exploitative and repressive because of its failure to recognise difference and its reliance on totalising belief systems.

The importance of discourse and language

These developments have contributed to new ways of understanding the self in context, which question the central assumptions of human nature and models of the person encoded in professional knowledge and derived from the modernist projects of sociology and psychology. Language is seen as central:

> An understanding of the part that language plays in the formation of human selves, human thought and human subjectivity underpins the postmodern perspective. (Howe, 1994: 521)

Instead of being described as a tool that simply reflects objects, language is seen as mediating and constituting all that is 'known'. Reality is not just obtrusive, but is also embedded within interpretation and 'language games' (Lyotard, 1984), so that 'truth' is a product of language. We cannot transcend the influence of interpretation and assume that reality is simply waiting to be discovered; it is constituted and constructed within language.

If it is the way in which language is structured that provides us with the basis for our notion of selfhood, personal identity and the way in which we relate to social 'reality', a central part of such approaches is to look at the way language is structured, used and accomplished in any situation. It is in this sense that the notion of discourse becomes key. For while such approaches give particular weight to the linguistically constituted character of reality, it does not mean that discourses are 'mere words'. 'Discourses' are structures of knowledge claims and practices through which we understand, explain and decide things. In constituting agents, they also define obligations and determine the distribution of responsibilities and authorities for different categories of person, such as parents, children, social workers, doctors, lawyers and so on. A discourse is best understood as a system of possibilities for knowledge and agency that makes some actions possible while precluding others. It is a system of possibility that allows us to produce statements which are either 'true' or 'false'.

Thus, whereas modernity assumes that increasing knowledge of the real world produces power, postmodernity reverses the formula, recognising that the formation of particular discourses creates contingent centres of power, which define areas of knowledge and truth claims, and frameworks of explanation and understanding. Those with power can influence language and discourse and can therefore influence the way in which life is experienced, seen and interpreted. However, because there is a range of different contexts, cultures and discourses available at any one time and place, there is also a plethora of different meanings, knowledges and truths available and many experiences and interpretations of self and identity. Notions of plurality and difference are widespread. Thus we should proceed on the recognition that language does not simply reflect or mirror objects, events and categories existing in the social and natural world – it actively constructs those things. Words do not simply describe things, they do things and thus have social and political implications.

Implications for practice

It has been suggested, however, that the implications for politics, policy and practice of such perspectives are at best ambiguous and at worst undermine many of the central values and principles of social work itself. Similarly, they may neglect the salience of issues of inequality in a simple celebration of difference. Postmodern perspectives have been criticised for being overly relativistic, nihilistic, negativistic and anarchistic, failing to recognise the importance of agency and resistance, and overturning the past in a way that does not take heed of the positive and progressive elements that have previously gone on under the umbrella of social work (Smith and White, 1997). Such criticisms indicate that social work must be wary of such perspectives, for it is essentially a practice where decisions have to be made and practitioners have to act. Although practitioners need to develop a critical reflexive awareness, they must also feel sufficiently confident to act. The contemporary challenge for social work is to take action, which demands that we have made up our mind, while being open-minded.

In this respect, Rosenau (1992) provides an important contribution in characterising postmodern perspectives along a continuum from the sceptic to the affirmative postmodernist. Although it is difficult to accommodate the sceptic perspective, with its nihilistic stance on truth and other absolutes, within social work, the emphasis of the affirmative postmodernist on 'truth redefinition' rather than 'truth denying' is potentially much more suggestive. Rosenau's interpretation of an affirmative postmodern vision demonstrates that, while it cannot offer truth, it is not without content. It is interpretative and its focus is receptivity, dialogue, listening to and talking with the other. It reveals paradox, myth and enigma, and it persuades by showing, reminding, hinting and evoking rather than by constructing theories and approximating truth. It is suggested that our focus should be narrative, fragmented fantasies and different stories. Social work takes on the guise of persuasive fiction or poetry.

Such an approach demonstrates that postmodern perspectives are not necessarily bleak or antisocial work but provide novel and creative insights that clearly talk to a number of themes and approaches which have been associated with social work for much of its history. It almost suggests that social work could be (re)interpreted as being postmodern all along. Many social workers will identify with approaches that blur the difference between fact and fiction, history and story, art and science (England, 1986), and which take the view that what an individual perceives or experiences as their reality is *the* reality, but a reality capable of change in an endless variety of ways.

There are now a number of attempts to develop and apply the positive elements of such an approach explicitly to social work practice. In the process, a number of themes and issues are illustrated that are of wide application and can be developed further in different contexts. Uncertainty is seen as central, for, as Pozatek (1994: 399) suggests, 'the acknowledgement of uncertainty is an essential element of the postmodern practice of social work' and such a position can push workers to make the effort to understand a service user's experience. A position of uncertainty is seen to represent a more respectful approach to cultural difference, as certainty and objectivity are an illusion. Social workers should not expect, therefore, to know in advance what the outcomes of interactions will be. They can, at best, only trigger an effect. A position of uncertainty means that social workers will approach each situation respectful of difference, complexity and ambiguity. Words are understood by clients according to how they have constructed the reality embodied in the interaction. It is thus essential for practitioners to be aware of this and construct, through dialogue with the client, a shared understanding and reality which they agree is a representation of their interaction. It is an approach which recognises that language is crucial for constituting the experiences and identity of both the self and the interaction, and which takes seriously the diverse elements of power involved. It is similarly serious about notions of partnership and participation, and potentially enables the views of service users to be prioritised. This is not to say, however, that such issues are self-evident and clear-cut. A commitment to uncertainty, indeterminacy and unpredictability will reinforce social workers' continual attempts reflexively to consider what they are doing, why and with what possible outcomes.

Sands and Nuccio (1992) have similarly identified a number of themes central to postmodern perspectives that can be drawn on in practice. Thus, rather than think and act according to 'logocentrism', assuming that there is a singular fixed logical order which is 'real' or 'true', practitioners need to recognise that there are no essential meanings. Definitions and interpretations are historically contingent and context bound and hence fluid. Similarly, logocentric thought promotes thinking in terms of binary opposites – male/female, black/white, adult/child, true/false – which are seen as mutually exclusive, categorical and hierarchical rather than interdependent. Such categories are usually embedded in language in a way that privileges some experiences and marginalises others. It is thus important explicitly to recognise the important, but fluid and changing nature of difference, so that the oppressed and devalued can have a voice and we can think and act in terms of both/and relational terms.

One way to recover suppressed meaning is through the key postmodern operation of 'deconstruction', whereby phenomena are continually interrogated, evaluated, overturned and disrupted. Deconstruction is a way of analysing texts, language and narratives that is sensitive to contextual dimensions and marginalised voices. The process of deconstruction recognises that, while multiple discourses might be available, only a few are heard and are dominant, these being intimately related to the dominant powers/knowledges. When one deconstructs, one does not accept the constructs as given but looks at them in relation to their social, historical and political contexts. Constructs are 'problematised' and 'decentred'. Through deconstruction, the presumed fixity of phenomena is destabilised, and the perspective of the marginalised can be given voice. It involves, among other things, helping people to externalise the problem, examining its influences on their life, reconstructing and liberating themselves from it. The notion of possibility (O'Hanlon and Beadle, 1994) recognises that things can be changed. A vision of possibility can be used to mobilise people's potential and competence, and can empower them to reclaim and redefine who they are and how they want to act.

However, we should not assume that postmodern perspectives are concerned with giving suppressed subjects a voice in any simple way. The notion of 'subjectivity' is itself complex. While, within a logocentric tradition, the individual is autonomous and (if healthy) integrated and has an essential subjectivity, identity, personality, this is not the case with postmodern perspectives. In the latter, subjectivity is precarious, contradictory and in process, constantly being reconstituted in discourses. Accordingly, the subject is multifaceted and speaks in many voices, depending on the sociocultural, historical and interpersonal contexts in which it is situated.

It is perhaps the emphasis on language and its intimate relationship with knowledge and power that provides the most distinctive message for practice arising from postmodern perspectives. A focus on social work as text, narrative and artistry, as opposed to social work as science, moves centre stage. Whereas science looks for explanations and causes, the story or narrative approach is intent on finding a meaningful account. As Howe (1993) has demonstrated, via his in-depth analysis of studies of what clients say about what they value from counselling and therapy, it is the latter that is important. Talking not only helps people to understand their experiences, but also allows them to control, reframe and move on. As Howe (1993: 193) states:

there are no objective fundamental truths in human relationships, only working truths. These decentred contingent truths help people make sense of and control the meaning of their own experience. This is how we learn to cope.

Such approaches emphasise process and authorship. An open-minded engagement with people's stories and the possibility of helping them to re-author their lives using more helpful stories can be both an empowering and respectful way of understanding situations and bringing about change.

Constructive social work

These ideas have been built upon in terms of the development of constructive social work (Parton and O'Byrne, 2000). The term 'constructive social work' was chosen for two reasons. First, to demonstrate a positive, strengths-based approach, and, second, to reflect the postmodern, discourse and social constructionist theoretical perspectives which inform it. The constructive approach, developed by Parton and O'Byrne, emphasises process, plurality of both knowledge and voice, possibility and the relational quality of knowledge. It is affirmative and reflexive and focuses on dialogue, listening to and talking with the other. Social work practice is seen as a specialised version of the process by which people define themselves, participate in their social worlds, and cooperatively construct social realities. It underlines both the shared building of identity and meaning that is the basis of effective practice, and the positive results for service users that stem from the approach.

Constructive social work is concerned with the narratives of solutions to problems, and with change; instead of providing the practitioner with information about the causes of problems, so that they can make an expert assessment and prescribe a 'scientific' solution, the service user is encouraged to tell the story of the problem in a way that externalises it, giving more control and agency and creating a new perspective on how to manage or overcome it. These narratives construct the future and anticipate change; questions encourage the service user to identify exceptions to the apparently overwhelming nature of problems – situations where they have done something that made a positive difference. Constructive social work develops techniques and thinking associated with 'solution-focused' (de Shazer, 1985, 1991, 1994; Miller, 1997), 'narrative' therapy (White and Epston, 1990; White, 1993), 'possibility' (O'Hanlon and Weiner-Davis, 1989; O'Hanlon, 1993; O'Hanlon and Beadle, 1994) and the 'strengths' (Saleeby, 1997) perspectives. The approach attempts to provide questions that elicit clear goals about what the service user wants, in their own words, and which involves them in doing something in the immediate future that can launch a new beginning. The practitioner's mode of address is one of 'curiosity and respectful puzzlement' (Parton and O'Byrne, 2000) at the service user's unique way of making things better, rather than expertise in fitting an intervention to a need. Service users are encouraged to repeat successes, to identify solutions as theirs and as steps to the achievement of their own goals.

Service users are invited to tell their stories using the cultural resources of their communities – local language and interpretation of the problem and the origins of their oppression and exclusion. The language of oppression, domination, subjugation, enslavement and recruitment is used in order to try and establish how the problem is dominating the person. The service user is then encouraged to distance themselves from the problem and to give it an unpleasant name, using their own metaphors. It can then be 'externalised' and 'politicised', in terms of the forces operating against empowerment and achievement in society, in terms of style, appearance, class, gender, race, ability, family relationships or whatever. The approach aims to defeat the stereotypes of the blaming official organisations, and offers service users new ways of giving an account of their situation in which their agency becomes central, and they begin to take control. This reduces conflict between the practitioner and the service user and prepares the ground for cooperation in trying to reduce the influence of the problem, and constructing possibilities and solutions. None of this reduces the accountability for mistakes, offences or the abuse of others, although it may challenge beliefs about more fundamental issues of self-worth and the potential for change. Thus, a key aspect of the approach is that it encourages service users to retell their stories in terms of courageous opposition to their disadvantages and heroic resistance to their problems.

Conclusion

In this chapter, I have attempted to outline a number of approaches and perspectives that have emerged over recent years which explicitly draw on and use ideas and concepts associated with postmodernism and social constructionism. In doing so, a range of creative, critical and challenging possibilities have been opened up – not only in terms of how we can understand and analyse contemporary social work but also in providing positive contributions to practice itself. In doing so, such approaches can be seen as being particularly pertinent to developing and refining the notion of reflective practice. As Imogen Taylor (1996: 159) has suggested, reflective practice and reflective learning may be conceptualised 'as a response to postmodernism, as a positive and creative approach to the prospect of living with contingency'. In a world of uncertainty and rapid change, reflective practice offers the possibility of developing strategies for learning how to learn and how to practise in a self-conscious way. The concern is less with developing our knowledge than with developing and deploying our capacities for reflexivity and action.

For further discussion of postmodernist perspectives, see Chapter 17, and for the wider 'ideas' context of social work, see Adams et al., 2009a, Chapter 6.

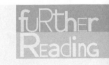

Fawcett, B., Featherstone, B., Fook, J. and Rossiter, A. (eds) (2000) *Practice and Research in Social Work: Postmodern Feminist Perspectives*, London, Routledge. This wide-ranging and lively book considers a range of key issues and possibilities in response to the question of what it means, practically, to research and practise from a postmodern feminist point of view.

Gorman, K., Gregory, M., Hayles, M. and Parton, N. (eds) (2006) *Constructive Work with Offenders*, London, Jessica Kingsley. Contributors from a range of settings draw on constructive approaches to critically reflect on the current state of policy and practice with offenders and demonstrate ways of working that emphasise the importance of working with strengths, being creative and being critically reflective.

Leonard, P. (1998) *Postmodern Welfare: Reconstructing an Emancipating Project*, London, Sage. From a critical perspective founded in Marxism and feminism, draws on elements of postmodern deconstruction to consider the current state and future of social work and welfare more generally.

Parton, N. and O'Byrne, P. (2000) *Constructive Social Work: Towards a New Practice*, Basingstoke, Macmillan – now Palgrave Macmillan. Provides a detailed critical approach to practice that explicitly draws on concepts and insights derived from social constructionism, postmodernism and narrative perspectives.

Taylor, C. and White, S. (2000) *Practising Reflexivity in Health and Welfare: Making Knowledge*, Buckingham, Open University Press. Provides an in-depth analysis of the idea of professional reflexivity, drawing on social constructionism and discursive psychology. Explores how knowledge is used in professional practice, and how it is made and generated in everyday encounters.

Dedication

This chapter was originally drafted and planned with Wendy Marshall, who died on 26 March 1997. It is dedicated to Wendy's memory and her considerable contribution to social work education and practice. She is much loved and missed.

Part 3

DEVELOPING CRITICAL PRACTICE

INTRODUCTION

We move on in this part of the book to explore the main areas of social work practice. Chapter 1 explored what is entailed in becoming critical. This has set the scene for the book. Part 1 has tackled aspects of the values that inform practice. In Part 2, we have seen the range of social work theories and approaches on which social workers draw. In Part 3, we move on to consider how critical practice develops in different fields of practice.

We begin by examining what it means to sustain a critical approach in practice (Chapter 21). Then we consider in turn, chapter by chapter, a series of basic areas of practice: safeguarding children (Chapter 22); fostering and adoption (Chapter 23); working with looked-after children and young people in residential care (Chapter 24); family-based practice (Chapter 25); youth justice (Chapter 26); safeguarding adults (Chapter 27); care management (Chapter 28); mental health practice (Chapter 29); physical disability (Chapter 30); learning disability (Chapter 31); work with older people (Chapter 32); end-of-life care and bereavement work (Chapter 33). These chapters are linked by exploring what critical practice means, awareness of the issues involved in developing a critical practice and where appropriate, highlighting its capacity to transform social work.

Being a critical practitioner 21

Chapter overview

This chapter delves into what is entailed in becoming a critically reflective practitioner and argues that the complexity, uncertainty and unpredictability of people's problems require critically reflective social work. We deal in turn with the concepts, contexts, perspectives, process and applications of critical reflection in practice.

Concepts: being and doing 'reflective and critical'

In this chapter we continue the process we began in Chapter 1 of this book. We take the same topic here, but instead of viewing it conceptually from above, we go into its application. In order to reach applications, however, we do need to revisit the concepts and theoretical aspects in more detail than previously.

Critically reflective practice is a concept that is sufficiently plastic and open-edged to be allied with any one of many theoretical perspectives, yet is sufficiently firm to be able to support an in-depth process of inquiring practice. While this seems to be an ideal situation, it actually makes the situation of critically reflective practice somewhat problematic, situated as it is among the ever-expanding wealth of literature on social work theories, approaches and practice. Fook and Gardner (2007: 128) acknowledge a diversity of perspectives and understandings of the concept of critically reflective practice, a lack of consensus, experience of it as being rather uncertain and its outcomes often somewhat difficult to predict.

Having said that, there is widespread acceptance among qualifying social work programmes and individual academics and practitioners of the value of developing reflectiveness and criticality in practice. Yet the idea of being a critically reflective practitioner is more appealing and less challenging to students and practitioners than carrying it out in practice. At the same time, there is a danger of adopting the 'talk' of critical reflection without recognising that it is not, and should not be, detached from theory.

We shall come to the words 'critical' and 'reflection', but before this we need to acknowledge the notion embedded in many texts, namely that 'reflectiveness' is a state of being as much as something you do.

What do the words 'reflection' and 'critical' mean in practice? Doing reflection critically is not at all the same as reaching an understanding of it. Reflection may seem straightforward because it is the same word used in everyday speech to mean 'thinking about' or 'considering'. However, the extensive literature on reflective practice makes it clear that the process of acquiring knowledge and understanding from reflection is complex and demanding.

Critically reflective practice combines two quite distinct aspects of being a practitioner – being reflective and being critical. Is there any real difference between being reflective and being critical? Surely, if we are reflective, this entails being critical? This is not the case, as we can see by identifying some key questions associated with different activities related to evaluation of practice: reflection and critical reflection (Table 21.1).

Table 21.1 Some key questions associated with reflection and critical reflection

Reflection	What happened?
	How did it compare with previous experience?
	How did I do?
Critical reflection	How well did I do?
	What could I have done better?
	What could I have done differently?

In the context of working with managers, Oldham (2002: 3) suggests that the term 'critical reflection' may be a tautology. She uses Cowan's (1998) distinction between analytical reflection – 'How do I do it?' – and evaluative reflection – 'How well can I do it?' – as the preliminary to arguing that evaluative reflection is critical 'in the sense of exercising discernment and making judgement' (Oldham, 2002: 3). Oldham (2002: 3) adds that 'without such critical evaluation it would be difficult to complete the reflective process, and for the learning from reflection to result in action and improvement'.

Good social work requires critically reflective practice

The different professions working with people in the human services vary according to the weight they give to different components of the professional task and social work occupies a special position. In this chapter, we do draw on some literature beyond social work. However, social work deals with the specialness, the uniquely demanding – complex, unpredictable and uncertain – nature of some people's problems. Inevitably, these characteristics tend to mean that the more demanding cases are referred by other professionals to social workers. So doing social work well means doing it critically. Also, social work shares with other health and social professions the well-articulated notion of the reflexive cycle that links thinking and action.

This overlaps with the three domains that Brechin (2000) identifies as essential for successful caring work: critical action, critical reflexivity and critical analysis. Although distinct, these are inseparable components of critical practice. Inevitably, because critical thinking will use the experience of action and its outcomes to inform further thinking, critical practice is a cycle in which thinking is bound up with action. There is widespread acknowledgement, also, that critical theory and practice entail identifying and challenging injustice and power structures (Dalrymple and Burke, 2006; Thompson, 2006; Jones et al., 2008b). Accepting this, according to Fook et al. (2000: 212), reflectivity 'is about uncovering unintended assumptions which flavour (and often determine) practice, in order to improve practice by bringing it in line with intended theory'. Critical reflectivity also entails 'uncovering assumptions about power relations, in order to make practice more egalitarian and emancipatory'. We bear this distinction in mind as we construct the components that comprise the expertise of the critically reflective social worker.

Is critical practice also 'critical best practice'?

Jones et al. (2008b) have combined the notions of criticality and best practice in critical best practice (CBP). This is a brave attempt to move forward debates about social work by replacing what they call a widespread deficit model of practice with a best practice that aligns the radical element in social work with the best of what is practical, incorporating managerial, practitioner and user perspectives alongside social work theories. Jones et al. (2008c) maintain that doing this enables CBP to be skilfully supportive, therapeutic, authoritative and also able to challenge existing power structures.

According to Harry Ferguson (2008: 15), the 'critical' element of practice reflects how social theory is brought to bear in an analytic way and is 'the key reason why such practice can be regarded as 'best'. It is also 'best' in the sense that it promotes positive learning about social work 'by setting out examples of best practice; that is, outlining and analysing instances where it is argued that what social workers did was done well'. Best practice, apparently, is not synonymous with evidence-based approaches and 'what works', because it incorporates more than just outcomes, by focusing not only on what is done but how it is done (Ferguson, H. 2008: 27).

In the same volume, Ferguson (2008: 18) has raised the key question about critical best practice himself, in debating whether 'the notion of CBP seems like a contradiction in terms. For how can one be critical of something that is best?' His response is that CBP sets out examples of how critical practice can be done well; it is not perfect practice, but it is practice that acknowledges complexity (Ferguson, H. 2008: 33).

This brief summary enables us to see that critical best practice aspires to many of the goals we set out in Chapter 1 of this book and goes some way towards some of the detail set out in this present chapter. CBP highlights the value of pursuing the goal of criticality in practice, but because of the inherent contradiction between achieving 'best' practice and maintaining a constant 'criticality', the term 'best' unfortunately is somewhat of a misnomer, not least because it:

- indicates a correspondence with the 'best practice' of managerially dominated practice
- implies that perfection is already attained or is attainable.

Its preferred title would be 'good practice' or 'excellent practice', in other words, anything except 'best' practice. The critical practice we develop in this chapter, in my view, should merely claim it is preferred rather than it is best.

Contexts

Practice is affected fundamentally by different contextual factors. These are rooted in the policies and laws governing services for children, families and vulnerable adults. The character of providing organisations has a huge impact on practice as well. Arrangements for procuring, commissioning and contracting services set the context for day-to-day practice. Services are likely to be provided by a variety of statutory, voluntary and private agencies, organisations and groups. Since the 1970s, critical commentary has identified those features of social work organisations that induce certain responses in practitioners. Simpkin (1983) pointed to the alienation experienced by practitioners, and the consequences of managerialism in the 1980s onwards in terms of the powerlessness experienced by professionals in more regulated and proceduralised work conditions have been well documented (Clarke et al., 1994). The varying arrangements for providing services affect the work conditions of social work practitioners in different ways and we can identify three overarching factors affecting them: stress, uncertainty and complexity.

Stress is a major feature of the working environment of social workers and its nature, consequences and the responses to it have been researched extensively. Much of the literature is concerned with identifying how practitioners can find ways of coping with stress (Balloch, et al., 1995; Thompson et al., 1996; Davies, 1998).

Uncertainty is a feature of work in organisations faced by many practitioners. It particularly arises in social work where the cases are complex, the problems are unpredictable and the range of possible outcomes is not clear. A tension exists between the inherent uncertainties involved in practice and the strategies adopted by organisations in managing it. One of the main strategies is to try to reduce uncertainties by 'playing safe', that is, by managing risks. In some settings, risk management may dominate to the extent that decisions about cases are made more on the basis of minimising risk than benefit to the service user.

Complexity is an integral feature of much social work. Complexity arises in different ways:

- through the diversity, range and depth of people's problems
- because of the different roles required of the practitioner
- through different organisational arrangements for managing services
- because of the variety of multi-professional teams

- through the tasks associated with working in partnership with people who receive services and their carers
- through the range of different disciplines, substantive knowledge and skills on which practitioners draw in their work.

Perspectives

In social work, a perspective is a theoretical viewpoint, or a direction from which one regards a concept, approach, process or activity. Fook and Gardner (2007: 69–73) identify four main perspectives on critical reflection: reflective, reflexive, postmodern/deconstruction and critical social theory. Using this as the base, we can work out the general features of each perspective (Table 21.2).

Table 21.2 Four important perspectives on critical reflection

	Reflective	Reflexive	Postmodern/ deconstruction	Critical social theory
Theory	Implicit in practice	Ourselves and our contexts affect our practice	Dominant discourse masks multiple perspectives and realities	Power and subordinate as well as dominant beliefs are socially constructed
Professional practice	Practice is amenable to reflection	We are researchers and research tools	Our practice (including how we think and use language) questions how we support dominant interests without realising it	We examine how our actions may undermine the interests and perspectives we want to support and we develop ways of resisting and challenging them
Applications (particular usefulness)	We act as a tool to evaluate practice, carry out research into practice, develop practice theory	We act self-consciously as researchers with an understanding of how we influence the knowledge we create and our own beliefs	We excavate assumptions, views of a single 'truth', omitted perspectives, construction of identities, categories of theories, related knowledge, problems and assumed 'solutions', providing a range of different views of problems or situations	We act to develop emancipatory research and practice to challenge systems, structures and processes which sustain the interests of more powerful individuals and groups

Source: Based on Fook and Gardner, 2007: 69–73

Ideally, through reflection, we should be able to reach the point of developing our own practice from one of these major theoretical perspectives. Let us review the first two of these briefly, so as to fill out the theoretical concepts and perspectives embedded in each. We comment on postmodernist and critical perspectives in Chapter 1.

Reflective perspective

The aim of reflective perspectives is to focus attention systematically on what is happening and to pose questions that alert the practitioner to the learning from experience which is taking place.

Reflexive perspective

This is where we return to an aspect hinted at in the opening stages of this chapter – the presence in the concept of critically reflective practice of 'being' as well as 'doing'. We could summarise the literature by asserting that critically reflective practice is about a state of being as well as, or more important than, a commitment to doing. Reflexivity is a concept that connects with this idea because it recognises the importance, the relevance, of the person we are to what we do. The key to understanding reflexive perspectives is to grasp the contrast between two views:

- the 'positivist' view that knowledge is an objective reality out there waiting for the researcher or the practitioner to grasp it and understand it
- the reflexive view of the researcher or practitioner who recognises that a person who perceives social phenomena cannot be detached from them, but responds to them and this response has to be taken into account when carrying out practice and/or research.

Process

The processes of reflection and critical reflection in practice are dealt with particularly clearly by Schön and Fook, so we do focus on them in this chapter, mainly because they give illustrations of how students and practitioners work with practice teachers, mentors or coaches to understand and learn from experience. The most noteworthy feature of this work and the ever-growing literature around it is that we need particular skills in order to engage in critical reflection. Building on the work of Atkins (2000) and FitzGerald and Chapman (2000: 10), who write for a broader professional group including social workers, nurses and other professionals, our list includes expertise in:

- imaginative speculation
- creative thinking
- learning how to think rather than what to think
- self-awareness
- thinking about experiences
- describing experiences
- critically analysing situations

- synthesising experiences and learning
- developing new perspectives
- evaluating the learning gained and the learning process.

We consider two main phases of learning and practice development below: pre-qualifying and post-qualifying.

Pre-qualifying: educating the critically reflective practitioner

Initially, we can learn something useful from the literature on how professionals make the transition from pre-qualifying learning to qualified practice. We can understand professional practice more adequately once we have briefly visited the preparation for qualification. Pease and Fook (1999) make a strong case for us to deconstruct and reconstruct what goes on in social work practice, with reference to critical perspectives. Fook et al. (2000) have studied in detail the processes of pre-qualification and entry into the first years of qualified practice. The purpose of referring to it here is to expand our understanding of what is entailed in critically reflective practice. These authors point out that the terms 'deconstruction' and 'reconstruction' normally are used in conjunction with postmodern or poststructural perspectives. Their position is that they take on board reflective, feminist, experiential, postmodern and poststructural thinking in their analysis (Fook et al., 2000: 212). They liken deconstruction and reconstruction to 'a critical reflective process whose aim is to redevelop practice theory in the light of reflection' (Fook et al., 2000: 213). This 'provides a theoretical framework which guides deconstructive analysis towards aspects of behaviour, thinking and structural arrangements which support undesirable power relations' (Fook et al., 2000: 213). So, deconstruction from a critical perspective uncovers the inequalities and discrimination; reconstruction can reformulate practice theory and develop 'new conceptualisations which are more equitable' (Fook et al., 2000: 213).

Why is it so important for the not yet qualified practitioner to develop this critical approach? It is because this enables the person 'to recognise multiple perspectives, as part of the ability to work with multi facets of the whole context' (Fook et al., 2000: 213). So this critical approach enables the practitioner-to-be to appreciate multiple perspectives on a given practice situation and the reality that they may be not only diverse but contradictory and ever-changing.

Traditionally, the knowledge base for professional practice might have been assumed to be relatively stable and fixed, whereas the reality nowadays is that the knowledge base is in a state of flux (Fook et al., 2000: 214) (Table 21.3). The process of education and professional training should enable the emergent critical practitioner to 'locate themselves, their personal interpretations, experience and behaviour' (Fook et al., 2000: 214) in relation to this context of constant flux. However, as we indicated above, our critical stance enables us to locate within this ever-changing context the core of structural inequalities such as poverty, as well as the unjust exercise of power, which are structural features of many societies in the West as well as in developing countries.

Table 21.3 Traditional and critical postmodern perspectives on knowledge base

Traditional perspectives	Postmodern perspectives
Knowledge base is fixed, simple, unified and always the same	Knowledge base is adaptable, subject to constant change, complex and multifaceted

Source: Based on Fook et al., 2000: 214

Post-qualifying: what is the profile of the typical critical practitioner?

In criminology, there is a fashion for employing people to produce profiles of typical offenders. Let us look at this situation in reverse – at the profile of the typical critical practitioner working with any person who uses social work services. What makes up the profile of the critical professional? We can look back at the research carried out by Fook et al. (2000) into the development of professional learning to the point where practitioners can demonstrate expertise. They summarise their theory of learning for expertise as follows:

> Professional expertise involves the ability to create knowledge from experience in context, and the ability to transfer this knowledge to different situations. Our theory of professional expertise is thus a theory of contextual knowledge development, in particular the development of learning around procedural skills which are readily transferable across different contexts. *Expertise*, in this sense, is *context relevant*, but *not context dependent* – it is learnt in context, but what is developed is knowledge which allows this learning to be applied successfully in new and diverse situations. Expert knowledge is, therefore, generalisable because of its contextuality. It is *contextual*, rather than *context-free*. (Fook et al., 2000: 198)

Drawing on their expansion of this statement, we can define this person as aspiring to demonstrate the following seven characteristics in their practice, even if not always achieving this:

- criticality
- reflexivity
- contextuality, that is, this person ensures that the entire context of the worker and the person who uses services is present whenever there is work done with them
- connectedness, that is, this is a person working with the entire context, rather than with some aspects of it
- ability to transfer knowledge and skills to different situations
- ability to create their own ideas, that is, the ability to generate knowledge
- ability to develop theories, that is, able to create understandings based on their own critical reflections in and on their practice.

Contextuality is a key component of the expertise of the critically reflective practitioner. This is because it enables the practitioner to work in conditions of uncertainty.

In this event, contextuality means that the practitioner can transfer knowledge – 'knowledge of', that is, substantive knowledge based in different disciplines, and 'knowledge how to', that is, skills – to different circumstances. This can apply to existing knowledge applied to new contexts or new knowledge applied to existing contexts.

We shall now revisit Schön's work on the actual detailed practice of reflection, because this is one of his strengths.

Reflecting on practice

Inside this simple phrase 'reflecting on practice' is a multifaceted concept. Schön comes close to analysing the heart of the process of reflecting as we practise in his concept of reflection-in-action. According to Schön (1991: 129), the basis for reflection-in-action is that the practitioner:

- approaches each case as presenting unique practice problems, which are not immediately obviously given and can't be dealt with using standard theories or techniques
- does not seek a standard solution to these problems, often presented with controversy about the best means, about which problems to tackle and what role the practitioner should take
- seeks to distinguish the particular features of the problematic situation and design an appropriate response. The practitioner finds the situation problematic and so has to reframe it before proceeding.

Schön (1991: 129–30) breaks down the concept of reflective practice. He distinguishes reflection-in-action, which entails reflection as the action proceeds, from reflection-on-action, which is essentially retrospective. Reflection-in-action entails identifying new aspects of the situation and considering them while proceeding with the action, and is a way of responding to the above-described problems. Rolfe et al. (2001: 23) describe reflection-on-action as the process by which we change information into knowledge. However, as they admit, reflection does not only do this, but also 'challenges the concepts and theories by which we try to make sense of that knowledge' (2001: 23). According to Schön (1991: 137), the reflective practitioner adopts three particular approaches:

1   Bringing past experiences to bear on the unique problems presented by the person.
2   Using reflection creatively to develop new ways of perceiving these problems.
3   Creating new opportunities to experiment in reframing the problems, that is, trying to secure a fit between the person's problems and the way of framing them.

Schön relates practice to a model of research. He describes practice as distinctive from research, however, in that it is associated not just with understanding the person's situation but in bringing about change that potentially is transformational. The notion of making connections is vital to this, between the person's experience inside practice and outside it (Schön, 1991: 147–8). Termination of the process of practice occurs when the practitioner (and, one assumes, the person worked with) perceives changes judged to be 'satisfactory' (Schön, 1991: 151).

Schön crystallises the definition of reflection-in-action while discussing aspects of management and introduces the useful notion of the 'reflective conversation'. Reflection-in-action:

> consists in on-the-spot surfacing, criticising, restructuring, and testing of intuitive understandings of experienced phenomena, often it takes the form of a reflective conversation with the situation. (Schön, 1991: 241–2)

This idea of the reflective conversation is important. It has already surfaced when Schön (1991: 166–7) brings in another important distinction between reflection-in-practice and traditional experimental research. The research takes place and is finished, but the reflective conversation continues alongside the practice. This enables the practitioner to vary the reflection-in-practice according to the context and specific knowledge of other practitioners.

Reflective responses to management situations cannot be reduced to techniques. The manager has to be sensitive not only to the uniqueness of each situation but also to the presence of uncertainty and change. Schön regards reflective practice as having some characteristics of an art – an idea we encounter again below in the writing of Fook. Practice as art has two meanings according to Schön:

- as intuitive judgements and skill, the feeling for data, events, phenomena and action called 'knowing in practice'
- practice reflection on the context of action.

Putting Schön in perspective

We have reached the point where we can put Schön's notion of reflective practice in perspective. It is sufficient to encourage us to engage with the difficult task of thinking about our practice, but it is limited in the following ways:

- It is a descriptive theory of what we as practitioners consider rather than what we should do next.
- It is stronger on ideas about how to develop a perspective on, or framework for, our practice than on ideas about how we can locate our practice in its various contexts – of social science theories, policies, laws, organisational procedures, professional approaches and so on.
- It is rich in ideas about how we as practitioners should 'be' and develop, but sparse in ideas about how to translate 'being' into 'future actions'.
- It encourages us to reflect on where we are now and where our practice is, but does not require us to 'think outside the box', push the boundaries of our practice towards the unknown, the new, the transformation of present realities.

A fifth shortcoming arises not from Schon's ideas but from how they are often used. This limitation is a corruption of the notion of reflective practice, by regarding it simply as meaning recalling or revisiting it. I often read students' 'reflective diaries' and find they are nothing more than diaries of what has happened. The reflective element is hardly present or absent altogether. In other words, to attach the main elements of reflective practice to our practice as though it is simply another technique for recording what we have done is to run the risk of practising unreflectively.

Critical practice involves reflectiveness, but transcends it. One of the contributions of feminism has been to challenge the assumption that women should be content with achieving equal opportunities in a man's world, rather than changing this world. Reflection is apt to stop short of challenging in this way. Reflective practice contributes to critical practice but of itself is not sufficient. Reflection on its own views the situation unchanged, whereas critical practice is capable of change. Reflection on the situation as it is does not achieve transformation. Critical practice offers the prospect of transformation by not being bound by the status quo. The critical practitioner is capable of being deeply involved in a situation, while being detached from it and viewing it from an independent vantage point, bringing to bear on it contextual, theoretical and conceptual understandings. Thus, the critical practitioner can be both insider and outsider and can move between these positions.

There is a need to engage critically with the notion of reflectiveness and move beyond it. Criticality goes one stage beyond reflective practice by engaging with what we do next. Criticality is concerned with what lies beyond – the implications of our current reflection for future practice.

From reflective practitioner to critically reflective practitioner

So we move on now to identify the additional characteristics of the critically reflective practitioner, whom Fook et al. (2000: 180) refer to as the 'expert practitioner', that is, the practitioner who demonstrates 'expertise' beyond just exercising 'routine practised ability'. Not everybody would go along with the term 'expert', which is logically linked with the use of 'expertise', but to some conveys the image of a member of an elite group. However, substituting another word doesn't change the distinction they make between the 'experienced' practitioner and the 'expert' practitioner.

We can present the comparisons that Fook et al. (2000: 179) note with the work of Collins and Eraut in a tabular way (Table 21.4). Professional practitioners can expect to face both well-defined and ill-defined problems, and one of the characteristics of these is that they are unlikely to have control over when and how they occur and how they are defined. The expert practitioner needs to develop the ability to respond quickly and although there is evidence from research that it can take ten years to accumulate sufficient expertise to achieve 'international performance in a wide range of fields' (Fook et al., 2000: 180), the length of time it takes to build up the necessary experience to achieve this cannot be guaranteed. The quality of the experience – both learning and practice – during this period is the key factor, rather than the length of the experience. Expertise does not necessarily follow from any number of qualifications, levels of achievement or years of experience, but refers to a quality of practice.

Table 21.4 Competent, experienced, excellent and expert practice

Experienced practice	Expert practice (Collins, 1990)
Routinised and intuitive because has been internalised	Innovative and creative
Competent practice	**Excellent practice (Eraut, 1994)**
Proficient when working with well-defined problems within routine procedures	Displaying excellence with ill-defined problems in non-routine situations
Less qualified and experienced	More qualified and experienced

Essentially, the expert practitioner is reflexive, has the ability to think creatively, takes risks in conditions of uncertainty and exercises expertise in practising contextuality and connectedness. Rojek et al. (1988: 5) observe that critical practitioners need to be able to deal creatively with uncertainty rather than simply following prescriptions. The idea of 'transferability' is relevant here. The expert practitioner is able to make connections and exercise contextuality because of transferability. This is a feature of expert practice that is linked with these other different aspects. It is an aspect of contextuality and connectivity, since transferable practice makes connections and locates practice in its wider context. Transferability also relates to theories of and for practice. It indicates a way of using theories. It reflects confidence in using knowledge, both procedural and 'how to' knowledge. Critically reflective practice involves us in four key aspects of engagement (Table 21.5).

Table 21.5 Key aspects of engagement in critically reflective practice

Engaging with ourselves	Reflexivity
Engaging with knowledge, skills and understanding in more than one setting	Transferability
Engaging with boundaries between domains of being, learning and doing	Holism
Engaging relevant perspectives/settings/disciplines/approaches in practice	Contextuality

There is a detailed discussion of these aspects in Fook et al. (2000: 170–95). Table 21.6 develops a comparative analysis of the circumstances of less experienced and expert practitioners respectively.

Table 21.6 Less experienced and expert practitioners

	Inexperienced	Expert
Relations with context	Isolated from contextuality	Connected/contributing to/ constructing and changing
Relations with practice situation	Objective/apart from/above/ passive observer	Integrating/making links with
Reflexivity	Not open to self-awareness	Uses self in work with others
Degree of engagement with users	Intervention in/on users' lives	Involvement with users and carers
Extent of empowering practice	Service delivery focus	Empowering people focus
Relations with rules/ procedures	Following procedures	Creative practice – multi-level work, use of reflexivity
Extent of power to act	Disempowered practitioner	Empowered practitioner
Interconnectedness/ connectivity	Isolated and relatively powerless	Interconnected – gives sense of agency, potency and responsibility
Relations with values	Bound by compliance to inflexible rules	Subscribes to higher level values
Change orientation	Concerned with maintenance of people and services	Committed to bringing about change, at all levels

Applications: what it means to practise critically

Let us return to our initial discussion of critically reflective practice at the start of this chapter. We implied that the critical reflectivity lay in the analysis of the situation, discovering structures of inequality and unfairness in the distribution and exercise of power. What is the point of analysis if we don't use it? The next step is to argue that critical practitioners do something about this, in developing practice that is empowering and emancipatory, in order to challenge these injustices and aspects of oppression. This is the inescapable logic of developing connectivity and contextuality.

We can infer from the previous discussion that, by definition, because expertise moves the practitioner beyond routinised, procedural rule-following, there is not one expert way to do all social work. The critical practitioner has the knowledge and confidence to question and the expertise to match appropriate (practice) actions to the appropriate circumstances at the right time. Because practice situations are unpredictable, it follows that the practitioner develops the confidence to make different kinds of judgements in differing circumstances about how to proceed.

Theoretical perspectives are essential tools that are likely to enable us to develop our critical grasp of social work. Dipping into the literature on inclusion, we can see from the work of Clough and Corbett (2000: 145) how from this initial viewpoint our progress towards 'becoming' critical practitioners is likely to go through the following five stages:

1   *Links:* We begin by making links. We examine our own biography and discuss with other people their own biographies. We identify how our own history through life experience and general work experience connects with the specific field of social work practice.

2   *Ground clearing:* We do some personal 'ground clearing', that is, we recognise that our views – how we regard our world – give shape to our theoretical perspective. More than this, it is not what goes on, but how we interpret it, that affects us.

3   *Accept ignorance, uncertainties and change:* We relax and learn to live with our uncertainties about some topics and our ignorance of others. We have noted that as we discuss and read, our ideas are constantly developing. We accept that it is 'normal' to change our theoretical perspective as we read, learn and develop.

4   *Self-critical scrutiny:* We develop the habit of subjecting our practice and our views to self-critical scrutiny. This is a more sustained process than 'ground clearing' and recognition. It entails a systematic examination of our own intellectual and emotional connections with, and responses to, what we are doing. It involves us analysing these, as far as we can.

5   *Manage tensions and complexities:* We grapple with the complexities raised by this process and we learn to manage the tensions. Realistically, this is the best we can do, accepting that we cannot resolve tensions and we cannot abolish complexity. These are both inherent in the subject matter of our studies and practice. They are what Clough and Corbett call a 'natural process of intellectual growth, not a weakness'. We accept that this process is untidy and may be painful. It is also unending. The further we delve into it the more complex it may seem to become.

We can try to summarise at this point what critically reflective practice is not and what it may potentially provide in practice (Table 21.7).

Table 21.7 Clarifying the potential applications of critically reflective practice

What critically reflective practice is not	What critically reflective practice may offer
Critically reflective practice is not: ■ negative comment ■ learning gained through therapy ■ critical feedback ■ criticism	Critically reflective practice can offer: ■ more than one way of understanding practice ■ holistic accounts of practice ■ entry to developing practice theory ■ a way of designing and carrying out practice-based research

It is worth bearing in mind that critical reflection on practice and researching practice are close neighbours. Critical reflection is likely to cross and recross boundaries between doing, evaluating, thinking, researching and doing again; in the process, it is likely to encourage practitioners to take more responsibility for developing more accountable strategies for both research and applications to practice.

Table 21.8 sets out the main components of an agenda for developing our critically reflective practice. This consists of four main aspects: developing a critical culture in the organisation, developing an infrastructure to support critical practice, developing the practice of criticality and developing a research-minded critical practice.

Table 21.8 Developing our critically reflective practice

Developing a critical culture in the organisation
Cultivating a culture of critical practice
Open exchange of opinions
Non-judgemental, no-blame culture
Developing an infrastructure to support critical practice
Management forum
Mentoring
Co-supervision
Practice forum
Developing the practice of criticality
Considered risk-taking
Purposeful innovation
Creativity
Developing a research-minded critical practice
Evaluative and exploratory
Multi-method, not just methodological variety
Qualitative as well as quantitative
Posing many questions/problems from different/competing perspectives

Conclusion

This chapter has explored in some detail the journey from being an experienced to expert practitioner, from reflectivity to critical reflectivity. We have set out the reasons – basically, the complex, uncertain and unpredictable nature of people's problems – why social work must have critical practitioners. We conclude that we should be developing in ourselves, and encouraging in others, a practice that is thoughtful, questioning, properly hesitant, critical and self-critical. We should encourage a style of reflection and action that does not follow the majority line and refuses to take the easy route. We should applaud practice that takes risks purposefully in the interests of empowering people who use services. Critical practice should be creative and courageous. Critical practice may be the only practicable and ultimately safe response to some of the more difficult – complex and unpredictable – cases that social workers face. It should be mainstream practice for all social work agencies and practitioners.

For further discussion of the practicalities of preparing for practice, see Adams et al., 2009a, Chapter 25, and for perspectives on handling complexity and uncertainty, see Adams et al., 2009c, Chapter 2.

Fook, J. and Gardner, F. (2007) *Practising Critical Reflection: A Resource Handbook*, Maidenhead, Open University Press. Helpful and up-to-date source of thoughtful material on critically reflective practice.

Schön, D. (1991) *The Reflective Practitioner: How Professionals Think in Action*, Aldershot, Ashgate. Useful source of relevant, if dated, material, particularly on reflective practice.

Thompson, N. and Thompson, S. (2008) *The Critically Reflective Practitioner*, Basingstoke, Palgrave Macmillan. Introductory text that marries discussion of theory with practical strategies and skills.

Safeguarding children 22

Critical practice can be sustained in the fraught field of safeguarding children if workers constantly reflect on how their work is measuring up to their vision and values, use knowledge proactively but tentatively as working hypotheses, and openly negotiate the various imbalances of power.

Chapter overview

EXAMPLE

The critical practitioner

We met quite by chance that day in the college car park. I (JP) was on the way to my office and Peter was arriving for the first day of a post-qualifying childcare course. Ten years ago we had spent a lot of time in each other's company. We were both active trade unionists, involved politically and intent on making a positive difference through social work. Changes in both our lives, domestic, work, political, had taken us in different directions. On the odd occasions that we met, we exchanged a few words, but on this occasion, we agreed to meet later that day and 'catch up'. When we did, we talked about a lot of things including why Peter was doing the course. Unusually, he had stayed in frontline practice. Not unusually, he often felt overwhelmed and dragged down as he struggled with the crises and chronic difficulties that beset the families he worked with, particularly where safeguarding children was an issue. Over the years, he had used courses as a way of re-energising himself. He was on this one to see if there was any new thinking around that could help him develop in a useful way his critical perspective on the steady stream of government initiatives that he and his frontline colleagues were constantly being told they had to keep up with.

I was not surprised to hear Peter's reason for coming on the course. He had always resented and resisted what he saw as the distortion of social work with families by the 'protocolization' of practice (Munro, 2004). I was more surprised that he had also held on to what had been our shared view that a searching, critical perspective was the best way to inform the under-standing, decisions and actions of practitioners. For us, critical theory had never been 'a God too far' (Cohen, 1975) – a retort that in some form or other has greeted every attempt to kindle critical engagement within social work, whether from a Marxist, feminist, black or postmodernist perspective. Critical theory, to borrow a phrase from Price and Simpson (2007: 4) in their promotion of sociology for social work, 'prises open the contradictions'. For me, that unmask-ing of the taken for granted in a way that reveals its hidden dynamic is a core responsibility of a social work academic. For Peter, it was a part of being able to cope with the daily grind of practice.

Safeguarding children from abuse and neglect based on a critical perspective demands constant questioning: not only of personal actions, both the worker's own and those of their colleagues, but also of structural constraints and opportunities, organisational and societal. Most importantly, it requires a critical questioning of the relationship between personal action and those structural opportunities and constraints – criticism not in the sense of blame but as the development of informed judgement on which to base effective action. While time away from direct practice may be useful for reflection and preparation, critical questioning can only really be addressed in the context of the day-to-day delivery of services. This is not an easy task, especially in an area as fraught and demanding as safeguarding children, but it is possible. It requires consistently coming back to three questions:

- How is practice measuring up to the worker's vision and values?
- What working hypotheses are being tested in practice?
- How is the balance of power being negotiated?

Values: measuring up to a vision

In getting beneath the surface of safeguarding practice, a critical perspective makes explicit the vision and values that constitute the broad ideological context and the personal ideology of practitioners. The challenge is for practitioners:

> to locate themselves, as fully conscious participants, within arenas where understand-ing and action will be contested, [which requires them] to develop a conscious ideological position of their own. (Spratt and Houston, 1999: 315)

Peter used to debate the difference between values and ideology and why the former got a good press while the latter was generally viewed with suspicion. In a dated but still useful discussion of ideology and power, Therborn (1983: 15), a Marxist sociol-ogist, notes:

> The operation of ideology in human life basically involves the constitution and pattern-ing of how human beings live their lives as conscious, reflecting initiators of acts in a structured, meaningful world.

He makes it clear that ideology is neither a rigidly imposed world view nor 'false consciousness' – meanings often associated with the term. Indeed, it is more than just sets of ideas. Ideologies are expressed in the way in which a social worker dresses, the furnishing of an interview room or the holding of a case discussion in a family's sitting room, rather than a social services office, as much as it is expressed in the ideas that hold sway at a case conference.

The dominant ideologies within the societal context and the organisational structures in which social work practice take place are neither intrinsically right nor wrong, accurate nor inaccurate. The ideas and practices of existing ideologies, and how they are expressed, endorsed or challenged in the personal ideology of individual workers, provide the meanings required to engage in life as social actors. These meanings express contested views – not only of how the world is, but also how it should be and how it could be. Although no longer politically active, Peter still held to a socialist view of the world. Even in the way he dressed, you could see he was holding out against 'the suits' of public sector managerialism. He was still angry about how the years of New Right Conservatism had undermined confidence and pride in the welfare state and in particular in what it had done for generations of children. He resented the 'unholy trinity' of factors (Ayre, 2001: 888) that had shaped practice with children and families following the inquiries into the tragic deaths of Victoria Climbié, Jessica Chapman and Holly Wells:

- the aggressive public pillorying of those the mass media deemed responsible
- the evermore detailed recommendations for implementation by overburdened welfare agencies
- the issuing by central government of increasingly prescriptive practice guidance.

Peter's initial optimism on the election of New Labour had given way to despondency that market-oriented economics were driving the social agenda inspired by a 'New Authoritarianism' imported from the US (Jordan and Jordan, 2000). While there were ambitious plans for tackling child poverty and social exclusion, these seemed predicated on meeting economic rather than social justice targets (Social Exclusion Task Force, 2007). He did, however, draw confidence from the way that the United Nations Convention on the Rights of the Child of 1989 (UNCRC; www.unicef.org/crc/) had established itself as the touchstone for policy and practice in all aspects of child welfare, including safeguarding. This was apparent in the development of cross-governmental strategies, such as *Every Child Matters* (DfES, 2004), aimed at promoting children's best interests through focusing on outcomes that every child should expect to achieve.

For Peter, the UNCRC provided a global vision for children that was immediately relevant for him in its bold assertion of three key principles:

- children's rights to be available without discrimination of any type (Article 2)
- children's best interests to be a primary consideration in all actions concerning them (Article 3)
- children's views to be sought and taken into account in all matters affecting them (Article 12).

He welcomed the appointment, in each of the UK's four nations, of commissioners for children and young people charged with promoting the rights of children as enshrined in the UNCRC. In addition, Article 19 of the Convention sets out in two paragraphs the obligation of states to protect children from all forms of maltreatment perpetrated by parents or others responsible for their care, and to undertake preventive and treatment programmes in this regard. Article 34 states in a single paragraph the child's right to protection from sexual exploitation and abuse, including prostitution and involvement in pornography. These were aims that Peter believed he was directly involved in pursuing through his safeguarding work. The UNCRC gave expression and status to his beliefs and developed them further in relation to promoting children's active involvement in determining their own lives.

Article 5 of the UNCRC also sets out the duty of states to respect the rights and responsibilities of parents and the wider family to provide appropriate direction and guidance to children in the exercise of their rights. It asserts in a preamble that:

> the family, as the fundamental group of society and the natural environment for the growth and well being of all its members and particularly children, should be afforded the necessary protection and assistance so that it can fully assume its responsibilities within the community.

For Peter, this balancing within the UNCRC of authority, responsibility and rights between state, children and families, which can also be found in the Children Act 2004 for England and Wales and related legislation within Scotland and Northern Ireland, reinforced his view of the state's enabling and resourcing responsibilities. It also reinforced his personal values. A critical perspective requires a capacity for self-criticism, which includes putting core personal values under scrutiny. A simple way to do that is for the social worker, either as an individual or as part of a group, to complete the sentence: 'Promoting the safeguarding of children expresses my/our belief that …'. For Peter, this would prompt statements such as:

- every child is a unique human being and their individual wishes and feelings must be respected
- the best interests of the child must always be the primary consideration of the adults they depend on
- children's views about their situation and what should happen to them should be listened to
- children have the right to a childhood free from all forms of abuse, neglect and exploitation.

But it would also prompt other value statements attaching rights not only to children but also to parents, the state and social workers themselves:

- parents have rights through their responsibilities to their children
- wherever possible, children should be brought up within their own families
- parents are individuals who deserve respect for their rights and the range of needs and strengths they have

- the state should be the ultimate guarantor of every child's right to safety and protection
- staff are individuals with needs and rights as well as being workers with authority and responsibilities.

Peter's experience had taught him that values are not neat, safe, 'feel good' phrases but challenging guides to action within particular circumstances. He had also found that some values, which may be regarded as of equal importance when considered in the abstract, compete against one another when applied in practice (McLoughlin and Pinkerton, 1995). Peter was constantly having to make judgements about the relevance and relative weighting to give to his different values according to the circumstances. This was not a weakness in his practice but one of 'the everyday creative accomplishments of professionals on the ground' (Spratt and Houston, 1999) as they engage in the social construction of their world.

Promoting the vision and holding to values consistent with the UNCRC is not just the responsibility of individuals like Peter. In signing the Convention, governments go beyond just declaring what 'should be' for children. They are also making a statement about what 'could be' and their regular reporting to the UN Committee is the means to monitor their progress in making it so. Among the many ways that governments have to express their commitment to the Convention is the work of staff who have responsibility for safeguarding children. Enabling workers to engage with every case as an expression of the Convention's vision for children at risk is an obligation of government. This requires that agencies and staff, families and neighbourhoods are provided with the necessary resources to identify and assess children at risk and to provide appropriate prevention and intervention programmes. Staff should not hold themselves responsible for failure to meet needs where resources are not made available by those with the power and authority to do so. A critical perspective draws attention to where the power to effect change actually lies (Parton, 2005). This is not to say that resource allocation is not the business of practitioners but rather to clarify that their responsibility can only be within the limits of their power. While they can exert pressure through collective action in trade unions, pressure groups, professional organisations and political parties, organisationally and structurally power over major resource allocation lies elsewhere.

Knowledge: testing working hypotheses

Peter's dogged optimism was based on his calculations and hopes for change. In delving beneath the surface of phenomena, critical theory assumes nothing to be constant. For social workers with safeguarding responsibilities, as in any other area of practice, change and how it is managed through defining and redefining needs and services dictates the circumstances in which they pursue their vision through practice. Change is absolutely central to any understanding of the present nature and future role of social work (Campbell and Pinkerton, 1997). It structures the context and is the focus for social work in safeguarding children. Social workers are expected to minimise the danger to children while maximising their welfare (Munro, 2002), but with the change management of risk goes uncertainty.

The history of child protection shows a number of stages on the way to the present day weakness in professional self-confidence (Corby, 2005). First there was the recognition during the 1970s of child abuse as a major issue for social services, represented by the tragic milestone of the Maria Colwell inquiry report. During the 1980s came the promotion of an assertive child protection as the dominant service response. This was first stoked by the findings of the various child death inquiries, such as Beckford, Henry and Carlisle, but then severely questioned by the reports into overintrusive intervention, such as Cleveland and Orkney. Growing concern about an overproceduralised child protection system was brought to a head in the 1990s with the publication of *Messages from Research* (DH, 1995a). From that review of the findings of 20 government-commissioned research projects, it was clear that however efficient the closed, professional child protection system might be, it was not effective. It was overidentifying children as being in need of protection and failing to respond appropriately to the varying types of need identified. The system was failing even on its own terms. In the wake of the Victoria Climbié tragedy in 2000, the focus shifted to one of promoting a culture of accountability for the safeguarding of children both within and across organisations (DfES, 2006). Following the events in Soham in 2002, there has been a renewed focus on the identification and management of adults who pose a risk to children. Workers, like Peter, who were always uncomfortable with the dominance of a narrow child protectionism, are now supported by the *Every Child Matters* agenda, with its assertion of the importance of interagency working in support of children and their families (DfES, 2004). They now find themselves better placed to retrieve something of their preferred style of practice as 'resourceful friends' (Holman, 1983). But this cannot mean a full return to the loose, enabling, problem-solving of the past. Change is not a circular movement.

Thanks to the years of preoccupation with child abuse and child protection, there is now a substantial and still growing literature that will ensure no return to the days before the 'discovery' of child abuse and the growth of complex child protection systems. Professional practice and academic study within social work, medicine, history, sociology, philosophy, social policy and psychology have all contributed to a much fuller understanding of abused children and their families and how best to respond to them. Work carried out within the English-speaking world of North America, the UK, Ireland, Australia and New Zealand is increasingly informed by European and international material (Harder and Pringle, 1997). It becomes evermore difficult for anyone, especially busy practitioners like Peter, to keep fully abreast of all this material. There is a growth in publications, particularly from government, which aim to systematically draw together practice experience. Organisations such as the Social Care Institute for Excellence (www.scie.org.uk) and Research in Practice (www.rip.org.uk) exist with the aim of bringing research to practitioners as and when they need it, using developments in new technology.

It is important to recognise, however, that while Peter is keen to draw on this burgeoning knowledge base, he does not see this as ferreting out the one right technical answer for solving the problem of any particular case he is involved with. The drive to develop a formalised and prescriptive approach to the identification and management of child protection issues is 'often seen (by practitioners) as a device for protecting management from outside criticism rather than for protecting children from abuse' (Munro, 2002: 2). Part of Peter's resistance to procedure-driven practice is his conviction that people's lives are too complex to fit neat administrative responses – especially in an area as socially and emotionally fraught as safeguarding children. Peter's practice is informed not by an illusory 'scientific certainty' but by 'working hypotheses'. These are based on knowledge that is only in part made up of the messages on needs and services coming from the literature and research and are at all times open to challenge and modification.

Certainly the critical practitioner needs an understanding of how child abuse and child protection express the dynamic interactions within social systems and how these play out for individuals within the context of established patterns of human growth and development. To understand abuse, Corby (2005: 131) has helpfully suggested three main groups of perspective:

- *psychological theories:* these focus on the instinctive, psychological qualities of individuals who abuse
- *social psychological theories:* these focus on the dynamics of the interaction between abuser, child and immediate environment
- *sociological perspectives:* these emphasise sociopolitical conditions as the most important reason for the existence of child abuse.

Each has its own strengths and weaknesses, which Corby usefully rehearses. The danger in all of them for the critical practitioner is that of reductionism. Sociobiologists' preoccupation with genes should no more be dismissed out of hand than the feminist concern with patriarchy, but neither should be seen as providing the total picture.

One thing that is made clear by the literature is the complexity of the dynamics of child abuse and the response to it. Attachment theory may provide a convincing and detailed explanation of the process whereby abuse and neglect can be derived from, and transmitted through, poor adult–child relationships (Howe, 2005). Both psychodynamic theories (Bower, 2005) and behavioural approaches (Macdonald, 2001) engage with and explain intra- and interpersonal dynamics and suggest intervention aims and strategies. Marxism, feminism and postmodernist explanations bring the structures and relations of power into clear view (Parton, 2005). But none of these theoretical perspectives is sufficient alone. Nor is it possible or even desirable to integrate them into a unified theory. They provide the basis for uneasy amalgams that usefully inform working hypotheses about what is at issue for the individuals caught up in child abuse.

Precisely because of the complexity and lack of a single uncontested theoretical base, these hypotheses must be explored and open to challenge in order to be discounted or confirmed as useful in any particular situation. This requires another type of knowledge – knowledge of the particular history, characteristics and aspirations of the individuals involved. In order to gather that knowledge, it is important to avoid 'typification' (Marsh and Fisher, 1992: 38; Dattalo, 1997). This is where, often encouraged by agency procedures, relationships between social workers and service users are defined by routine responses that place service users into pre-existing, fixed, typical categories. This has been further encouraged by the increasing emphasis on the multidisciplinary and interagency response to the risks being experienced by children. The drive from policy makers for professionals to work together more closely for the protection of children (for example DfES, 2006) suggests a view that professionals choose not to work together for the better protection of children. Such a view lacks any understanding of the intricacies of responding to the complexities of child abuse and neglect. Peter recognises that errors made by individuals are often the result of contextual factors that shape how different professionals communicated with one another. But refusal to reduce individuals, workers and service users alike, to either the victims or villains of child abuse or to being the heroes of child protection has always been the hallmark of Peter's practice.

Skills: negotiating within a context of inequality

At the core of the skills of social work lies building, maintaining and realising the potential for change within relationships. The centrality of the relationship, 'that dreaded idol of traditional social work' (Leonard, 1975: 53), holds true for the critical practitioner. Power is what fuels relationships. What is distinctive about the work of a critical practitioner like Peter is that the power differentials expressed within relationships are openly acknowledged. Drawing as much on his political and trade union experience as on his casework, Peter has always prided himself on being both aware and 'up front' about inequality in power. He assessed it, he acknowledged it and he worked with it – whether it was the power imbalance between adult and child, male and female, white and black, between worker and service user, among service users, or within and between social workers and their managers.

In child protection work, the relationship between worker, parent and child is generally tightly circumscribed by legal and procedural requirements. The power and status imbalance is firmly with the worker who is advantaged as a representative of the state. It is also likely to be reinforced by the parents being disadvantaged by factors such as class, gender, race and age. It is not surprising that such imbalance can prompt resistance through the extremes of either withdrawal or violence. At the same time, it needs to be recognised that social workers not only exercise power over service users, but are also subject to the very power they are exercising. Peter talked of being carried along by the logic of child protection procedures he believed should never have been instigated; of supervising contact visits where he agreed with parents that this was not necessary, but still was bound by a management decision. Only when power was acknowledged could the imbalance be negotiated in a manner least likely to be oppressive. Peter applied the open approach to power, whether representing staff interests to management, ensuring that a parent was accompanied by an advocate at a child protection case conference or seeking the exclusion of a violent partner.

Power is a complex and contested concept (Hugman, 1991). It is expressed within both process and structure: 'social workers' power is expressed not only in what they do but what they are' (Harris, 1997: 29). Power is interactional and ubiquitous. The various aspects of the imbalance of power within child protection are based on social inequalities of class, gender, age and race and on the nature of state power. Social inequalities and oppressive state power are deep-seated within the social and political structures of British society (Ferguson et al., 2002). The shifting configuration of state, civil society and ideology provides the structural supports and constraints of all social work intervention (Campbell and Pinkerton, 1997). Child protection is no exception. Structural contradictions find expression in the dilemmas of care and control that are found in all childcare, whether provided informally within the social institutions of civil society, such as family and neighbourhood, or through the formal services provided by the state and the voluntary sector. Certainly, these dilemmas are particularly sharply experienced in child protection work, where ensuring the safety of children can require the naked display of state power, but they are not peculiar to it.

The inequality of power relations within child protection has been explored through the considerable work done on partnership (Holland and Scourfield, 2004). This work suggests that what is too often lacking is attention to the basic requirements for ensuring working relationships. Service users, like service providers, need written information, manageable practical arrangements, advice and emotional support. It is also the basic decencies of human relationships that have been stressed by service users. Advice from one group of parents with children deemed to be at risk included:

- use everyday language we can understand
- be realistic about how well you really know us and only write reports on us when you do
- don't put us 'under a microscope'
- don't come across as threatening and sticking too rigidly to rules and regulations
- deliver on what you say you'll do and don't expect of us more than you would of anyone else in our situation (Pinkerton et al., 1997).

Children value social workers who listen, are available and accessible, non-judgemental and non-directive, have a sense of humour, are straight talking and can be trusted (Butler and Williamson quoted in Bannister et al., 1997: 1).

Much of the problem with partnership working where safeguarding children is the central concern lies in the absence, confusion or difficulty in achieving agreement over what constitutes the shared goal of the worker and the family. It is crucial to be clear as to the mandate for working with families on particular goals:

> These goals may be agreed with the user because they are what the user wishes to work on, or they may be agreed with the client as a result of some external authority placing them on the client's agenda via legal proceedings. (Marsh and Fisher, 1992: 18)

That second mandate provides a difficult basis for partnership working but can be 'reframed' as part of a managed process of partnership (Pinkerton, 2000).

Like many practitioners, Peter is sceptical about the term 'partnership' – however reframed. Again drawing as much on his political and trade union experience as on his casework, he prefers the term 'negotiated agreements'. Negotiation permits all those involved, whatever their status, to signal their needs and wishes so that there can be a search for a common goal, even if this is only an accommodation between different views. It provides the means to pool resources to work together in achieving the desired outcomes. Successful negotiation can require the professionals involved to relinquish some power and status – something they can find difficult to do. This is not just out of a desire to be in control – the dominant reflex in any state functionary. It can also be hard for the professional to acknowledge that what they bring to any negotiation is only a contribution, and often a minor one, to the wider and deeper pool of resources that children in need and at risk require. As family group conferencing seems to be showing, many of these resources may be better accessed through informal networks (Marsh, 2008).

One other point stressed by Peter was that in negotiating and implementing agreements, it is important to accept that the unexpected will occur – sometimes involving gains, sometimes losses. This can be anything from a sudden shift in the dynamics between a mother and her alcohol-misusing partner, to a child reconnecting with an important adult, to a job move by a key member of an interdisciplinary child protection team. Accepting the inevitability of unpredictability allows practitioners to respond earlier and more flexibly when the unexpected occurs so as to take advantage of any gains and manage the impact of losses. Expecting the unexpected also reinforces the need to regard all outcomes as unfinished business – which is a way of saying that safeguarding children is a creative process. The best planned intervention will still need to be brought alive by the creative endeavours of all the individuals involved, service users as well as service providers.

Conclusion

As Peter and I talked, I felt reassured that the critical perspective I had held on to over the years was not some throwback to the illusions of more optimistic times. Uncertainty and complexity are now accepted as defining characteristics of safeguarding children. This was always the view taken by critical theory, with its capacity to get beneath the surface of certainty. A critical perspective was never a means of tidying up reality, shoe-horning it into a particular framework, but rather a way of opening it up to exploration, contest and change. Measuring up to vision and values, testing working hypotheses and negotiating the imbalances of power may not have the surface appeal of heroic child rescue or the cosy warmth of universal family support. But applying those three imperatives of critical practice will support solid commitment to children for themselves, an informed sense of social and psychological perspective and attention to the fundamentals of human communication. Together, it is those things that are most likely to nudge child protection slowly but surely towards its rightful place as a crucial but minor aspect of a child welfare system that supports children and their carers. A critical perspective offers practitioners like Peter, and others who see our function as supporting them in their work, the means to dig down and dig in for the long haul.

For further discussion of safeguarding children, see Chapter 5, and for safe-guarding adults, see Chapter 27.

www.everychildmatters.gov.uk   Website of the Department for Children, Schools and Families that sets out the policy context for the delivery of integrated children's services in England. There is a facility to register for updates and good links to government-funded research.

www.nspcc.org.uk/inform   Website of the National Society for the Prevention of Cruelty to Children that hosts summaries of research conducted by and on behalf of the organisation, and provides the facility to receive a free weekly update of news and developments relating to the safeguarding of children.

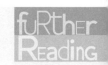

Corby, B. (2005) *Child Abuse: Towards a Knowledge Base*, 3rd edn, London, Open University Press. Well-informed, clearly presented and thoughtfully considered review of the existing multidisciplinary knowledge base covering the historical development, definition, extent, causation and consequences of child abuse.

DH/SSI (Department of Health /Social Services Inspectorate) (1994) *The Challenge of Partnership in Child Protection: Practice Guide*, London, HMSO. Through a clear statement of the principles of good practice in partnership, detailed discussion of how these can be applied at different stages in the child protection process and a useful set of team and individual exercises, this remains a useful resource for skilling up for negotiating child protection.

Doyle, C. (2006) *Working with Abused Children: From Theory to Practice*, 3rd edn, Basingstoke, Palgrave Macmillan. Offers an insightful and wide-ranging introduction to direct work with children who have been abused, giving attention to children's own perspectives on their abuse and to issues of diversity.

Hulme, K. (1985) *The Bone People*, London, Hodder & Stoughton. Booker Prize-winning novel focusing on the strange and uneasy relationships linking a solitary artist, a lost boy she befriends and his abusive stepfather. Powerful representation of the violence, raw humanity, ambivalence and confusion in situations of abuse.

Parton, N. (2005) *Safeguarding Children: Early Intervention and Surveillance in a Late Modern Society*, Basingstoke, Palgrave Macmillan. Offers a clear, invigorating and theoretically sophisticated commentary on child abuse and child welfare policy, explaining how changes in philosophy and intervention have been informed by cultural, economic and political contexts.

Wilson, K. and James, A. (eds) (2007) *The Child Protection Handbook*, 3rd edn, London, Baillière Tindall. Comprehensive book providing an informative and accessible account of child protection practice in three sections: understanding child abuse, managing the process of safeguarding children, and interventions in safeguarding children.

23 Fostering and adoption

Chapter overview

This chapter explores what critical practice in fostering and adoption involves, by looking at fostering and adoption in their current contexts, considering the critical application of research to practice and exploring the dilemmas and tensions in practice via a practice area pertinent to both fostering and adoption: 'safe caring'.

Social workers in the fields of fostering and adoption hold both children's and families' lives in the balance. Critical practice is essential to enable each family to facilitate the best possible start in life for an individual child.

Fostering and adoption practice in their current context

Fostering and adoption are two separate areas of practice governed by separate legislation and policy. However, they also have many similar features. They are both primarily concerned with enabling a child, in need of a family, to be placed in a new family, either temporarily or permanently. It is not within the remit of this chapter to outline the legislation and policy governing fostering and adoption but rather to concentrate on practice. This is not to suggest that knowledge of legislation and policy are not crucial for critical practice but rather that there is insufficient space within this chapter to cover these areas. Coverage of the legislative framework can be found in Brammer (2007) and Braye and Carr (2008). At the time of writing, fostering practice is underpinned by the Children Act 1989 and 2004 and the *Fostering Services: National Minimum Standards: Fostering Services Regulations* (DH, 2002a). The legislative framework underpinning adoption practice has been overhauled in this decade by the enactment of the Adoption and Children Act 2002 and 2006 and the Adoption and Children (Scotland) Act 2007 as well as the national adoption standards (DH, 2001a).

The placement of children with substitute families involves the recruitment of carers, assessment, matching children to carers and training and support of carers and children. There is a symbiotic relationship between fostering and adoption practice and social work practice with children and families, as fostering and adoption are dependent on the quality of work undertaken with birth families and networks as well as children. For a child to be adequately matched with a substitute family, there needs to have been a thorough and accurate assessment of the child's needs, personality, history, attachments, likes and dislikes and health and educational attainment. If the assessment was lacking, there is a much higher likelihood that the child will be misplaced and the placement will be likely to break down. The quality of the work done in trying to retain the child within their own family is also of great consequence to the fostering and adoption process, as well as to the child's future ability to make sense of the disruption to their life.

The processes of long-term fostering and adoption have become much closer as changes in adoption patterns have materialised. In England and Wales, the number of adoptions of infants under one year old dropped dramatically from 1968, when 75 per cent of all adoptions were of infants, to 1991, when that percentage had dropped to 12 per cent (Triseliotis et al., 1997: 15). Currently, the majority of adoptions are in relation to children in public care, whereas in the past this was not the case. This has meant that social workers have to make complex assessments as to whether or not the needs of a child in public care would be best met through being adopted or through long-term foster care. This assessment is not simple, involving the consideration of the prognosis of finding a suitable adoptive family who would be able to take on board contact arrangements for the child as well as their troubled and complex history. The critical practitioner would hold in mind that there are currently benefits and costs to both options (Sinclair et al., 2007). For example, adopted children and families often find that post-adoption resources and support are not always forthcoming, leading to serious difficulties for families caring for children with troubled pasts and multiple needs.

Recruitment

Adopters and foster carers are 'ordinary' members of the community. They come in all forms with different histories, cultures, strengths and weaknesses. Over recent decades, most fostering and adoption agencies have become more inclusive in who they recruit. The Adoption and Children Act 2002 was a clear marker in this dynamic, making it possible for same-sex couples who weren't in civil partnerships to adopt jointly, thus bringing them in line with married couples, same-sex couples in civil partnerships and unmarried heterosexual couples. The stereotypical, white foster mother with husband out at work and birth children washed and scrubbed is still being recruited as an invaluable resource, but she has been joined by many other carers of different races and cultures as well as single carers, gay carers and some carers with disabilities. However, despite these changes, the traditional picture of the foster carer, shown in a Scottish study, still prevails and numerically they are still the majority (Triseliotis et al., 2000). Given the changing nature of children placed in foster placements or for adoption – they are older than they were and have more complex needs – there may be a tension between what the 'traditional' carer had to offer and what the current child needs. We need to revisit who we are recruiting as carers to make sure that they have a secure sense of self and are resilient, so that they can withstand the personal and public exposure of self that inevitably arises from caring for children (Nutt, 2006).

Assessment of carers

Once recruited, all carers have to be assessed. The National Foster Care Association UK Joint Working Party on Foster Care's code of practice (1999a) and national standards (1999b) as well as the national minimum standards (DH, 2002a) provide some clarity in respect of aspects of fostering and specifically in relation to assessment. Prospective carers have to undergo a lengthy and rigorous assessment process and a number of checks to ascertain if they will have the potential to care for other people's children in their own homes. Nearly all agencies use the British Association for Adoption and Fostering's 'Form F' as a framework for this assessment.

The nature of adoption and fostering is now so diverse (Wheal, 2005) that it is often the case that the same carer may be suitable for one fostering project but not for another. For example, someone may be able to offer a considerable amount to a sexually abused seven-year-old child but not meet the criteria for a multidimensional treatment foster care scheme (DfES, 2007) or a support care scheme (Brown et al., 2005). Some adoption applicants would make excellent concurrent planning prospective adopters for a two-day-old baby but not for a troubled ten-year-old child.

Matching children and families

The *Looking After Children: Assessment and Action Schedules* (DH, 1995d) and *The Framework for the Assessment of Children in Need and Their Families* (DH/DfEE/Home Office, 2000: 17) offer frameworks for assessing and recording children's needs, attainments, wishes, 'social presentation, family and social relationships, identity, emotional and behavioural development, education and health'. *The Looking After Children: Assessment and Action Schedules* for a child being placed from within public care should also record the child's 'care' history.

If the carer's assessment has examined in detail what the family or individual has to offer as well as their limitations, theoretically it should be possible to 'match' a child with a placement with the optimum chance of success. In a number of voluntary and independent projects, 'good enough' matching is possible, because some agencies have a number of carers ready to take children. Unfortunately for many local authorities, it is recognised that there is a shortage of carers, so that the sensitivity of matching is likely to be significantly blunted and reduced to 'who has space'.

Matching should involve consideration of the child's needs, wishes, abilities, age, race and ethnicity, care plan, and their need for contact with their own family. Thoburn (1994: 63) noted the range of placement types, emphasising the enormous range of placements that are needed, from 'short-term "shared or relief" fostering right through a whole range to adoption', in order to satisfy the varieties of care plans. For critical practitioners to make good enough matching decisions and a placement for a child, there needs to be a range of carers available to meet the diverse needs of children needing placements.

Training and support of carers

Many agencies incorporate the Fostering Network's (2003) *The Skills to Foster* training programme into their assessment process. This gives the assessors the chance to see the applicants functioning in a group as well as seeing how they manage new information. Occasionally, through training, it becomes apparent that the applicants will not make appropriate carers or they decide themselves that they do not want to proceed. Training also is considered now by most agencies to be an essential aspect of support for carers. As new dilemmas arise, they can make sense of new information and try to apply it to their own circumstances. Training involves being in a group with other carers where similar and shared difficulties can be explored. Many agencies run carers' support groups. However, group support cannot be a substitute for individual supervision from a supervising social worker. Not all carers can take advantage of group settings and the confidential nature of much of what a carer may wish to discuss also means that group discussions sometimes have to be 'general'.

Agencies accept that training is their ongoing responsibility for carers who increasingly are caring for children with complex needs (DH, 2002a). This remains a tension between fostering and adoption, as the majority of adopters will not receive post-adoption training even though their needs may be as great as foster carers and the children they are caring for are often very to those in long-term foster care.

Support to carers is more than just training. Support is one of the laments of carers often feeling that they do not get enough. Fostering and adoption agencies vary in what support and supervision they offer. One theme emerges – the actual or perceived lack of support or appropriate support is a major contributory factor to why carers cease to have children placed with them (Triseliotis et al., 2000). Lack of good quality support and supervision are contributory factors in poor placement outcomes (Sellick et al., 2004; Sinclair, 2005). For the critical practitioner who is aware of this, there is a tension as a result of the current recruitment and retention crisis in social work. 'Support' is one of the first things to receive less attention when an agency is under pressure, ultimately leading to disruption for some children's placements. Instability for children in public care is of national concern. Reducing the number of moves for looked-after children as well as emphasising permanence for children is rightly a primary focus of *Care Matters* (DfES, 2007). Given that children have entered the public care system because it was deemed to be in their interests, Jackson and Thomas's (1999: 41) finding that 'research consistently points to a high level of instability and change for the majority of children in the care system when compared to children who remain with their own families' has to be of grave concern.

Children also need to be supported in placement. They are often in need of ongoing effective social work to enable them to make use of the placement, to sustain meaningful relationships, where appropriate, with their own families as well as, again where appropriate, form attachments to their new family. They may need many years of support to 'recover' from previous trauma. The children will need a consistent and effective social work input to make sure that their needs are being met and their voice heard. Support for a child and supervision and support for a carer are delivered by separate social workers. Often they need to be liaising with education and health professionals in order to maximise the chances of the placement achieving stability and success as well as making sure that the health and educational needs of a child are met.

The quality of the recruitment, assessment, matching, training and support contributes to the successful outcome of placements and bettering of outcomes for children in public care and those who need to be adopted. Critical practice is integral to bettering outcomes at each stage of the placement process but it is also reliant on sufficient resources.

Critical application of research to practice

Later than some professional groups, social work has entered the world of evidence-based practice. This is an arena where critical practice has to be alert and vigilant. The mechanistic application of theory or research findings to an individual placement scenario could be as damaging as theoretical and research ignorance. As Jackson and Thomas (1999: 5) write: 'The truth is that research is about generalisations but practice is about individuals.' Practitioners need to be aware of theoretical perspectives and relevant research findings, hold these in mind and apply them thoughtfully to the individual circumstance and individuals with whom they are working. This necessitates the practitioner being research literate, able to form effective relationships to enable a full assessment to be made and then use their own critical thinking to assess whether or not some specific theory or research applies to a particular case. The practitioner needs sufficient confidence to remain flexible in relation to the application of 'evidence' to practice and focused on the individual child's interests.

Research literacy

Current practitioners are in the fortunate position of having a number of accessible and user-friendly research reviews available to them (Berridge, 1997; DH, 1999a; Jackson and Thomas, 1999; SCIE, 2004; Sellick et al., 2004; Sinclair, 2005). Texts that focus on the experience of the looked-after child (Fahlberg, 1994; Cocker and Allain, 2008) can also help practitioners to remain child focused. However, for the practitioner to make sense of this material, they need to be research literate. By this, I mean they need to have the capacity to understand research findings as well as research outcomes, thus being able to make sense of the researcher's interpretation of the data. They need to understand a sufficient amount in relation to research methods to make sense of whether or not a specific research design was sufficiently rigorous to deliver findings that were valid (see Adams et al., 2009c: Ch. 26).

◇◇◇◇ CaSE EXaMPLE ◇◇

Tania had been a 'child in need' from age two, when her maternal grandmother, with whom she and her mother lived, had died. Tania's mother, Jane, was a crack cocaine user and Tania's grandmother had undertaken the total care of her. Tania and Jane had then moved into Jane's boyfriend's flat, where she lived for five years. She had been cared for minimally by Jane but had received affection and intermittent physical care from the boyfriend's sister, Sarah, who was a neighbour. The family lived on income support and, by any criteria, Tania suffered from neglect. She attended her primary school intermittently and her health visitor had had to work hard for her first immunisations to happen.

The primary school head had referred Tania several times to social services but they had not visited, as concerns were vague and unsubstantiated. Jane's crack habit increased, as did Tania's neglect, neither receiving any help. Sarah visited on Tania's eighth birthday to find Jane unconscious and Tania sitting in a urine-soaked bed feeding herself baked beans out of a tin. Sarah managed to get Jane admitted to hospital and Tania was accommodated that evening and placed with short-term foster parents.

After an initial and core assessment by the local authority, it became apparent that Jane vehemently did not want Tania to return home and Sarah, although wanting to remain involved, could not care for Tania. Neither Jane's boyfriend nor Tania's father could be traced. The social worker for Tania, being mindful of the need to assess Tania's degree of attachment to significant people in her family of origin (Fahlberg, 1994; Howe, 1995) through a process of careful observation, noted that there was a significant attachment between Tania and Sarah. Sarah was involved in the care planning for Tania, but Jane was not, despite valiant attempts by Sarah and the social worker to involve her.

After seven months and a number of court hearings resulting in a care order, it was decided that a permanent substitute family should be found for Tania and that contact should be maintained with Sarah. The placement team had three families available. The social worker needed to keep in mind the following research findings:

- The success of a placement lessens as the child's age increases at point of placement (Quinton et al., 1998)
- Outcomes for children are improved if contact is maintained for the child with significant people (Sellick et al., 2004)
- If the placement family has a child very near the age of the child to be placed, the prognosis for success is poorer (Jackson and Thomas, 1999).

According to the above, Tania, now eight years old, was more likely to experience disruption than if she had been one year old. However, she may have had a number of 'protective factors' in her favour, for example she was attached to her grand-mother and Sarah, which might mean there was a better prognosis for her attaching to a new family. It would be important to find a family that would encourage her contact with Sarah and help to maintain that attachment. It would also be better if she could be placed in a family with no children near her own age.

However, two of the families available to take children were reluctant to main-tain regular contact permanently between Sarah and Tania and the other had a nine-year-old son. Tania urgently needed a family, as her short-term foster family were migrating to Australia and she would experience further disruption if she were offered another short-term placement.

Critical social work has never existed in a predictable, stable world of ideal resources. By the nature of practice situations, the practitioner is often choos-ing the least damaging option. This practitioner met the family with the nine-year-old son, as it was her belief that it was of paramount importance that Tania maintained the relationship with Sarah as her one remaining attachment. As a result of the thorough assessment and good observational skills of Tania's social worker, the importance of this relationship had been recognised. On visiting the family, the social worker was struck by the matu-rity and confidence of the nine-year-old son as well as the inclusive warmth of the family and its openness. When she returned to visit Tania, the frailty and lack of self-esteem of the child overwhelmed her in comparison to the foster family's son. She knew that either the foster son's confidence and matu-rity would give enough space to Tania for her needs to be met or that she would feel inadequate by comparison. However, she was also cognisant of the fact that outcomes in relation to human beings and their relationships with others are often unpredictable and unknowable. Even the best informed crit-ical and reflective social worker cannot predict the future. Much practice is about well-informed leaps in the dark.

Tania was placed with the foster family. Both children attended the same school in different years. Sarah visited weekly and Tania stayed with her for a weekend every month. Her new family formed a strong attachment to Tania as she did to them. As Tania became more settled and attached to the family, competition and conflict increased between the son and Tania. However, the practitioner worked with the family, including encouraging Tania to focus some of her increasing energy into judo, at which she excelled. After a year, the foster siblings were able to express feelings for each other and the competitive nature of their relationship decreased. Tania's social worker remained involved, helping Tania, Sarah and the family to secure the placement. After three years in placement, the family applied to adopt Tania, with the approval of Sarah and the consent of Tania's mother. Her father still could not be traced. Tania, post-adoption, continued to see Sarah every week and stay the monthly weekend. All parties had managed to be open enough to enable Tania to have a second start in life while maintaining what was important to her, her previous attachment to Sarah.

The social worker, through her awareness of the relevant research, as well as consideration of the unique and specific aspects of the case, had made a statistically risky placement, which she believed stood a good chance of permanence.

Dilemmas and tensions: 'safer caring'

When the National Foster Care Association published *Safer Caring* in 1994, it was much needed as a practice guide. The rate of allegations by children against carers had been increasing rapidly and some research showed that the majority were in relation to sexual abuse (National Foster Care Association, 1994). It was an area of uncertainty that provoked considerable anxiety. The extent of allegations against carers and actual cases of abuse have been difficult to measure accurately (Nixon, 2000). The rise in numbers was likely to be linked with adults being more ready to listen to children, resulting in them being more likely to divulge abuse than was the case in the past.

As is sometimes the case with subjects that raise anxiety in social work, there was the occasional overzealous reaction to the increase in the number of allegations. For example, in the National Foster Care Association's (1994: 24) helpful guide, when advising carers to think carefully about their lifestyles in order to lessen the likelihood of allegations, it said: 'make sure that your family, and children joining your household, have a dressing gown and slippers as well as nightwear'. I, for one, have been left puzzled as to how 'slippers' were going to help. However, Slade's (2006) more recent publication is realistic and informative.

When recruiting and assessing carers, agencies usually integrate safer caring into the assessment and training processes. This involves helping families to reflect critically on their lifestyles in minute detail and think about how a child coming into a family might feel about, and interpret, that lifestyle. Inevitably, caring for a child, new to the family, requires practical as well as emotional adjustments to keep the family and the child safe. This does not involve simply helping carers to lessen the likelihood of allegations being made against them, but also involves practical matters, for example fire precautions and so on.

Why is this is an area of dilemma and tension? Because, as in any area of practice that raises high levels of anxiety, social workers sometimes lose the capacity to think critically and can, as a result, fall back on mechanistic procedural processes or 'blame' one party, neither of which are in children's interests.

Drawing on training that I have run over six years with carers, work as a consultant in relation to complex cases involving allegations and as a foster panel chairperson, I have developed a simple model of categorising children's allegations. As with any model, it is only a guide and is in no way prescriptive or fixed. I have seen a pattern of allegations that fall into four groups:

- *Actual:* the event described by the child happened
- *False:* the event described by the child did not happen

- *Perception of the child:* resulting from past experience and other factors, the child misinterprets the behaviour of the carer
- *Behaviour of the carer:* resulting from the impact of the child's behaviour and the dynamic between the carer (or the carer's household) and the child, the behaviour of the carer (or member of the household) is affected.

Many allegations fall into the last two categories and often overlap. Agencies regularly approach investigations of allegations through 'child protection procedures', throwing up the dilemma of, at the same time as investigating thoroughly, holding in mind that occasionally children make allegations about events that have not happened. The reaction to a 'false' allegation, which causes such agency and placement difficulty, can be to blame the child rather than consider the meaning of the allegation. Allegations are powerful tools for children who can feel as if they have, and often do have, little or no access to power or control over their own lives. They may want to move from a placement and know no constructive way to voice their wishes. The child's social worker has to contain the anxiety generated by an allegation. The practitioner, at the same time as offering appropriate support to the family or directing them to such support, needs to focus on the best interests of the child making the 'false' allegation. In one case, a young person made the same 'false' allegation against two carers before he was helped to disclose that the 'actual' incident had happened within his own family several years previously.

Placing children with troubled pasts in new families inevitably stirs up complex and difficult feelings for both the child and the family. The tension as well as the dilemma is making sure that carers are properly supported through the processes of investigation, while continuing to support and work with the child. To be a critical practitioner is to be able to 'hold in mind' a number of differing and often conflicting matters, feelings and dynamics at the same time; to retain the capacity to 'think' under pressure and to remain child focused. Once an allegation has been made, there is the potential for 'splitting' (one party becoming the 'goody' and the other the 'baddy') and the practitioner needs to hold on to complexity and the 'whole' in the child's interests.

Conclusion

Since the important work of Rowe and Lambert (1973), which identified the extent of drift and stagnation for children in public care, there has been a re-emphasis on trying either to return children as quickly as possible to their families of origin or to place them permanently in a substitute family either through adoption or fostering. However, we have made poor progress in creating stability for children in public care, many of whom have had an unacceptable number of moves between foster families (Jackson and Thomas, 1999; DfES, 2007).

We currently have a shortage of carers to place children with and many troubled and upset children to place. The government has tried to tackle the situation partially via *Care Matters* (DfES, 2007), which has released monies to tackle the problem. However, resources are not the only consideration. The quality of the social work being done, in assessing children's needs, in the recruitment and assessment of carers and the matching of a child with a family, is fundamentally important. These social work processes are dependent on the practitioner's capacity to think and practise in a critical fashion. This entails an awareness of self, theory, research, skills and values; to enable the analysis of dynamics, facts and processes in the interests of children. For a child to be separated from their birth family is a traumatic, life-changing event. Those professionals responsible for children in public care and in need of adoption owe it to them to practise in a critical and reflective manner; to get it 'right enough' to enable them to have a stable remaining childhood within a family where they can develop their potential to the full.

For further discussion of looked-after children, see Chapter 24, and for the context of policy and practice, see Adams et al., 2009a, Chapter 22.

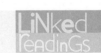

www.fostering.net   Fostering Network

www.baaf.org.uk   British Association for Adoption and Fostering

DH (Department of Health) (1999) *Adoption Now: Messages from Research*, Chichester, Wiley. Useful outline of key research findings in relation to adoption.

Jackson, S. and Thomas, N. (1999) *On the Move Again? What Works in Creating Stability for Looked-after Children*, Ilford, Barnardo's. Review of research looking at stability for looked-after children.

Sellick, C. and Thoburn, J. and Philpot, T. (2004) *What Works in Adoption and Foster Care?*, Barkingside, Barnardo's. Review of current research findings.

Sinclair, I. (2005) *Fostering Now: Messages from Research*, London, Jessica Kingsley. Review of current research findings.

Wheal, A. (ed.) (2005) *The RHP Companion to Foster Care*, Lyme Regis, Russell House Publishing. Collection of papers covering areas relevant to foster care.

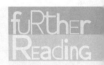

24 Looked-after children and young people in residential and foster care

Chapter overview

This chapter focuses on the transformative potential of four fundamental elements of critical practice in residential care: critical consciousness; critical reflexivity; critical awareness of the residential space; and relationships. It identifies a conceptual framework that highlights the context and boundaries of child-care work.

Critical practice in residential care

Recent policy has continued to define the need for listening, involvement and partnership with young people, while the reality for many young people often appears to be one of marginalisation and tokenism (McLeod, 2007). As Winter (2006: 59) suggests: 'it is likely that the very framework designed to put the child first will continue to at best constrain the voices of those it is interested in and at worst silence them'. In this chapter, we propose that critical practice has the potential to transform the structural constraints of childhood for individual children and young people in residential care.

Our understanding of critical practice in residential childcare contains four fundamental elements:

1 'A critical consciousness which is able to imagine the transformability of current social structures and work towards that' (Ferguson, 2003: 1007).

2 A critical reflexivity to develop relevant evidence that supports the transformation of negative impacts of current social structures to positive outcomes agreed with the individual child and reflects the diversity of children and childhoods (Taylor and White, 2000; James and James, 2004; Prout, 2005).

3 An awareness of complexity and the ecology of the socially constructed residential space, including all actors and actions within it, to facilitate children and staff working creatively and jointly with uncertainty (Hassett and Stevens, 2005; Stevens and Hassett, 2007).

4 Recognition that diverse needs can only be met through meaningful, consist-

ent, positive relationships, which implies that services should prioritise these and also find ways to help staff and looked-after children to use relationships positively (Gilligan and Akhtar, 2005; Jordan, 2006).

Within a critical practice framework, the needs of the individual child are not viewed as fixed, but as socially constituted and open to change (James and Prout, 1997). Such an approach distinguishes between the child as an individual and childhood as the socially constructed space that children occupy in relation to adults, recognising that there is not one childhood but many (James and James, 2004). In relation to looked-after children, it distinguishes between the residential place (the physical institution) and the residential space (the social construction of what happens within the residential place), the boundaries of which are far wider than the place (Massey, 1995; Stevens and Hassett, 2007).

We draw on the following case example to illustrate some of the issues that child-care workers encounter when attempting to work effectively with a young person while fulfilling policy agendas.

CASE EXaMPLE

Kirstie is a 15-year-old girl of dual ethnicity who was accommodated at the request of her mother and herself when she was 14. Her mother said she was unable to cope with Kirstie and was concerned about self-harming behaviour that seemed to be getting worse. Since becoming looked after, she has had three placements in residential units within eight months and consequent changes of school. Each placement has broken down in response to violence against other resident children. Kirstie has been pleased to move and easily makes new friends with peers. She relates well to adults, but as peers rather than adults. Each placement has resulted in an escalation in Kirstie's disruptive, violent and self-harming behaviour, culminating in a court appearance and two hospital admissions. In her current placement, Kirstie became involved in selling sex. A further placement is now being sought in the private sector at a cost of approximately £3,500 per week.

Developing a critical consciousness and reflexive use of the knowledge base

In this case, the priority must first be to work with Kirstie's disruptive, violent and self-harming behaviour; to make her and others in the residential space safe. But rather than merely responding or reacting to her disruptive behaviour, it is the carer's responsibility to further Kirstie's wellbeing. Critical care work would require the residential worker to be conscious of the structures that influence this behaviour and to build trusting relationships as a prerequisite to helping Kirstie to explore her feelings. Young people value professionals who find the time to build a sustained relationship with them, one in which they can trust, feel safe and be listened to (Whiteford, 2005). Gender, ethnicity and age identities will be central.

Kirstie's racial identity can be a positive lever for change. For example, in a similar case, Jones and Waul (2005: 38) describe an intervention that identified 'using every resource available to children' to reinforce their strengths. They involved the (white) mother closely and took a team approach that ensured the child had access to positive black role models across as many areas of his life as possible. This may not be appropriate for Kirstie and it will be important to explore racial identity with her and understand the competing discourses for children of interracial parentage (Barn and Harman, 2006). Additionally, gender differences in offending behaviour, both in terms of level and type of offence, are also acute. Females who offend can be deemed to be doubly deviant, having transgressed laws and stereotypes of appropriate female behaviour. This may potentially lead to a cumulative constellation of disadvantage The critical practitioner will need to reflect on their own and others' understanding of Kirstie's violent behaviour, which is more likely to be viewed differently by virtue of the fact that she is female and 'black'.

Power relationships between adults and children are often played out within the residential space. These are inherently unequal and most children are emotionally, physically and financially dependent on adults. Children are not authorised, in the same way as adults are, to speak within their own discourse. They are only 'heard' if adults sanction the sense of it; if adults decide that their feelings and wishes, statements and communications are meaningful and in their best interests. A structural constraint of childhood is a lack of control over resources to cope with, minimise or change life situations (James and James, 2004). The means available for young people generally to access money are restricted. This situation can be worse for looked-after children who often lack access to the family resources available to children living in the community. Kirstie may perceive sex work and accessing money as the only realistic way for her to achieve any level of independence and autonomy (Phoenix, 2003). Practitioners working with 'streetwise' children such as Kirstie are therefore left to bridge the gap between normative childhood expectations and lived experience that are often at odds – a reality that can leave practitioners feeling powerless too.

These issues can only be addressed within relationships of genuine concern and trust. While professionals might argue that Kirstie is in need of protection, she should also be engaged with as an autonomous individual with her own ideas and biography. Such exchanges can be complex and highly challenging and the agendas are likely to be individual in nature and content. A successful intervention with Kirstie will require the dedication of practitioners with time, a repertoire of interpersonal skills, an ability to critically apply the evidence base and to work with risk and uncertainty. With reference to the self-harming behaviour, for example, immediate decisions must be made as to whether Kirstie should be allowed to have access to sharp instruments and whether her wounds should be sympathetically tended to. Busy A&E departments can make short shrift of teenage girls who present with these kinds of injuries, and preventive policies often involve ensuring no access to potentially damaging objects (Bracken and Thomas, 2000). Evidence suggests that an alternative practice approach is to respond in a non-judgemental but sensitive way that allows the young person to build up trust while retaining control over their own body to do what they want. This approach, carefully managed, has been demonstrated as effective (Spandler, 1996).

Kirstie's sex work also presents risks. A critical appraisal of these risks, however, reveals how 'the risks that young people in prostitution are exposed to are "transformed" into risks to the agencies. Equally, the "responsibilities" that agencies have for their young charges are "transformed" into responsibilities that the young people have to leave prostitution' (Phoenix, 2003: 158). Practitioners must therefore acknowledge this shift in responsibility with Kirstie. Drawing on a complexity framework, Hassett and Stevens (2005) have developed a model of risk management and assessment based on spatial analysis and complexity that has been used in training nearly 200 childcare workers to develop safe care practices. In line with complexity theory (Geyer, 2003), Stevens and Hassett (2007) take a non-linear approach to risk, moving away from notions of cause and effect to take account of system boundaries, which are always open to change, attractors – factors that impact on the system – and fractals – decreasing or increasing replications of the form of the risk. We consider that complexity theory may be useful to critical practice because it offers the practitioner a framework that recognises some aspects of our physical, biological and social worlds as orderly, for example the need to eat, school and public transport timetables, some as disorderly, for example environmental events and fire, and some as a blending of the two, or complex, with emergent, less foreseeable outcomes. This enables practitioners and managers to accept the uncertainty inherent in practice and for children and young people, the uncertainty inherent in their lives, and to understand how they might engage with it for better (jointly defined) outcomes rather than pretend it is not there or can be solved through linear measures, such as better procedures, abstinence, taking away sharp instruments and so on.

Jones and Waul (2005) underline the importance of working with policies and procedures that must be compatible with a philosophy of care in order to develop and strengthen residents and staff. This entails having a good understanding of the needs of all within the residential space and a dynamic understanding of its ecology; factors that are constantly changing over time and influence the space. To do this, residential carers can become reflexive research practitioners (Taylor and White, 2000) on behalf of children in their care, drawing on critical evidence appraisal skills (Ferguson, 2003). Furthermore, in order to challenge structural disadvantage, they can also help develop some of these skills in the child residents, enabling young people to become critically reflexive of their situation and using data-gathering skills to work with young people to help them see and even challenge the structural causes of their trauma and exclusion. For example, a young woman with an eating disorder can be empowered to understand and take action against the media in her own way through writing, blogging and social networking. Staff can enable young people to connect corporate agendas with personal suffering, such as exploring the commercial roots of smoking and alcohol addictions (Prilleltensky and Prilleltensky, 2003).

Intervention that emphasises adult control can exacerbate the feelings of disempowerment that can underpin self-harming behaviour. Thus a further issue for the critical practitioner is the extent to which they can allow their power to be restricted and controlled by the child facilitated, and an understanding of how powerlessness can shape the responses of those who are marginalised (McLeod, 2007). This is relevant to issues such as 'passive' (on behalf of) or 'active' (by) advocacy with looked-after children (Boylen and Wyllie, 1999), confidentiality (on behalf of or with) (Wattam, 1999), involvement in decision-making/mediation (given information or participation) to name a few. From an adult's position, such as Eekelaar's (1986), giving children control could be viewed as damaging. The practice challenge is to take risks, to allow the child to retain control while encouraging less damaging behaviour, as in the self-harm example above. In doing so, practitioners need to empower themselves, have the confidence to take risks and know that they will be supported. Thus, critical and challenging practice requires a high level of skills, a sympathetic organisation and a supportive practice environment, which makes an explicit commitment to work positively with uncertainty and ambiguity (Parton, 1998a).

Consultation, involvement and rights

The United Nations Convention on the Rights of the Child (UNCRC) (see Chapter 22) offers a baseline standard for all childcare systems: the UN is adamant that the Convention must be interpreted as a whole and not taken piecemeal. Some may take issue that the UNCRC does not go far enough, viewing it as an adult interpretation of childhood. A rights framework can be helpful in practice, offering broad checks and balances, discussion points and underpinning principles (United Nations, 1989). However, Kirstie's current priorities may be significantly different to those of professionals and carers assigned to or involved with her case, with Kirstie striving for perceived independence and autonomy and professionals seeking to manage and/or control her behaviour to keep her safe. This difference underlies the contradictions within a rights framework. Eekelaar (1986) has argued the importance of taking a long-term view in relation to children's rights, proposing that the duty of adults who care for children should be less about rights in the present and more about adult responsibility (see Chapter 22; Adams et al., 2009a, Ch. 19). Quite simply, would Kirstie thank her carers for promoting her right to freedom of association, for example, if this leads to sex work that as an adult she may claim she should have been protected from? The balance between Kirstie's struggle for autonomy, its relation to risk-taking behaviour and a worker's duty of care is highly complex.

It may be thought that involving children/young people in decision-making processes is a further step towards enabling control to rest with them (see Adams et al., 2009a, Ch. 19). Most local authorities have accepted the case for participation; however, there are numerous demonstrations of how tokenistic models of participation (Kirby et al., 2003a; Mason and Fattore, 2005), such as inviting children to adult-led meetings, still dominate practice. Undoubtedly, Kirstie will have been invited to participate in preparation for and involvement in the review process, but she would have had little input into the agenda, the invitees, the timing or the venue. In review meetings, personal information about the child, their behaviour and relationships is often shared without the right of veto by the young person. Far from experiencing such meetings as representing listening, involvement and partnership, children often report feeling humiliated. Additionally, involvement in the review process may, for some young people, stand in contrast to their limited autonomy in everyday decisions about their care and where and how they spend their time, hence increasing the sense of tokenism and pointlessness some feel about this process. Hart's (1992) 'ladder' displays levels of children's participation. At the bottom are forms of 'non-participation', where children's involvement is marginal and tokenistic, with adults retaining control. At the top are child-initiated and controlled projects in which adults play a less significant role. A critical practice framework would work consciously with children at all these levels, making the reasons for the stage of participation clear and negotiating involvement with the child, where appropriate identifying boundaries and constraints and working jointly to overcome them.

The UK Race Relations (Amendment) Act 2000 places a general statutory duty on all public bodies to eliminate unlawful racial discrimination and promote equality of opportunity and good relations between persons of different racial groups. However, some have raised questions about the ability of the state child protection system to meet the needs of children from black and minority ethnic populations and their families. For example, Humphreys et al. (1999) suggest that, despite the best intentions of many individual workers, discriminatory policies and practices are perpetuated at an organisational level (see also Gilligan and Akhtar, 2006). At worst, fixed ideas about difference and sameness can lead to racism or simplistic stereotyping (Gunaratnam, 2003). The critical practitioner will need to understand and respect Kirstie's, her mother's and their own personal cultural context in order to advocate on their behalf. Within the residential space all must be encouraged to adopt proactive and reflexive anti-racist behaviour that explicitly addresses the effects of inequality and discrimination (Jones and Waul, 2005) and the hybridised nature of racial identities (Modood, 2007). This space extends to the local community, school and other sites relevant to the children placed in the home.

Organisational context

There are a number of factors influencing the organisational context of critical practice in residential care. Among them are an undermining of social work practice over the past two decades and residential childcare in particular, which has meant that residential childcare is no longer a positive choice (Crimmens and Milligan, 2005). In addition, the number of children and young people in the care population is falling but the levels and complexities of the needs of those within it continue to rise (Berridge and Brodie, 1998).

Previous neglect of the 'looked-after' childcare system has been addressed by New Labour through a range of policy initiatives targeting the poor outcomes of looked-after children. The White Paper *Care Matters: Time for Change* (DfES, 2007) is set to address the gap in outcomes between looked-after children and their peers. The consultation process for *Care Matters* revealed that many children who are looked after would have preferred to stay with their parents or family. *Every Child Matters* (DfES, 2003) places emphasis on early intervention as a means of reducing the numbers of children needing to be looked after. Services that can provide intensive home-based support can be effective in enabling children to remain in their own homes. These include interventions to address adolescent and parent conflict, the overrepresentation of unsupported single parents and comprehensive, accessible, community-based child and adolescent mental health services.

The residential space extends to community resources that strongly influence how and whether children begin care careers. If Kirstie and her mother had been offered a tailored, intensive, home-based support package, it is possible that the need to be looked after would not have arisen. This is not a linear relationship, however. Resources can be understood through a complexity framework; shortages at the level of the meta-organisation (government, the economy) are replicated through different levels of the organisation (the local authority, the regional office) down to the individual worker and child. Along the way, choices are made according to a whole range of influences involving political and personal choices and local events and relationships. Disorder may impact through a highly publicised tragedy – the death of a child in care, for example, or sudden flooding of a region – which will influence the way in which resources are allocated. In the complex resource system, there are ways in which critical practice can assist by imagining transformability, using critically reflexive evidence, for example using selective in-depth case studies to argue for resources, demonstrating resource use through patterns of care careers and indicating how resources might be differently distributed, and working across the ecology of the residential space. Residential childcare is not restricted to the residential place (its physical geography); the residential space also reaches to the immediate community and the spaces occupied by those who act within the residential place – social workers, health workers, educators, community and faith groups and more.

In contrast to many other parts of Europe, UK social work has been ambivalent about the necessary skills/training and education base needed for effective work with children. The White Paper *Care Matters* (DfES, 2007), which aims to radically improve the care system, explores the use of pedagogy as a means of improving the care experiences of children and young people. In many European countries, pedagogic theory informs training and children's service provision and provides a coherent theoretical framework:

The pedagogue has a relationship with the child which is both personal and professional. S/he relates to the child at the level of a person, rather than as a means of attaining adult goals. This interpersonal relationship implies reciprocity and mutuality, and an approach that is individualised but not individualistic. (Moss and Petrie, 2002: 143)

It can be argued that the process of developing relationships of trust becomes problematic in an arena where practitioners are required to comply with instrumentalist and procedural agendas (see also Chapter 22). The bureaucratisation of the care system has created an environment in which relationships are pursued as a means to fulfilling an outcome-led agenda.

National care standards have been implemented, bringing some positive gains for children and staff. However, the downside of greater accountability and standardisation has been the introduction of the 'audit culture' (Munro, 2004), targets and performance indicators that without critical reflection and creativity can consume staff time and become ends in themselves. Thus, at the same time as need is increasing, childcare policy and guidance appear preoccupied with the 'surface' managerial agenda of outcomes and accountability at the cost of the 'depth' of feeling, thinking and relationship (Howe, 1996).

Within a culture of criticism in social work, ambiguity and the unknown have become increasingly hard to live with (Parton, 1998b). Practitioners are concerned that any intervention not officially sanctioned or approved may be open to misinterpretation and hence criticism. Such criticism could have serious professional implications for any individual social worker. Unambiguous directives have also become increasingly attractive to practitioners who can feel more confident with clearly defined objectives and targets. This leads to the development of defensive practice, which fails to address either the needs or the root cause of children's difficulties. The performance indicators set by *Quality Protects* (DH, 1999b) do not necessarily accord with the priorities of children and young people in the care system. Research has confirmed that children value positive relationships with their carers, continuity, reliability and availability, confidentiality, advocacy and doing things together (Bell, 2001; Munro, 2002; Whiteford, 2005). While some of these concur with the current outcomes agenda, the majority have a clear focus on the processes within the residential space – ways of relating and organising time and human resources.

Evaluating the success or failure of childcare programme outcomes using blunt measures such as exam results, movement and ethnicity can be inappropriate for some service users and too general to accommodate diversity. Hence, while it is perfectly possible to compensate for long-term disadvantage, it is essential to recognise the challenge of the task (Clough et al., 2006). A pedagogic approach again might prove valuable here, in that a

> central tenet ... is to reject universal solutions and accept a multiplicity of possible perspectives, depending on personal circumstances, particularly dynamics and events and sources of support. (Cameron, 2004: 145)

Critical practitioners would do a great service if they could turn their attention on how best to measure or reflect traditionally non-scientific concepts, such as meaning, trust, enjoyment, hope, nurturing, feelings, emotion and other features yet to be recognised, in ways that might be open to evaluation, that is, demonstrating their value.

In doing so, they must be supported by access to information (including research, current and relevant policy) along with regular and supportive supervision. It has been argued that supervision has increasingly been hijacked by an instrumental agenda, used to ensure that procedures have been followed rather than as a forum for workers to explore their practice (Blaug, 1995). Developmental supervision is essential to critical practice, providing the practitioner with the opportunity to be reflexive and manage anxiety in the context of creative solutions.

Conclusion

The critical practitioner needs to develop reflexive 'defensible' rather than defensive practice, adopting interventions that are informed by, and also progress, research, theory and experience. The current evidence base cannot be accepted uncritically if children and young people are to be genuinely engaged in a participatory practice. Thus, a foundation skill for critical practice is the ability to understand, scrutinise and appraise the knowledge base. So much of what has been taken for granted as 'best practice' is actually founded on little more than opinion and dominant ideologies of the time. Calls for an evidence base to childcare work mean that multi-method research and its implementation through a critical and reflexive lens must now be an intrinsic and constant feature of practice. This evidence must be able to reflect the uncertainty and complexity that is an inevitable part of human interaction and decision-making.

In this chapter, we have suggested that the location of critical practice is not solely with the individual practitioner or child; it is located in the structures and organisation of the residential space, supported by managers with confidence derived from a critical appraisal of the knowledge base. We consider that this can be approached through a conceptual framework that highlights the context and boundaries of childcare work, as illustrated in Table 24.1.

Table 24.1 Conceptual framework for critical childcare practice

Context	Boundaries	Critical practice
Individual	Child's individual needs	Understanding, negotiating, meeting need, particularly for identity, safety, trust and health
Immediate	Extent of adult control Degree of participation Boundaries of imposed regulations and regulators	Negotiating inclusion (active/passive, partial/complete) Critical research and evaluation Prioritising relationship and process
Wider social	Ideologies of childhood (immaturity, incompetence, innocence, dependence) Sources of difference and diversity (ethnicity, gender, ability, size, sexuality, age, class) Sources of regulation and control (risk society, mixed economy of welfare)	Skill building for social inclusion Deconstructing childhood Valuing diversity Promoting positive parenting Critical qualitative evaluation Community engagement

For further discussion of fostering and adoption with looked-after children, see Chapter 23, and for further work with children and families, see Adams et al., 2009c, Chapter 4.

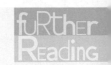

Blaug, R. (1995) 'Distortion of the face to face: communicative reason and social practice', *British Journal of Social Work*, 25: 423–39. Explores the changes in social work practice using Habermas's theory of communicative action. Offers some innovative ideas for social work that is practised in a bureaucratic and managerialist culture.

Brechin, A. (2000) 'Introducing critical practice', in A. Brechin, H. Brown and M.A. Eby (eds) *Critical Practice in Health and Social Care*, London, Sage. Explores the idea of critical practice and reflects the working challenges and dilemmas of practitioners to frame a three-way concept of critical practice. Suggests that critical practitioners are integrating analysis, reflexivity and action as they work and develop on a daily basis and are striving to establish and hold to principles of openness and equality.

Crimmens, D. and Milligan, I. (eds) (2005) *Facing Forward: Residential Child Care in the 21st Century*, Lyme Regis, Russell House Publishing. Useful collection of contributions focusing on the current policy context, difference and diversity, the voice of children and young people, group care theory and practice, educational attainment and offending, with practice examples.

Shaw, I. and Lishman, J. (eds) (1999) *Evaluation and Social Work Practice*, London, Sage. Provides a useful overview of the debates concerning what can constitute evidence for practice and helpful guidance on evaluation and empowerment, qualitative approaches to evaluation and different theoretical positions including feminist evaluation. Presents an informed and relevant challenge to performance culture.

Stevens, I. and Hassett, P. (2007) 'Applying complexity theory to risk in child protection practice', *Childhood*, 14(1): 128–44. Outlines complexity framework and despite a focus on child protection draws on work in residential care and describes training for residential workers.

25 Family-based social work

Chapter overview

This chapter considers the implications for family-based social work of the welfare policy context and recent research. It looks in particular at family group conferences as a model of family-centred practice.

Historically, social work with families in child welfare has been primarily concerned with therapeutic interventions that sought to achieve a change in family dynamics that had been assessed to be inadequate or appropriate. These interventions sought to enable the safe care of children and to promote better parenting. Social work texts argued for the importance of professional intervention in the treatment of the family as a 'dysfunctional' grouping presenting specific risks in relation to child rearing (see, for example, Dale et al., 1986). However, changes in the UK legal framework for children's services during the 1980s and 90s saw the emphasis begin to shift to one of debates about family involvement and participation in the services that their children received. Writers such as Thoburn (1992) and Marsh and Crow (1998) explored the research and practice possibilities of partnership and participation with families. It is this more recent framework of family involvement in the welfare plans for their children that informs the critical thinking for the discussion within this chapter. This framework for the analysis of family-based social work means that the chapter will not include a comparison of, or commentary on, effective models for professional intervention in family functioning. Instead, it considers the more recent discourses concerned with family engagement evident in Labour's child welfare policies, and the resulting implications for policy and social work practice.

The chapter sets out an overview of the policy and legal context for practice, and reflects on the implications for social work of this context. A brief summary of some of the research that provides evidence for the importance of maintaining family connections in achieving good outcomes for children is provided. The chapter goes on to use the model of family group conferences as an example to explore the tensions and challenges in adopting whole family approaches in social work with children and families. The chapter concludes with a critical reflection on practice and the future implications for social work in this setting.

Understanding families

There is a substantial body of literature that documents the structures and forms of family life and provides evidence of the increasing complexity of 'family'. With this diversification of form have come various implications for childhood and child rearing (Hill and Tisdall, 1997). Child and family social workers face particular challenges given these demographic trends:

> Yet while there are many commonalities about the ways in which people construct their family life, there is nothing set about the family as such ... There are many different families; many different family relationships; and consequently many different family forms. (Allen and Crow, 2000: 21)

One implication for this chapter of the data gathered about family life is the difficulty in defining the term 'family'. The evidence of changing structures and arrangements suggests the need for a broad definition that allows the range of forms to be recognised. Within the ensuing discussion, the term 'family' is therefore used to refer to the child's extended network – not merely the primary carers – and does not propose a specific structure or form. Evidence from a recent literature review (Morris et al., 2008) suggested that many family-based services are actually concerned with parenting, and as Gilles (2005) points out, in reality, are indeed concerned with mothers. This chapter avoids this confusing use of 'family', preferring to conceptualise family as a broad term inclusive of a wide network. Consequently, this discussion takes a critical stance in relation to methods of practice that perceive the family as a homogeneous grouping with common weaknesses or strengths shared by all. Instead, in this analysis for critical practice, family is seen as a rich and varied mix of resources, strengths and difficulties and the analysis aims to consider how practice can develop accordingly.

The work of the CAVA (Care, Values and the Future of Welfare) project (an Economic and Social Research Council group established in 1999 to develop a research programme on changes in parenting and partnering and the implications of these for future social policies; www.leeds.ac.uk/cava/aboutcava/aboutcava.htm), which explores how families conduct their lives, as well as the structures and arrangements for doing so, provided an important insight into contemporary family life. As Williams (2004) describes in her text *Rethinking Families*, research throughout the 1950s, 60s and 70s explored the structure and functioning of families and considered how the nuclear family as a social institution had changed and adapted to meet the demands of a modern society. She suggests that, more recently, research has been framed by 'family practices', concerned with examining how families live their lives, rather than who constitutes 'the family'. The CAVA research project looked at the practical ethics that are important to people in negotiating change in their family lives and personal relationships. The evidence showed people's desire to negotiate the 'proper thing to do'.

The study revealed that when working through their family life dilemmas, for example divorce, separation and work, practical ethics are revealed for adults and children:

> These are the ethics which enable resilience, facilitate commitment and lie at the heart of people's interdependency. They constitute the compassionate realism of 'good enough' care. They include:
>
> - fairness
> - attentiveness to the needs of others
> - mutual respect
> - trust
> - reparation
> - being non-judgemental
> - adaptability to new identities
> - being prepared to be accommodating and
> - being open to communication. (Williams, 2004: 74)

This analysis of family life is important in considering the social work task. Essentially, the empirical data suggests that families want to 'do right' by other family members and consequently will work hard to ensure that family life is supportive. Powers (2007), in her study of families surviving urban deprivation, also noted the key role that family members played in supporting child rearing and parenting, and in supporting children with their relationships with the surrounding physical and social environments. This evidence of the ethic of care frameworks adopted by families suggests that past approaches in social work that have argued for the existence of dangerous families and the absence of a capacity for care and protection may not represent the lived experiences of many families – including families who are marginalised and undergoing traumatic change and in need of social work services.

The legal and policy frameworks

In the decades leading up to the introduction of the Children Act 1989, social work practice with families ranged across a continuum from perceptions of families as needy and inadequate to concepts of families as dangerously dysfunctional. The emergence of research during the 1980s began to question the usefulness of this approach. The evidence of the increased use of formal powers in relation to children (Parton, 1991), coupled with the research that clearly indicated significant shortcomings in corporate parenting (DH, 1991), helped to form the backdrop to the introduction of the Children Act 1989.

Set within this 1989 legal framework were expectations about the principles underpinning child and family social work. Specifically, the Children Act makes clear that:

- where possible children are best brought up within their families
- families should be supported in this task where difficulties emerge
- compulsory intervention must rest on evidence that such action is actively preferable to no formal court order being made.

To achieve the preferred outcome of children being brought up within their families, the Children Act implicitly and explicitly expected professionals to develop working partnerships with families. While the term 'partnership' was confined to the accompanying guidance and regulations, duties within the Children Act to consult, inform and support families formed a framework for practice that renders some form of family involvement a legal requirement:

> The development of a working partnership with parents is usually the most effective route to providing supplementary or substitute care for children. Parents should be expected and enabled to retain their responsibilities and to remain as closely involved as is consistent with their child's welfare, even if that child cannot live at home either temporarily or permanently. (DH, 1989a: 8–9)

Part III of the Children Act 1989 lays out the framework for preventive and supportive services and in doing so introduced new thinking to underpin support services for children in need. Such thinking substantially challenged the basis on which some services had been, and indeed are, provided. The concept of informal helpful support services for a child and their family provided as needed created real tension with the demands of resource management. As research by Aldgate and Tunstill (1995) illustrated, many authorities managed this tension by defining 'children in need' within narrow, acute criteria. Their research showed that for the significant majority of local authorities, children in need were defined by judgements that focused on risk and harm. By working with eligibility criteria that reflected this focus on risk, social work services continued to be based on crisis intervention. One effect of this framework that directed social work services only to those in acute need was to enable underlying professional concepts of 'inadequate families' to be maintained (Morris and Shepherd, 2000).

New Labour's term of office began during the implementation of the 1989 Children Act. The policies developed by Labour indicated a significant shift in the landscape for social work with families – and how families were viewed and responded to in policy discourses. The 1989 Act was the subject of considerable criticism – said to have failed both in the principles it adopted and the manner of implementation. A series of wide-ranging reviews was put in motion, the cross-cutting review of the policy action team (PAT) that considered children and young people at risk argued that:

> PAT believes the philosophy which lay behind the Children Act 1989 has never been put into practice for a combination of reasons:
>
> ■ the fact that the costs of crisis intervention fall on different budgets from those that might fund earlier preventative activity – and services that might fund earlier preventative activity would not receive any payback from it
> ■ the way the priorities for services for young people are set out in legislation and policy guidance, and the consequences this has for their deployment of resources and
> ■ professional cultures. (Home Office, 2000b: 37)

As Labour's policies developed, children's wellbeing was firmly located within a conceptual framework of social exclusion, and services were redefined as the means by which children could be supported to become socially and economically viable citizens. Fawcett et al. (2004) argued that this shift reflected what Giddens (1998a) proposed to be the 'social investment state'. That is, in making this shift, the policy concerns for children and families became those concerned with later citizenship and productivity and the reduction of poor outcomes arising from exclusionary experiences. The earlier focus on individual risk and harm changed, and as a result, families came to be positioned differently in child welfare polices. Instead of acting as co-architects of the particular services their children received (as the 1989 Act supported), the new emphasis on families was as a source of support for the social welfare policies concerned with addressing social exclusion and exclusionary outcomes.

This changing context enabled the emergence of a set of discourses about families that centred on the notion that there was a commonly agreed 'way of being' for families. Labour explicitly and implicitly portrayed 'good' families as hard-working families that shared a common approach to parenting and family life. Those who failed to embrace this normative model were seen as failing to engage with the opportunities afforded to them, and we saw a growing tendency within the legislation to punish failing families (Hill and Tisdall, 1997; Gilles, 2005).

This policy environment led to new legislation and guidance. The *Every Child Matters: Change for Children* (DfES, 2004) agenda saw the introduction of the 2004 Children Act and the *Care Matters* White Paper (DfES, 2007). Alongside this came the introduction of the Public Law Outline (Ministry of Justice, 2008) , with a focus on kinship resolution prior to proceedings and the amendments to the 1989 Children Act – such as the articulation of the option to provide accommodation for families within section 17 of the 1989 Act. The legislation within the youth justice sphere also addressed aspects of family life – including the opportunity to formally sanction families that failed to ensure that their children's behaviour was appropriate (The Crime and Disorder Act 1998). The 2007/08 publications within the *Think Family* Cabinet Office initiative also began to consider the barriers to family-based practice and service delivery and started to identify how new holistic approaches could be developed.

As a result of these developments, we saw a number of changes for social work with families. First, some family members (parents) were expected to become stakeholders in the Labour project of reducing social exclusion. Through a series of large-scale national preventive initiatives, parents were targeted as a way of disrupting children's trajectories and securing inclusionary outcomes. The Sure Start and Children's Fund preventive programmes sought to address poor outcomes for children through the engagement of parents, families and communities, although the extent to which they were able to do so is debatable, with empirical evidence suggesting that marginalised children and parents struggled to take up these services (National Evaluation of the Children's Fund, www.ne-cf.org; National Evaluation of Sure Start, www.ness.bbk.ac.uk).

Second, a revised approach to kinship care emerged as the shortcomings of existing public care provision continued to be evident. Through a series of amendments to existing legislation, fresh guidance and new legislation, Labour sought to enhance the use by social workers of the extended family to care for children (Ministry of Justice, 2007). This development is considered further in the ensuing discussion; however, the tensions within this policy should be noted. The families that come into contact with statutory services in this formal context are often the families that Labour sees as resistant to the prevention-based initiatives already described. Families that are situated in the policy discourses as failing and as reproducing disadvantage (Welshman, 2007) contain the networks that the kinship care policies seek to enlist in the care of children. Indeed, such families, despite their 'othering' in policy discourses about effective child rearing, are simultaneously the families that should be assisted to assume the care of children they are deemed to have failed. These contradictions are further complicated by the realities of families' lived experiences, which are often absent from policy discourses and representations, and families may not perceive their circumstances and experiences to be reflected in policy and practice (Morris et al., 2008).

Third, Labour has started to consider whole family approaches, based in part on the analysis of the limited impact of existing preventive initiatives. Here, the focus is on those families that are seen to be most at risk of social exclusion and traditionally these are the families that seek or receive social work services. The emphasis here is on addressing what are perceived as entrenched and multiple problems (Social Exclusion Task Force, 2007) with a highly targeted and at times punitive approach – such policy developments hold significant implications for social work, which still seeks to practice within a value framework of respectful, participative engagement. The structural, material and attitudinal barriers faced by children, parents and families at risk of social exclusion are an important context for examining policy and practice responses to those considered to be 'difficult to reach' whether through mainstream or targeted services. Krumer-Nevo (2003) uses the term 'defeated families': families that are both defeated by their experiences and by the services that should be assisting them. This discussion has sought to consider how the changing policy context may make the social work task of engaging with defeated families more rather than less complex.

Importance of family connections

There is now a substantial body of research that explores the role and value of kinship networks for children. The outcomes of this research for the purposes of this discussion can be grouped around the themes of the emotional and psychological wellbeing of children, the impact on developing effective plans for children and the role in achieving good outcomes. Common to all this research and understanding is an acknowledgement that not all children can live within their families, nor can all families provide safe care. However, the value of maintaining kinship connections is apparent. Maintaining connections is not, as might be assumed, merely the promotion of contact. Maintaining connections can take a range of forms, such as letters, oral histories, family meetings, but the critical issue for practitioners is the creative thinking necessary to enable kinship connections to be respected. For children, their family can hold the means of understanding their identity and their heritage. While patterns developed within the family may not have been positive for the child, and indeed may even have been harmful, the family network still remains the key holder of the information about attachments, identity and heritage.

Empirical data also show that relatives remain the primary source of support for the majority of children. Research indicates that for many family members, times of particular need lead to increased contact with relatives and carers (McGlone et al., 1998). While the nature and pattern of this support varies according to need, economic circumstances, culture and ethnicity, the majority of children grow up within their kinship network. As established by Morrow (1998), children do not hold a rigid interpretation of family.

As social work has changed to reflect the impetus for integrated children's services and increased participation by those using the services, the role and value of families in planning for their children has been explored. Some aspects of practice have received considerable attention, such as child protection. Other areas such as family support have been less well researched. This may be a reflection of the professional anxieties involved in increased participation, areas of risk provoking more attention than areas of assumed cooperative practice.

Particular attention should be given to the experiences of children and families facing extensive barriers to participation and partnership. As research demonstrates (Bebbington and Miles, 1989), families in receipt of social work services are already facing economic and social disadvantage. The experiences of black and ethnic minority children living away from home highlight the extent to which professionally exclusive practices further exacerbate the oppression encountered (Ahmed, 2005; Hek, 2006). The take-up of family support services, such as family centre services, demonstrates that for many black and ethnic minority families the services provided are not accessible or participative (Butt and Box, 1998).

However, the conclusions drawn from the research exploring family engagement can be perceived as applicable to all areas of practice. Essentially, family participation is both possible and productive in the development of services to children. The more inclusive the approach to practice, the more likely that a child will either remain within their network, or will return to the network successfully (Bullock et al., 1998). Such practice demands changes in professional approaches, and may require new and different skills. It cannot be assumed that professionals hold the skills necessary to undertake social work with a family or to work in harness with a child's network (Morris and Burford, 2006). The following section explores one such practice model of family engagement, and highlights some of the professional challenges and dilemmas.

Family group conferences: an example of whole family approaches

Family group conferences (FGC) are a model of practice that places the child's family at the centre of any planning process, with professionals facilitating and supporting the work of the family. An FGC is, put simply, a significant change in 'the context for resolution' (Doolan, 2007). The scale and ramifications of this 'change in the context' should not be underestimated – few current child welfare services in the UK adopt anything resembling a 'whole family approach' (Morris et al., 2008).

The origins of this model lie in New Zealand – a country with its own family-based cultures and heritages. Importing the model to the UK in the early 1990s can be argued to have been divorced from an understanding of the model's radical social, political and cultural associations. The use of FGCs in New Zealand was embedded within a movement that sought to achieve social justice for Maori families who had lost their children into a white 'stranger carer' system (Burford and Hudson, 2000). The model was developed as a means by which Maori families could use social work services without the loss of right to care for their children. Likewise, in the US, the model is part of a political campaign that seeks to enhance the rights of minority and marginalised families and to deliver on issues of social justice, rather than simply to promote a means of planning to address the needs of a child and their family. The current UK developments in family group conferences pay little heed to this history of civil rights and oppression. Instead, the UK approach has largely been a pragmatic one – using the model, when this seemed feasible, to arrive at alternative outcomes to those currently achieved. But the dominant characteristic of the original model is a substantial shift in power – without this shift, there may be little to commend the use of FGCs as anything other than a process that might, on occasion, be helpful.

Considerable diversity exists in the form and the terms used for family decision-making. The review of the international evidence about the use and impact of family group decision-making (FGDM) found some 50 different types of family decision-making in the US alone (Burford et al., 2007). Therefore, there is considerable value in briefly rehearsing what a family group conference is, drawing on the basic model developed in New Zealand and imported to the UK. The following example illustrates the core features of the model and how the process works.

CASE EXAMPLE

A family group conference

Child A and Child B are both aged under seven and currently live with their aunt. The children's parents are both unable to care for the children because of enduring mental health problems and acknowledged concerns about keeping the children safe. The children's aunt is only temporarily in the UK – she leaves to return to her own children in four weeks' time. The extended family lives in the UK and South Africa. The FGC will need to involve all family members – both those who can attend a meeting and those who will need to participate remotely. The focus of the meeting will be an opportunity for the family to plan how best to meet the children's needs. The core features of the model are:

- Its primary purpose is to enable the whole family to formulate a plan to meet the needs of their child(ren)

- The term 'family' is widely defined to include all those within the child's network, for example blood relatives, family friends, significant others
- To arrive at a plan, families need:
  – adequate information about the professional assessments
  – an understanding of the professional statutory duties and responsibilities
  – descriptions of the resources available.

The FGC process is facilitated/managed by a coordinator, who should be independent insofar as they neither manage nor deliver services to the family. The aim is that the coordinator reflects family preferences regarding language, religion and/or culture, and should be the only person able to veto attendance by family members. Good practice suggests they should do so only on the grounds of risk of physical harm or attendance poses a risk to the wellbeing of the attendee. The nature of the process is inclusive, an assumption that all those identified are invited to participate – indeed it is in part the extended nature of the family participation that seems to encourage better outcomes (Marsh and Crow, 1997).

The core process of the model is:

- A need for a plan is identified – the need can range from support to protection
- A referral is made to an FGC service, a coordinator is appointed
- The coordinator maps out the family, beginning with the child and their immediate carers, alongside identifying those professionals who have a direct contribution to make to the planning meeting
- The coordinator facilitates maximum attendance from both family and professionals – issues of interpretation and translation are addressed, bearing in mind that the language of the FGC will be the family's chosen language. Date, venue and so on agreed with family
- The meeting is convened and where necessary advocates are present to support vulnerable family members. Children are assumed to be full participants but may find an advocate helpful
- The coordinator starts the meeting, facilitates information-sharing and enables family questions. The family is tasked with developing a plan, agreeing monitoring arrangements and contingency plans
- Private family time is held, all professionals withdraw
- The family presents its plan, the coordinator ensures agreement by all members, checks for clarity and ensures the plan is recorded. The professionals should agree principles and negotiate any resources, providing the plan does not place a child at risk of significant harm.

The model does not include the opportunity for professionals to guide the family plan or set the agenda and it does not assume minutes are kept of the meeting – the record of the meeting is the plan. The model is not an opportunity for the professionals connected to the family to complete a family assessment or for any statutory duties held by any party to be relinquished.

The recent developments in guidance for FGCs demonstrate the growing interest the UK government has in this approach. Initially, FGCs were promoted as a useful way of addressing any support needs that a child and their family might have, but were thought to be inappropriate for child protection procedures (DfES, 2006). More recently, the *Think Family* policy documents have identified FGCs as a means of offering a whole family approach to families with multiple and chronic needs.

In the 2006 review of care proceedings (DCA, 2006), FGCs were presented as an appropriate means of addressing matters that may otherwise result in proceedings – the hope here appeared to be that they would facilitate informal resolutions and reduce the need for formal interventions. The resulting promotion of the model of the Public Law Outline seems to fit within this framework and, it could be argued, is linked to attempts to better exploit kinship care opportunities. The *Care Matters* White Paper (DfES, 2007) also promotes the use of FGCs, and supports a programme of training to develop the necessary professional skills. So, in essence, central child welfare policies have increasingly adopted FGCs as a useful social work tool:

- to facilitate early intervention service delivery
- to bring forward alternative resolutions
- as a means of managing formal processes to reduce delay.

The endorsement of FGCs within UK policy and guidance holds within it a series of unresolved contradictions. The tensions created by the adoption in guidance of FGCs as cited above are:

- The model is a family-led approach to problems, but the professional interpretation of the problems, indeed, what is recognised as a problem, may not echo those problems identified by the family. If the professionally defined problems are the only ones a family is asked to respond to, the capacity of the model to achieve change may well be limited.
- Like any planning model, FGCs are only as good as the information they rest upon. Sadly, using FGCs does not guarantee the quality of the assessments or information provided by professionals. They may simply make more evident their shortcomings as families question and explore the information they are given at the start of the meeting.
- If the agenda for a meeting is preset and is essentially 'who can care for child X if parent Y cannot?', this will inevitably influence attendance. The model's potential rests on harnessing the knowledge, resources and insights that a wide range of family members may be able to offer – irrespective of whether or not they can care for the child. To pin the use of the model to this agenda will, I suggest, hinder its potential for arriving at creative, helpful solutions.

A review of the research exploring FGCs and FGDM arrives at a series of themes:

- *FGCs are occurring in many different forms* – The review of the evidence nationally and internationally indicates the broad range of practices under the label of

FGC. Within the UK, the model has been piloted in a range of settings and adapted to reflect the needs arising from these settings, again indicating a diverse range of practices.

- *Not all FGCs are family-led decision-making processes* – This point follows naturally from the above point – extended consultation may well be welcome, but in itself is not a family-led planning process. Such approaches are evident in situations where, for example, families are not left alone to plan in private or where minimal family participation is encouraged. The resulting outcome should not be described as a family plan, or presented in formal settings as the result of an FGC, but existing practice suggests this may occur (Morris and Burford, 2006).

- *Emerging UK-specific practices may start to change the overall empirical understanding of the impact of FGCs* – The evidence from recent UK evaluations suggests that the drive to embed the model within existing practices and polices may be resulting in amended practices that significantly alter the basic principles and characteristics of this approach. Specifically, there is trend towards professionals setting the family a series of questions that the family are asked to respond to in their private planning time (Morris, 2007). These questions may or may not reflect the primary issues the family feels it is facing, and there is empirical evidence of these questions being used as an opportunity to complete a shortfall in the assessment.

- *Most families produce safe, appropriate plans* – The reviews of the research evidence have a consistent theme – families are able to plan for their children and this process of engagement produces evidence of significant engagement of family members in the wellbeing of their children. Families are positive about this approach, while realistic about the difficulties they may face in trying to plan together. Families also experience this approach as culturally responsive and an intrinsically different way of working with them, facilitating a greater use of their knowledge and resources.

- *Evidence of reduced need for formal intervention and increased kinship care, formal and informal* – FGCs do support a greater level of care of children within their extended network, and reduce the need for formal state intervention. However, less is known about the longitudinal outcomes of this approach and whether family plans are sustained in the medium to long term. Indeed, some evidence suggests that the maintenance of plans, by families and professionals, can be difficult. Family life changes, initial goodwill may evaporate and professionals may not honour their original undertakings.

FGCs are one example of the ways in which social workers can engage with families.

Conclusion

Whole family approaches in social work are seemingly in a period of renaissance. The existing splits between services (adult/child or by type of need) are unable to respond effectively to the multiple and complex needs that may cross generations or networks (Morris et al., 2008). This analysis, and the evidence of the limited impact of some existing provision, has provoked a review of how families are responded to by social care and social welfare provision. While the above discussion has explored one model of whole family approaches and the potential it offers, this resurgence of interest in families also brings with it some unease. The basis for the Labour government's political and policy shift towards families lies in the conceptual framework of inherited or transmitted deprivation. This link to previous understandings of failing families as dysfunctional and hard to reach runs counter to the values framework for social work practice and may result in families being the subject of intervention rather than participants in achieving change.

Existing social work practices demonstrate a growing capacity for service user partnerships. Our understanding of families from empirical data and analysis suggests that they are sources of support and guidance. The challenge for social work lies in identifying and adopting approaches that capture the strengths of families, despite a political context that may stigmatise and alienate marginalised families. Underpinning examples of innovative practice developments are complex issues of professional attitudes and values (Brown, 2007). Central to the critical development of inclusive social work practice are core values about the worth and value of service user input (Morris and Shepherd, 2000). In seeking to take forward new approaches to working with families, social work will need to reflect on the uneasy union between its values framework of challenging oppression and inequalities with a policy discourse that marks out marginalised families as pathologically weak and unwilling or unable to take up the opportunities presented.

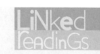

For further discussion of aspects of social work with children and families, see Adams et al., 2009a, Chapter 22 and Adams et al., 2009c, Chapter 4.

www.americanhumane.org   The website of the American Humane Association: National Center of Family Group Decision Making offers a leading resource for information about family decision-making. Seeks to promote family decision-making and therefore does have a bias towards this approach.

www.frg.org.uk   Family Rights Group. Leading UK-based web and agency resource on family involvement in child welfare policy and practice, includes a dedicated FGC section and seeks to promote family engagement by professionals.

Henricson, C. and Bainham, A. (2004) *The Child and Family Policy Divide*, York, Joseph Rowntree Foundation, www.jrf.org.uk. Explores the current adult/child divide within UK service provision, and identifies the difficulties and challenges this presents.

Morris, K., Hughes, N., Clarke, H. et al. (2008) *Think Family: A Literature Review of Whole Family Approaches*, www.cabinetoffice.gov.uk/social_exclusion_task_force. This literature review considers the evidence nationally and internationally and explores the emerging theory and practice.

Williams, F. (2004) *Rethinking Families*, London, Calouste Gulbenkian Foundation. Draws together the CAVA research project findings as they relate to family life, and offers important insights into family approaches to the resolution of difficulties.

Youth justice and young offenders

26

This chapter argues that a critical understanding of the youth justice system and knowledge of international conventions are needed for effective work with young offenders. It makes its case based on a philosophy of putting children first.

Chapter overview

CASE EXAMPLE

John is 15 years old. He is currently on remand in a private remand centre over 200 miles from home. John has a short history of committing minor offences and has been subjected to a number of interventions. Many of John's problems are linked to difficulties he has experienced with school. Since starting secondary school, John has been the subject of bullying. A child of normal abilities and performance in primary school, John's schoolwork has since deteriorated and he often plays truant.

John's first offence, a minor act of criminal damage, was committed when he was 13, for which he received a police reprimand. Two months later, John was arrested for an act of minor criminal damage, committed while he was truanting from school. The police gave him a final warning and referred him to the youth offending service (YOS). John's YOS worker involved him in an offending behaviour programme designed to tackle his lack of respect for other people's property. John did not seem interested and failed to complete the programme. During the school holidays, John was involved in two antisocial behaviour incidents: underage drinking and throwing stones at houses. He was reported to the antisocial behaviour unit and received a warning letter.

After the school holidays, John's reoffending continued, again while he was truanting from school. John was arrested for shoplifting from a sports store. He had been under surveillance for some time, being suspected of theft by store detectives on previous occasions. John was prosecuted and given a referral order by the youth court. The YOS, police and the sports store were represented on the youth offender panel. Two magistrates participated as community representatives. John attended with his parents. During the panel, John talked about his problems with school and bullying. He explained that he had taken the sports shoes, which were later recovered, to try to 'fit in' with other kids.

The panel agreed a programme for John comprising the sending of a letter of apology to the sports store manager, parentally supervised after-school-only visits to the shopping centre, 15 hours community service and a requirement that he attend school. Monitoring quickly showed that John breached the programme's requirements. His truanting continued but, more seriously, John reacted negatively to the punitive and restrictive elements of the programme.

Following the panel, John's truanting and offending escalated. On his 15th birthday, John was arrested for shoplifting and bailed. One week later, John's school contacted the police, as he was found in possession of a knife. The school suspended him. The police arrested him for carrying an offensive weapon. John explained that he carried the knife because he had been threatened by other boys and wanted to protect himself. He was prosecuted and remanded in custody.

John is now on remand in custody. He was interviewed in custody by YOS bail support staff who assessed him as unsuitable for a bail support programme due to previous non-compliance. YOS staff recorded, however, that John appeared isolated in custody, had not received visits from his parents and had reported being bullied and afraid. Consequently, John was made subject to special supervision by custodial staff.

Critical practice could have prevented John's situation. A critical practitioner would not have subjected John to an offending behaviour programme without holistically evaluating his behaviour. The youth offender panel should have dealt with the school problems more effectively and information from YOS partner agencies, for example the antisocial behaviour unit and police, could have been shared at an early stage to enable appropriate interventions to be deployed. John's YOS worker did raise his non-attendance at school during the panel, but expressed frustration at the way in which the YOS sought only to deal with offending behaviour instead of engaging effectively with other agencies, involving them in focused, problem-solving approaches. YOS staff believe bullying is prevalent in schools but that sometimes attempts are made to hide the problem to protect the school's reputation, with limited anti-bullying programmes being implemented.

Throughout John's short teenage years, no one has listened to his story, taken his problems seriously or acted constructively to improve his situation. A lack of critical practice has failed John. Interventions have focused on John's offending, failing to address the problems underlying his behaviour. Instead, John has been perceived as a problem and an offender: the system has responded to him accordingly. As a result, John, an average 15-year-old child, sits alone and afraid in custody awaiting his fate.

The youth justice system in England and Wales has been completely overhauled by a raft of legislation that has left no area of the system untouched (see, generally, Goldson, 2000; Pickford, 2000). The range and extent of these reforms make a detailed, critical analysis beyond the scope of one short chapter (but see Goldson, 1999, 2000; Muncie, 1999; Goldson and Muncie, 2006). Indeed, it would be a mistake to embark on a path of critical practice in a piecemeal and ad hoc manner, as this would subsume critical practice within the boundaries of the government's agenda, and critical practice must, at times, step outside these boundaries. This chapter will discuss reform of the youth justice system and develop an approach to critical practice that is grounded in an understanding of the youth justice system, international conventions and a children first philosophy.

The politics of juvenile crime

Throughout history, no area of public policy has attracted such sustained interest and controversy as crime, and none more so than juvenile crime. In recent times, we have become accustomed to the politicisation of juvenile crime, and, all too often, particular juvenile offenders. The politics of juvenile crime, it seems, fuels the rhetoric of governments and political parties as they compete to capture the popular punitiveness of public opinion and electoral success (Pitts, 2000).

Doing something about juvenile crime is a constant feature of national politics. This 'doing something' inevitably leads to policies and calls from government to intervene more seriously and earlier into the lives of young people who have offended – the 'nipping offending in the bud' mantra. However, critical practice, initiated, developed and extended through local networks of juvenile justice practitioners, has a long and important, although chequered, history (see Thorpe et al., 1980; Haines and Drakeford, 1998). The need for critical practice is paramount. No matter how clever the government thinks it is, no matter how much it believes that it should steer and local agencies should row (Pitts, 2000), no matter how many tactics it seeks to employ to ensure local compliance with central policy, there is an enduring need and capacity for local agents to shape and mould national structures into local practices.

Intervention, intervention, intervention

Although a common-sense view might be that policies towards juveniles who have offended are generally tougher and more punitive under a Conservative than a Labour administration, this has not necessarily been the case in recent decades. It is true that the Conservative administration from 1979 to 1997 ushered in some overtly punitive measures, and it would be quite wrong to attribute the 'Thatcher years' as child friendly (Haines, 1997). In criminal justice terms, however, the Conservative administration quietly sanctioned and gradually adopted most of the practitioner-led developments, which resulted, among other things, in a significant growth in diversion from prosecution and a reduction in custodial sentencing (Haines and Drakeford, 1998). These major trends overlaid some other notable practices. During the 1980s and early 1990s, there was no evidence that that system was net-widening (Bottoms et al., 1980) or up-tariffing – intensive community-based supervision was being effectively targeted at the so-called 'heavy end' young people who would otherwise receive a custodial sentence (Bottoms, 1995). Thus, other lower tariff disposals remained important sentencing options. The conditional discharge, for example, remained a popular sentence of the court and an effective disposal in terms of low reconviction rates (Audit Commission, 1996).

High rates of diversion from prosecution, popular and effective low tariff sentences, properly targeted intensive supervision and low rates of custodial sentencing, plus no evidence of an increase in the amount or seriousness of juvenile crime were, therefore, the characteristics of the juvenile justice system as it operated under the Conservative government prior to the election of the Labour administration in 1997 (Haines and Drakeford, 1998). The type of work with young offenders promoted during this period (Haines, 1996; Haines and Drakeford, 1998) was based on professional knowledge about the effectiveness of different types of intervention, including the potential for inappropriate interventions to have negative short- and long-term consequences.

New Labour and youth justice

While one might expect to find a more interventionist core at the heart of Labour policy, one might also expect this interventionism to reflect a more child-oriented than offender-oriented character (Pitts, 2000). In just over a year after election, the Labour government enacted the Crime and Disorder Act 1998 – following the White Paper, *No More Excuses: A New Approach to Tackling Youth Crime in England and Wales* (Home Office, 1997) – which ushered in the major elements of its reforms of the juvenile justice system. The very title of the White Paper was to give an important indication of Labour thinking and policy. In his introduction to the White Paper, the home secretary said:

> An excuse culture has developed within the youth justice system. It excuses itself for its inefficiency, and too often excuses the young offenders before it, implying that they cannot help their behaviour because of their social circumstances. (Home Office, 1997: 2)

This statement is significant in a number of important ways.

1 It demonstrates the policy of the Labour government to discredit the youth justice system and portray any claims for success in organisational, administrative or professional terms as obfuscations of the underlying realities.
2 This undermining of the 'old youth justice system' represents an attempt to establish a discontinuity with the past, thus creating the opportunity for the Labour Party to fashion the new youth justice in its own image. Thus, the heavy baggage of those who operated the 'old' system did not need to be unpacked and examined, it was simply to be left behind.

3   It indicates that the government was not going to tolerate offending behaviour or those who 'made excuses' for it.

The strength of these anti-child (even if they are offenders) attitudes was both necessary and problematic for the Labour government – necessary because of the Labour Party's emerging interventionist philosophy and the need to manage the perceptions of the fear of crime, but problematic because of its anti-child sentiments and the contradictions with the broader social inclusion agenda. The contradictions and consequent bifurcation are clear:

> To put it more bluntly, current youth crime policy appears equally committed to preventing the social exclusion of children and young people at risk and increasing the exclusion of those who go on to offend. (Anderson, 1999: 83)

The resultant confusions, caused by competing political objectives, have led to a professional and morally undesirable outcome:

> By drawing the less problematic young people into an extended social control network at an earlier age, Labour has revealed how a logic of 'prevention' and 'risk management' is quite capable of being used to justify any number of repressive and retrograde means of dealing with young people in trouble. (Muncie, 1999: 59)

Whatever the contradictions and conflicts, the moral or ethical vicissitudes of the Labour Party, its policy for youth justice is 'held together' by the official objective for the youth justice system of preventing offending by children and young people. Furthermore, the Labour government has shown a determination to have its policies put into practice. To this end, in September 1998, it established the Youth Justice Board (YJB) for England and Wales, whose responsibility is to ensure that the policy, philosophy and practices of the new youth justice are implemented speedily and fully. Although, as a quango, the YJB has few formal powers, it has a considerable amount of money at its disposal to 'pay for' the development of 'desirable' practices in the new multi-agency youth offending teams (YOTs) and it has produced and promulgated a series of guidance documents evidencing effective practice in a range of youth justice interventions (Stephenson et al., 2007).

Since its creation, the YJB has set about ensuring that the Labour government's policy for youth justice is implemented. Strenuous efforts went into ensuring that local areas established YOTs in the manner envisioned by the YJB. Fervent endeavours have been applied to the development and implementation of new practices in these YOTs. The YJB has made use of every opportunity and mechanism at its disposal to ensure that a new system is created in the image it intends. In short, from its inception to its implementation, the new youth justice is a top-down venture. It is thus important to unpick, a little, this broader context in which youth justice practice is now managed and conducted.

The managerialist approach

The postmodern approach to crime and offenders is centred on the management of insecurity in the present, not the guaranteeing of security or the promise of a better future (see Finer and Nellis, 1998). Are we just to accept this as the inevitability of our modern culture, or do we believe in the capacity of individuals to shape and reinterpret macro-social structures in (sometimes different) micro- or local practices? It is our capacity to give light to this latter possibility that drives critical practice.

The framework in which we struggle to manage caseloads on a daily basis, or within which we try to create space for new or fresh thinking, is not normally one of our own making, but rather it is imposed from above. In the area of crime, and crime prevention in particular, Pitts and Hope (1998) have argued that a central government policy has been superimposed on what remain essentially local criminal justice agencies. Thus, in Britain, local actors have found themselves operating within different agencies struggling to compete in an imposed interagency framework, which did little to meet the daily work needs of staff and, more seriously, at best only tenuously made any positive impact on the lives of local people, whether they had committed offences or not (Haines, 1996). This brief discussion is important because it highlights the central characteristics of the British government's approach to policy development and implementation. Thus, the establishment of YOTs, the new framework of youth justice, the setting of objectives for the system, the development of administrative/professional tools, and the measurement of performance and so on have not been the product of local discussion, debate and action, but rather have been and continue to be imposed by the government and the YJB in an ongoing, ever-changing and increasingly prescriptive manner. The most significant problem that this approach gives rise to is the tendency of YOTs to take, as their primary reference point for the organisation and delivery of services, the national YJB and not those communities which the teams serve.

Critical practice, therefore, begins from an understanding of the institutional context of youth justice and the implications of the choices that are made within this broader context. There are important connections between structural and organisational factors and the services that YOTs provide and, perhaps more importantly, the manner in which these services are provided. Processing a child through a final warning, recommending a referral order and running a youth offender panel, completing an ASSET assessment and supervising a child following a period in custody can be undertaken with different objectives. A team can pursue these activities because they comprise government policy, legislative requirements or because they are prescribed by national standards, key elements of effective practice (Stephenson et al., 2007) and the 'scaled approach' (see www.yjb.gov.uk), or these activities can be conducted to promote the best interests of the child in a manner consistent with professional knowledge and objectives (see Case et al., 2005). These differing approaches are in tension and it is essential that practitioners understand these tensions and are clear about their objectives in planning and undertaking interventions.

The criminology literature is redolent with publications exploring and explaining the vicissitudes of managerialism (Peters, 1986; Feeley and Simon, 1992; McWilliams, 1992; Vanstone, 1995; Haines, 1996, 1997; Brownlee, 1998) and the pursuit of policy objectives through increasingly intrusive administrative control measures. Ranged against this is professional knowledge, which often appears weaker or less certain, but in reality is simply more complex, as it deals with the real lives of real people and not simply organisational processes. In modern criminal justice systems, therefore, critical practice is rooted inevitably in professionalism.

Reconnecting with the past

Critical practice also begins with what we know. We have already noted how a central characteristic of the Labour government and the YJB's strategy for implementing the new youth justice discredited previous practice and the professional knowledge that supported it, in order to disconnect the new (managerialist, administrative, policy-driven) future from the old (professionally based) past. Critical practice, therefore, must take as an important starting point an appreciation of what we already know about young people, the social conditions that shape their behaviour and the effectiveness of interventions and reconnect this knowledge with current practice.

Such a call is not an anti-government statement, but a recognition that there are times when professional knowledge supersedes government policy and that to act professionally is not always the same as compliance with administrative requirements. How and when can we make the decision about when it is appropriate to act in such a manner? In part this decision is based on the accumulated knowledge of what works in working with young people. Intervention must be based on solid, grounded, professional practice knowledge. But there is also a higher calling, and it is to this we must turn.

Fundamental principles for positive critical practice

Any attempt at an international comparison of youth justice practices will demonstrate the differences between systems across countries (Mehlbye and Walgrave, 1998). In the modern world, however, countries no longer operate solely within the boundaries of the nation-state, but increasingly there is an international context that structures the behaviour of all countries. International texts concerning the special treatment that should be afforded to children, including juvenile offenders, have been developing over the past 100 years or so. The 1924 Geneva Declaration of the Rights of the Child stated that particular care must be extended to children. This sentiment has been echoed in a range of international conventions (see, for example, Haines, 2000). The 1985 United Nations Standard Minimum Rules for the Administration of Juvenile Justice – often referred to as the Beijing Rules – state that as a fundamental principle, the aim of the juvenile justice system should be the promotion of the wellbeing of the juvenile and that criminal proceedings (of any kind) should be conducted in the best interests of the juvenile. The Beijing Rules are not binding in domestic law, but the 1989 United Nations Convention on the Rights of the Child is legally binding on countries that have signed the declaration, and in Article 3, it includes the important statement that:

In all actions concerning children, whether undertaken by public or private social welfare institutions, courts of law, administrative authorities or legislative bodies, the best interests of the child shall be a primary consideration.

In this instance, the definition of 'child' is any young person under the age of 18 years, and the Convention makes no allowance for different considerations to be made in respect of some children who may be labelled as, for example, 'offenders' – all children are to be treated according to the same principle. The definition of 'a primary consideration' (as it appears in the English version of Article 3) is intended to be 'the paramount' or 'most important consideration' (as appears in Article 21). These international conventions, therefore, firmly establish the principle that any action taken as a result of an offence committed by a juvenile must be in the best interests of the child.

Providing a universal definition of 'best interests' is, of course, no simple matter and deciding whether a particular action is in the best interests of the child is complex. However, the Convention itself provides some further guidance in these matters. For example, children have the right to education of a positive nature, to give their views and have their views listened to, not to be separated from their parents (unless it is in the child's best interests) or to have access to their parents where forced separation occurs, to leisure time and recreational activities, and to be protected from maltreatment, hazardous forms of employment (including that which interferes with school or play) and other forms of exploitation. These provisions have been established to give special recognition to the status of childhood and in particular the notion that childhood is a period of transition before adulthood and the nature of these transitions must be understood and acted upon (see Coles, 1995).

In thinking about work with young offenders, therefore, we must start from thinking about youth and about linking interventions with young people in difficulty into the range of provisions or activities that exists for all young people. In other words, international conventions establish the principle that interventions with young people, including those who have committed an offence, should be based on the premise of 'normalisation'. Thus, normalisation is a fundamental principle upon which all interventions with young offenders should be based and, in fact, this means reversing the trend of criminal justice interventions that have been recently developed in youth justice.

In England and Wales in recent years, the thrust of developments in offender interventions has been towards the development of evermore specialist, targeted and focused programmes. This trend is exemplified most strongly in the probation service, which, under particular pressure from the Home Office, has concentrated on 'evidence-based practice' (Hope and Chapman, 1998), cognitive programmes (McGuire, 2000) and accreditation for staff to conduct such activities, but similar developments are increasingly characteristic of youth justice (see Stephenson et al., 2007). In this manner, staff are trained and programmes of intervention are developed that draw offenders away from the community and into closed, intensive, 'offender-oriented' and offence-focused activities. Even where the 'community' may be involved in such activities, as may be the case, for example, in young offender panels, it is not the offender or the young person that is inserted into the community, but representatives of the community are drawn into the closed programme.

Evidence from Massachusetts (Coates, 1981) has shown the value, in terms of reduced levels of reoffending, of programmes that are 'community linked', but the principle of normalisation urges us to go further. A fully operational normalised programme of interventions would eschew the provision of specialist activities for offenders. Instead, intervention would be based on (re)inserting young people into the full range of social and educational provision that exists for youth in general. This approach is no less specialist or challenging, but it requires a changed focus of intervention, away from intervening in the lives of young people and towards intervening in the mechanisms that link young people into social and educational services.

Such an approach is predicated on the exclusion experienced by many young people in trouble with the law. For example, local monitoring in Swansea has shown that 70–80 per cent of all young people made subject to criminal supervision orders were not engaged in meaningful daytime activities (Haines et al., 1999). For those receiving custodial sentences, the figure was in excess of 90 per cent. A survey of first-time offenders indicated that over 20 per cent of the young people were either absent or excluded from school. Over half the young people, or their family, were in receipt of services from the social services department. It was also clear that the costs of exclusion continued into life after school, with higher numbers of young people who were disaffected and disengaged from education, training and employment involved in chaotic use of drugs and alcohol and lengthier patterns of involvement in offending behaviour. Risk-focused interventions rarely target these challenging social circumstances experienced by young people, yet they remain central to critical practice.

A normalised strategy of interventions, therefore, is based on the promotion of social inclusion. The promotion of social inclusion is, in fact, an explicit policy of the current government, but, as this chapter has shown, it is difficult to visualise the principles or practices of social inclusion in the methods of intervention promoted by the government and the YJB. Youth justice policy has become increasingly politicised, which has not only led to vacillations in policy directions and the exploitation of youth for political advantage, but to the development of an approach to working with young people in difficulty that reduces social inclusion and promotes social exclusion. This is a strategy the research evidence suggests is not only likely to promote further deviance and reduce the chances for young people to develop a positive life course, it is also contrary to the principles of international conventions. Before concluding this chapter, therefore, it is necessary to revise the key concepts, enshrined in international conventions, that shape critical practice in youth justice:

- Interventions should be in the best interests of the child
- Offence- or offender-focused programmes should be avoided
- Work with young people, including those who have offended, should be based on the accumulated knowledge and experience gained through practice
- Practice should be guided by the principle of normalisation and the promotion of social inclusion

- Normalised and inclusive practice is characterised by:
  - *justice*, not only in a formal legal sense, but according to the principles of natural justice
  - *participation* of young people in the full range of social and educational provision for youth
  - *engagement*, giving expression to the right of young people to make their own choices and decisions and to be fully involved in all matters concerning them.

Conclusion

This chapter has not focused on the details of interventions with young offenders or the range of new measures and changes to the youth justice system introduced by the current Labour government. The proliferation of new measures and so on renders such an approach beyond description and would also obviate the articulation of an alternative practice based on a critical approach, which has been the central objective here. Instead, this chapter has focused on an understanding of the dynamics of youth justice and the principles of intervention from which and upon which critical practice can be built and measured.

The central theme of this chapter has been that critical practice is based upon the accumulated professional knowledge about the effectiveness of approaches and methods of working with young people. It has been argued, further, that this knowledge must be placed in the context of international conventions concerning the treatment of young people and the principles set forth in these documents. Therefore the challenge for youth justice is not to find ways of meeting targets for the development of new measures, but to develop these new measures in a manner that protects and promotes the best interests of the child.

For further discussion of work with young people who truant and offend, see Adams et al., 2009c, Chapter 5, and for drug users, see Adams et al., 2009c, Chapter 10.

Goldson, B. (2000) *The New Youth Justice*, Lyme Regis, Russell House Publishing. Comprehensive and critical review of New Labour's youth justice and youth crime strategy.

Goldson, B. and Muncie, J. (eds) (2006) *Youth Crime and Justice*, London, Sage. Edited collection from leading experts covering a wide range of youth justice topics.

Muncie, J., Hughes, G. and McLaughlin, E. (2006) *Youth Justice: Critical Readings*, London, Sage. Drawn from a wide range of published material, provides a good introduction and discussion of a wide range of youth justice issues.

Stephenson, M., Giller, H. and Brown, S. (2007) *Effective Practice in Youth Justice*, Cullompton, Willan. Edited rebranded collection of the YJB's guides for YOT practitioners on effective practice across a range of youth justice interventions.

Safeguarding adults 27

This chapter explores the mechanisms in place for safeguarding vulnerable adults against abuse, exploitation or neglect and reflects on progress towards coherent practice in this arena. On the way, it addresses important questions about the way terms such as 'vulnerability' and 'abuse' are being used and about the aspirations that are wrapped up in the notion of 'safeguarding'.

Chapter overview

The first comprehensive guidance on safeguarding adults was published by the British government in 2000 under the title *No Secrets: Guidance on Developing and Implementing Multi-agency Policies and Procedures to Protect Vulnerable Adults from Abuse* (DH, 2000b). It was issued as secondary legislation, under section 7 of the 1970 Local Authority Social Services Act, which made it incumbent on social services to act as the lead agency in coordinating local arrangements.

The emergence of this policy over the past 10 years has sent up many shoots, which include measures for:

- improving the sharing of information between agencies
- planning and conducting multi-agency investigations and implementing risk management strategies
- adapting court procedures so that they are more accessible
- tightening regulation
- barring unsuitable individuals from the social care workforce.

If it seems at first glance that these measures run counter to the overarching commitment towards personalisation and flexibility that is driving current service provision, a more careful analysis of what it is that vulnerable people are at risk of helps to set the record straight. Safety, for people who rely on social care services, should not be bought at the expense of autonomy but seen as an essential element within it. But the converse is also true because it is vital that increased personalisation and flexibility does not leave some vulnerable people exposed and out of their depth.

Who counts as a vulnerable adult?

In drawing a line around who was to be included within the scope of the new policy, the guidance drew on previous deliberations, including the Law Commission document *Who Decides?* (1997), which had been issued as part of the consultation leading up to the introduction of the Mental Capacity Act 2005. The concept of a 'vulnerable adult' was incorporated within *No Secrets* to establish a boundary around those adults on whose behalf additional assistance would be mandated. The definition has two elements, referring to a person over the age of 18:

- who is or may be in need of community care services by reason of mental or other disability, age or illness
- who is or may be unable to take care of him or herself, or unable to protect him or herself against significant harm or exploitation (DH, 2000b: 9).

This means that any potential user of social services is entitled to assistance in relation to abuse, while those people who also lack capacity to make their own decisions or take protective steps on their own behalf will warrant more proactive intervention to ensure their best interests are safeguarded. The definition therefore reflects both an eligibility element and a judgement about capacity and autonomy but this chapter demonstrates that these are not unproblematic concepts when applied in the context of abuse. Although we hope to create cohesive communities where differences can be respected, older people or those who have disabilities or mental health problems are sometimes targeted in ways that other adults are not, even where they are usually managing their daily lives without much input from formal service settings: so the strict eligibility criteria adopted by social services departments screen out people who are in many ways more vulnerable than other citizens.

Some people are failed because they do not present as stereotypical 'victims' and the fact that they may also pose risks to others cuts across a shared commitment to safeguard their rights. Punitive models sometimes leak into services and the way they are managed, including into the conduct of any physical interventions that are authorised. 'Vulnerable' adults include in their ranks, for example, those who might just be seen as cantankerous alongside others who have a long history of violence, and also takes in adults living out-of-control, on-the-edge, hand-to-mouth lives – even if these are rarely glimpsed behind a veneer of bravado and addictions so that others struggle to empathise with them. For example, a young man with learning disabilities, who was tortured and murdered as a result of a hate crime, had difficulties with alcohol that might have cut across a willingness to help on the part of responsible agencies (see Cornwall Social Services, 2008). Understanding of the Mental Capacity Act tends not to look at the impact of trauma, drugs or alcohol on decision-making or credibility, even though there is evidence that these get in the way of accurate assessment.

Assessing capacity in the context of abuse is also complex, since the law is based on the idea that decision-making is a rational, linear process, where information is used to weigh up the pros and cons of a decision and come to a view about how to proceed. The reality is often something more messy that happens in, and under the influence of, competing relationships and expectations and where decisions are taken in a force field that can include deception, oppression, undermining or violence. Abuse, in which people who are visibly different are specifically targeted and groomed, as in cases of sexual or financial abuse, particularly test this framework, because the abuser actively sets out to disguise their intentions or the nature of the interaction. But these are a minority of cases, most abuse is much more ordinary and understandable, and vulnerable adults can usually be helped to access mainstream sources of support or avenues for redress. With support, most vulnerable adults can take good decisions for themselves, but the capacity element of the definition has to be applied in a careful and sensitive way. Deciding to leave a violent relationship or complain about care from a service that you will continue to be reliant upon, or making an allegation against a care worker who comes into your home are all decisions that would test anyone, regardless of their mental capacity. Decisions also have to be taken in the wake of an abusive incident or relationship, for example the person may be asked to decide if they wish to report a crime to the police or pursue a prosecution, and these are likely to be emotionally fraught matters made more complex by trauma and distress. These decisions need to be tempered by public interest and acknowledge the difficulty created by threats and intimidation, as happens in domestic violence cases.

What is meant by the term 'abuse'?

'Abuse' is also a contentious term and many people do not like it as an umbrella description. As a term, it can seem to minimise very serious crimes at one end of a spectrum, while sensationalising more minor infringements and relationship difficulties at the other. Other more uncompromising terms have been coined, including the naming of some crimes as 'disability hate crimes', which more accurately describes a few, very high-profile cases but, when generalised to the plight of a carer who is at the end of their tether, is too clumsy and even counterproductive, in that it risks stigmatising people who are out of their depth rather than full of 'hate'. Its starkness may discourage people from coming forward to ask for timely help, or work against whistle-blowers who want to bring concerns out into the open in a helpful way.

One way of conceptualising abuse is to think of it as an inability to control one's own personal space and bodily integrity, and would apply to anyone who finds themselves invaded or intruded upon in their own home (see, for example, Royal Courts of Justice, 2008). Relationships that are based on violence or exploitation may be downplayed but interlopers who are drawn into the vacuum that exists in the often sparse social contact of vulnerable adults can too easily be characterised as 'friends' by services that are overstretched and glad to be able to back off in the untested belief that this is someone receiving 'care in the community'. Similarly, actions that people have been forced to engage in are sometimes too readily seen as valid 'choices'. The fact is that if you cannot say 'no' to something, you are not really saying yes to it either, and these issues of intimidation and exploitation need to be taken clearly into account in the way situations are assessed and risk is managed.

So there is an urgency about unpicking the range of abuses that occur and understanding their very different roots, which do not reflect only those few individuals who harbour malicious intentions towards vulnerable people, but the conditions in which many otherwise caring and diligent care staff tip over into abusive practice, or the pressures that can drive a previously loving family member, or partner, to collapse into neglect, or lash out in frustration.

Different forms of abuse and abusing

No Secrets (DH, 2000b) began the task of definition by identifying the types of harm that come within the purview of the term 'abuse', setting out distinct categories:

- Physical abuse
- Sexual abuse
- Psychological abuse
- Financial abuse
- Neglect
- Discriminatory abuse.

But this 'list' approach seems to have reached the end of its usefulness. A recent analysis of abuse cases reported to one large social services department (Cambridge et al., 2006) identified the fact that most cases involved 'multiple' abuse, so we need to look beyond the nature of each act for explanations or helpful subcategories that might signpost us towards suitable remedies or indications of seriousness or risk. It is as if the 'types' are like beads in a kaleidoscope that needs to be turned if we want to see the pieces fall into place and allow patterns to emerge.

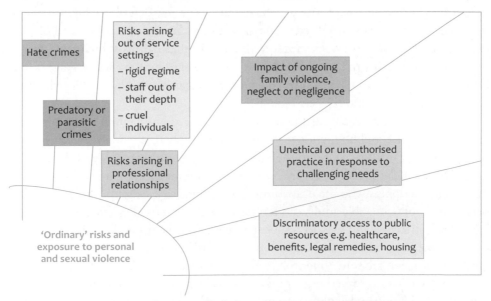

Figure 27.1 Constellations (not types) of abuse emerging from the literature

Source: Adapted from Brown and Seddon, 2003

Contextualising these isolated acts allows us to see them as the product of relationships and settings and thereby to forge more accurate explanations without deviating from a zero-tolerance stance. This 'map' also makes explicit the fact that service users are exposed to more harm than other people – they not only face 'ordinary' risks but additional sources of distress and in circumstances that make it more difficult for them to remove themselves or actively resist. It is not the case that abuse is purely a function of a person's impairment; just as disability arises out of social barriers and prejudices, vulnerability to abuse is more complex. But it would seem that being a member of a disadvantaged group involves more exposure to risk.

At the right-hand end of this continuum are abuses that are widespread and relatively low profile in the safeguarding world: discrimination against people on the grounds of age and/or disability is ubiquitous. It affects people's right to housing, employment and healthcare, including screening and clinical decision-making. Challenging needs and the need for intimate care demand clear boundaried practice and this is not always forthcoming in services. Difficult or aggressive incidents seem to invite retaliation, especially in the absence of a clear value base and professional narrative about the person's behaviour (see, for example, DH, 2003b). Intimate care is also a challenge, in that it involves stepping out of socially comfortable roles into space that is usually off limits: if carers are not helped to find ways of managing this, they may find it difficult to carry out these tasks respectfully, or to step back and re-establish appropriate distance when personal care tasks have been completed (Cambridge and Carnaby, 2006). A clear ethical framework is therefore required.

About half the abuse reported to social services takes place in the family (Cambridge et al., 2006; O'Keefe et al., 2007). It may be perpetrated by spouses, adult children caring for older relatives, or parents caring for adult children with disabilities. It may be an extension of ongoing domestic violence, or a role reversal fuelled by retaliation where there has been former abuse. Where domestic violence has characterised a relationship before one party became frail, it is likely that the dynamics will conform to other forms of gender-based violence. But sometimes family abuse represents a breakdown in an otherwise caring relationship, perhaps because the carer's situation deteriorates or their own difficulties escalate. A vulnerable adult has less scope for leaving when things go wrong in their family and this exacerbates family tensions and removes the most common form of resolution.

Abuse by people who are paid to be in the lives of vulnerable people tends to look different, depending on the power and status of the worker involved. Recent inquiries into some powerful healthcare professionals, especially in mental health services, eating disorder units and GP practices, uncover a pattern of arrogance and non-accountability that seems to license some workers to abuse, often through sexual exploitation but also in other departures from sound clinical practice (Halter et al., 2007). On the other hand, the literature about low-paid workers would suggest that they are sometimes motivated to abuse out of resentment, lack of knowledge or retaliation. When whole services sink into what is sometimes described as 'institutional' abuse, it may involve a mix of insensitive routines leading to rigid and impersonal care, and be compounded by a staff team that has not received appropriate training, support or supervision and therefore they do not know how they should conduct themselves, but also it may either allow or mask cruel individuals who do not stand out against the blurred backdrop of a poor service like the numbers in a colour-blindness test that cannot be seen.

Towards the left-hand end of the continuum, it is clear that the perpetrator's psychopathology and criminal intentions are driving the dangerous behaviour of a few individuals in cases that are universally condemned and morally unambiguous. Sexual and financial abusing often proceed from a deliberate process of targeting and grooming that might involve either deception or intimidation. Recent cases have also highlighted a more 'parasitic' (I am indebted to Dr Margaret Flynn for coining this term to draw attention to this particular form of abusive behaviour) mode of abusing especially where vulnerable people are living in, but cannot eject unwanted people from, their own accommodation, so that their space is taken over, their food stolen, their homes used to deal drugs or to store stolen goods and so forth. Hate crimes tend to take place in public places, and are often a product of peer group pressure and an escalation of antisocial behaviour, exacerbated by drink or drugs: the vulnerable person is targeted because they are seen to be visibly different and the behaviour is driven by the need to impress an audience of other young people, sometimes even recorded on a mobile phone as a trophy (see, for example, BBC news, www.news.bbc.co.uk/1/hi/england/tees/7002627.stm).

Thus abuse has no one cause or precipitating factor and needs to be analysed from a number of vantage points. Because it varies so much, there is a wide range of agencies and systems that need to be engaged on behalf of people at risk and it is extremely unlikely that vulnerable people or family carers will be able to find their way into the right systems or be able to trigger the right kinds of responses unless they are supported and signposted.

Why do vulnerable adults need a special framework?

Given that this is a number of separate agendas, what is the common ground that underpins the processes mandated by multi-agency policies and procedures? The evidence suggests that if vulnerable or stigmatised people attempt to bring these matters out into the open, they are more likely to be disbelieved or have their experiences downplayed (Dow, 2007; Flynn, 2007). Also their lives are more fragile and depend on relationships that are more often strained or conditional.

So ideally the safeguarding process should facilitate access to mainstream agencies, coordinate a range of responses in both the short term and over time, and it needs to augment and enhance the robustness of actions taken against perpetrators. The agencies concerned have different roles and remits in relation to both victims and perpetrators. As we know, the criminal justice system can only convict if there is a high level of proof that a crime has been committed by a named perpetrator but there are intermediary responses that can be called for if a prosecution fails, such as disciplinary procedures and sanctions, removal from a professional body, or additional scrutiny and feedback. These may be instituted as well as, or instead of, action within the criminal justice system and will be affected by the relationship between the perpetrator and the service user, their perceived culpability and the likelihood that they might harm the vulnerable person and/or others in the future. Moreover, action may need to be taken against an organisation rather than an individual if abuse has been at least in part caused as a result of corporate negligence or failure to uphold the 'duty of care'.

The relationship of individual workers to their employing agency is necessarily complex and governed by health and safety legislation. Workers who abuse may be acting outside explicitly stated guidelines, or they may be acting in the absence of guidance, training or knowledge about best practice. There may also be instances where workers are being asked to operate in ways that contravene natural justice and which they feel uncomfortable with, for example they may be asked to control and restrain people who might be engaged more positively if they are offered the right kind of support.

Despite these factors, it has been argued that vulnerable adults do not need a framework that separates them off from, or operates over and above, the mainstream responses to crime in our society. There are a range of agencies that exist to respond to all forms of violence, theft and fraud. These include statutory agencies such as the police, the NHS, housing or social care services, and voluntary bodies such as women's refuges, relationship counselling, family mediation or faith communities. People question whether the safeguarding adults framework (DH, 2000b) supplants these agencies, or removes from them the imperative to be open to all and find ways of reaching out to, and developing innovative ways of working with, vulnerable people. Does the existence of a special set of arrangements lead to vulnerable people getting a lesser response, or inadvertently to being seen as a 'soft touch'. This depends on whether the safeguarding process is posited as an alternative or an adjunct to these mainstream responses: *No Secrets* (DH, 2000b) very much aimed for the latter, so any slippage needs to be addressed in local multi-agency arrangements so that this stance is reiterated.

An important document encapsulating standards and offering examples of good practice, *Safeguarding Adults* (ADSS, 2005), made clear the need for this seamless continuum between the mainstream agencies and the safeguarding process, arguing for closer links with those agencies that exist for all adults whether or not they are identified as having additional vulnerabilities. The fact is that being the victim of violence or abuse always renders people vulnerable, and there is a strong evidence base suggesting that people with mental health problems are more likely to have histories of abuse in childhood or at the hands of partners than others, but that this root cause of their mental distress may get lost in the process of clinical assessment and diagnostic labelling (Jacobson and Richardson, 1987; Rose et al., 1991; De Zulueta, 1999).

So the field is complicated and given that some of the people involved may sometimes lack capacity to act in their own best interests, multi-agency protocols provide the mandate for agencies to share information on their behalf and coordinate actions across agencies and over a given time span. The decision-making process forges the links that a vulnerable person who has been abused may not be able to make on their own or identify, and identifies the most effective routes to take to restore their safety and/or the future safety of others.

What does it mean to 'safeguard' a person?

Safeguarding can be seen to involve actions at several stages in this cycle of vulnerability. Mostly, the aim is for 'primary prevention' that seeks to avoid abuse occurring from the outset and this is achieved by creating safe and well-boundaried services and practice underpinned by relevant and clear policies and guidelines, particularly in those areas of care that give rise to the most pressure or ambiguity for staff. Some areas of practice are just too ambiguous to be left to chance, where, for example, force is legitimised as a response to challenging behaviour, or intimate care offered (see Cambridge and Carnaby, 2006). Policies are not helpful if they talk in idealised terms without spelling out how practically to deliver good practice in the time, and with the resources, available. Guidance and training should be specific and make clear where the limits lie. Primary prevention may also be achieved by good recruitment and induction, and by screening those with a high risk of abusing out of the workforce.

But the evidence even from recent inquiries suggests that services that tip over into abuse or neglect drive complaints underground, and cover up bad practice so that it festers and worsens (Dow, 2007; Flynn, 2007). Creating safe routes for whistle-blowers and ways of inviting feedback in the context of inspections and reviews is one way of ensuring that any problems that do exist are brought out into the open in a timely way – this is 'secondary prevention'.

Lastly, we need to invest in 'tertiary prevention' for those individuals who have been harmed at the hands of those who should be caring for them, whatever the roots of that abuse. They are entitled to help in their recovery and support in seeking justice and redress just as any other citizen would be. Because their lives and social networks may be more fragile than others, vulnerable adults who have been victimised may also need help in shoring up their everyday lives for a while, so that the abuse does not set off a chain reaction of disadvantage and dislocation – as happens when people who have been victimised are summarily moved, lose contact with important people in their lives or suffer the concomitant loss of income or security.

Meanwhile, appropriate sanctions should be applied to individuals who have committed crimes or fallen into abusive ways of interacting, and appropriate regulatory actions taken to either improve or close failing services. This creates a difficult balancing act for safeguarding decision makers as they seek to provide input in good faith to services that have contravened agreed standards, while remaining alert to the possibility that the service will not be motivated to implement new ways of working or invest in safer practice. Switching tracks is the most difficult point in this trajectory, just as it is in a family where professional support seems to be tuned out or advice negated. Monitoring needs to build in points for review and reassessment with robust contingency plans if improvements are not evidenced. So support and sanctions should not be regarded as contradictory options but as twin planks in a properly orchestrated process of performance management.

Multi-agency working: overlapping but competing concerns

No Secrets (DH, 2000b) was directed towards local authorities and made it incumbent on social services departments that they take the lead in coordinating local arrangements. The document was very specific that this did not mean other agencies did not have a role to play but that they would be brought together by a single multi-agency protocol under the leadership of social services. Thus the first coordinator posts were largely forged within social services, usually from people with a background in either older people's services or in services for people with learning disabilities. Increasingly, 'safeguarding' across this divide has come to be seen as a specialism in its own right, and most authorities have dedicated posts to coordinate the process of responding to alerts, managing referral, conducting assessments and investigations, arranging and chairing case conferences and aggregating monitoring information. Their role usually includes providing input to a safeguarding adults board, which brings agencies together around the table to discuss issues (not individual cases), to identify training needs, and plan the delivery and dissemination of important information, changes in legislation, regulation and service development.

Multi-agency working requires collaboration at different levels – ranging from senior management through to the creation of strong alliances between practitioners directly involved with individual service users. At middle management level, the task is to liaise over specific cases and manage the sharing of information, the planning of an investigation/assessment and the decision-making process that takes place in a case conference. Liaising between specialist posts across agencies is difficult if these levels do not marry up or if geographical boundaries are not coterminous. For example, in some areas, the police have located this as a specialism alongside either child protection or domestic violence teams, whereas in others, it was seen as a generic expertise to be held by all police officers: these decisions affected liaison with specialist coordinators in social services on an everyday basis and the channels for delivery of training and managing information exchange were also compromised.

NHS colleagues have been hampered by a major reorganisation in the wake of the policy's introduction and it has taken a considerable time for the agenda within the different elements of the health service to emerge and be properly articulated. Safeguarding vulnerable adults is part of the remit of the National Patient Safety Agency, which exists to collate aggregate information about medical accidents and 'untoward incidents', but the clinical governance structures in each trust and professional regulation also play a role. The health remit might be defined as:

- *Managing concerns in long-term care situations* where people are effectively living within NHS premises, until such time as this kind of service provision is finally phased out.
- *Providing enhanced and individually tailored care to vulnerable patients* when they are receiving in- or outpatient treatment, which means marrying current initiatives such as those focusing on the Medical Council on Alcohol and the Dignity in Care agenda, making sure that people are helped to eat and drink and their views are sought.
- *Being alert to signs and signals that someone is being abused in their home, neighbourhood or workplace,* perhaps, for example, when they present frequently at A&E, ring emer-

gency ambulances to get help or present at their GP with bruising or distress as a result of domestic violence or sexual exploitation, which could be summed up as a 'vigilance' role – this involves being sensitive to the risk of diagnostic overshadowing, whereby new symptoms of abuse are misread and seen as a function of the person's disability, age or mental health condition. An example of this was described in a study of palliative care of people with learning disabilities, when one woman whose condition deteriorated as a result of infection postoperatively was assumed to be acting 'normally' for her even though care staff who knew her well were saying: 'This is not how she is usually, these are not symptoms associated with her learning disability but with her illness.'

■ *Combating discrimination against vulnerable groups,* whether this means age discrimination in clinical decision-making, or making cancer screening equally accessible to people with learning disabilities, which demands a more systemic approach to monitoring and advocacy.

■ *Providing treatment for people who have been abused*, which acts as tertiary prevention: and this means making sure that psychological therapies (for example through the IAPT agenda) are offered to all service user groups and that people with additional difficulties are not explicitly or implicitly screened out of talking therapies. This post-abuse work is a strand that has been least well addressed in the work so far, as *No Secrets* majored on incident reporting rather than prevention or recovery.

■ *Making generic safeguards equally accessible to vulnerable people and their family members* so that they can equitably report concerns, shape service improvement plans and activate the formal complaint system when they are the victims of what we could call 'ordinary' medical accidents or neglect.

■ *Continuing to regulate professions and settings* so that high standards are uniformly applied and maintained.

The responsibility for the quality of care in residential and nursing homes is shared between the contracts and commissioning departments of adult social services, individual care managers who may be spot purchasing specific care packages, and the regulatory body (currently the Commission for Social Care Inspection – CSCI), but these relationships have had to be adjusted at different points as workload and organisational responsibilities have been reordered. Regulators manage the standards at the point of entry to the market and seek to maintain quality through regular inspection and the negotiation of improvements, unless a service is so poor that it is deemed necessary to close it either immediately (which is rare) or over time if agreed changes are not delivered. Regulators have rights of entry, and of doing unplanned and unannounced inspection visits, and to seize pertinent evidence, but their role has changed to the point that the investigation is usually led from social services, with regulatory sanctions being called upon as a last resort.

The personalisation agenda will again throw organisational relationships into sharp relief as a whole new set of employment structures come into being outside the regulatory frameworks that have been set up. New, less formal arrangements may remain outside the requirement for criminal records checks and create new challenges in terms of training and supervision as individuals start to manage functions that were previously managed corporately. This has advantages as well as disadvantages. Certainly, safeguards need to be translated into these new arrangements, as evidence already exists to suggest that abuse is no respecter of informality (Flynn, 2007) and that the personal assistant role is not immune to power struggles, the need for specialist knowledge and expertise, or the potential for boundary violations.

National agencies also have important roles in relation to this agenda. The Office of the Public Guardian operates the Court of Protection, which will adjudicate difficult cases, provide oversight of the instruments designed to prevent financial abuse, and appoint deputies to make decisions on behalf of someone unable to do so in their own best interests, but also to challenge those holding these powers if they neglect or subvert their powers and cease to operate for the benefit of the vulnerable person.

Conclusion

It is a myth that understanding undercuts the commitment to prevent abuse; in contradiction to John Major's now famous dictum, that we should 'understand a little less and condemn a little more', the goal of safeguarding procedures is to understand as much as possible so as to prevent as much abuse as possible, and where this strategy fails, to create an effective backstop that leads to swift action that brings it out into the open and allows those responsible to help individuals who have been affected to recover. Condemning has a habit of driving things underground rather than stopping them, but understanding allows us to institute properly nuanced responses to abuse and abusers, maximising the potential for prevention and channelling lessons back into organisational learning for the future. The goal has to be that vulnerable people, as citizens, are properly assured of their rights and safety, whether they live in supported settings or independently in their own homes and communities.

For further discussion of issues regarding mental capacity and practice, see Chapter 7, and for working with the voluntary and community sectors, see Adams et al., 2009a, Chapter 24.

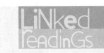

Brown, H. (2003) 'What is financial abuse?', *Journal of Adult Protection*, 5(2): 3–10. Demonstrates how abuse is not a one-dimensional matter and maps cases of financial abuse in terms of both financial gain and adequacy of care for older people who lack capacity to manage their own affairs.

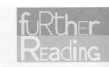

DH (Department of Health) (2003) *Independent Inquiry into the Death of David 'Rocky' Bennett:* An Independent Inquiry set up under HSG(94)27, London, HMSO, www.nscsha.nhs.uk/resources/pdf/review_inquiry/david_bennett_inquiry/david_bennett_inquiry_report_2003.pdf. Exemplary official inquiry, which dissects the minutiae of an incident that led to the death of this young African-Caribbean man while being restrained. It analyses the immediate and concrete things that went wrong, addresses the broader issues of institutionalised racism and demonstrates how these fed into the incident as it unfolded. The report began a process of reflection and positive action in relation to racism in mental health services and to restraint and its regulation.

Flynn, M. (2007) 'Unlearned lessons from the Health Care Commission's investigation into the service for people with learning disabilities provided by Sutton and Merton Primary Care Trust', *Journal of Adult Protection*, 9(4). Provides a comprehensive picture of institutional abuse and examines the many different factors that contribute to abusive practice in such settings and allow them to continue unchecked. Addresses the role of families and the importance of working with families and empowering them to complain in a timely way if they notice things are not right in services their relatives depend on.

Marsland, D., Oakes, P. and White, C. (2007) 'Abuse in care? The identification of early indicators of the abuse of people with learning disabilities in residential settings', *Journal of Adult Protection*, 9(4): 6–20. Draws out the features of abusive settings and makes explicit the early warning signals that emanate from failing services but which family members and professionals fail to act on. It assists in the articulation of what might otherwise be dismissed as 'gut instincts' and grounds such observations in the evidence base emerging from recent reports.

NHS Confederation (2008) 'Implementing national policy on violence and abuse: a slow but essential journey', Briefing, June. Explores the links between abuse in childhood or adulthood and mental ill health. Documents the evidence base for the link between sexual abuse and mental distress, and argues that assessment should always explore this as a contributing factor in mental ill health. Goes beyond identifying abuse to a consideration of how it should be addressed in services and remediated.

Saxton, M., Curry, M., Powers, L. et al. (2001) '"Bring my scooter so I can leave you": a study of disabled women handling abuse by personal assistance providers', *Violence Against Women*, 7(4): 393–417. Investigates the perceptions and experiences of women with physical and cognitive disabilities relating to abuse by formal and informal personal assistants. Shows how abusive dynamics can cross over into what are in other ways more empowering and life-enhancing models of care: designing stronger safeguards without undermining the hoped-for autonomy that underpins such models will be a challenge for social workers in the future as personalisation becomes the norm in social care service provision.

Tomita, S.K. (1990) 'The denial of elder mistreatment by victims and abusers', *Violence and Victims*, 8: 171–84. Presents a number of theoretical models that help us to understand how someone who is 'caring' for an older person can lapse into, and find themselves justifying, instances of abuse.

Care management 28

Care management has established itself as a distinguishable mode of intervention on the global social work scene and in the UK is the umbrella under which all social work with adults is now organised. Some argue that it has led to the demise of relationship-based social work, yet creative possibilities are emerging.

Chapter overview

Care management is a system for delivering health and social care services to adults, which is established across North America, the UK and Australasia and increasingly features in the systems employed in developed countries. It was formally introduced in the UK in 1993, following the implementation of the 1989 White Paper, *Caring for People* (DH, 1989b) and the National Health Service and Community Care Act (NHSCCA) 1990. Defined as

> any method of systematically linking the processes of identifying and assessing need with the arrangement, monitoring and review of service provision for adults (DH/SSI, 1991),

care management is at the heart of the 'new' community care. Codifying as it does changes in philosophy and political context as well as procedure and practice, the NHSCCA is regarded as a watershed piece of legislation in the UK, which has had a marked impact on social work with adults. This chapter examines the impact of care management on social work practice. Through close attention to the process of service delivery to the user, we shall explore a way forward for creative care management, infused with social work values and skills.

Social workers or care managers?

'We're not social workers anymore, we're just care managers' is the complaint commonly to be heard among practitioners. The following case provides a typical example.

---

* formerly Lloyd

case example

Mrs Grant is an 85-year-old widow whose nearest relative lives 200 miles away. She lives alone in the house she has owned for 40 years but has been socially isolated since her neighbour died a year ago. Following a fall at home in which she sustained shoulder and leg injuries, she was admitted to hospital and has recently been discharged to an acute rehabilitation unit. Prior to the fall, she had a low-level care package and reasonable mobility. However, since the fall, she is unable to stand and is in need of a wheelchair and hoist. The pressure on the social worker in the multidisciplinary team is to free up her place in the rehabilitation unit as quickly as possible. Mrs Grant is determined to return home. Combining information from the medical assessment with a review of the available services, the social worker considers that Mrs Grant could be discharged home if she were provided with a pendant alarm linked to 24-hour warden cover, an electric wheelchair, for which there is a six-month waiting list, and increased home and daycare.

Underlying this case is the question of whether a social worker needs to be there at all. What are the knowledge base and skills required in organising a package of practical support services? One of the earliest issues raised by commentators was the deprofessionalising influences in the community care 'reforms' and the overriding of professional judgement by bureaucratic procedure and managerialist imperatives (for example Cochrane, 1993; James, 1994; Sheppard, 1995; C. Clark, 1996; Lewis, 1996; Cowen, 1999). Lewis and Glennerster's (1996) study of implementation found some senior managers enthusiastically embracing the reforms, interpreting this enthusiasm as stemming from the new status afforded to them as developers and managers of locality information systems and plans. They found some frontline staff believing these new-style managers to be antipathetic to social work, with widespread agreement that the social work task was being redefined. A decade later, research finds social workers reframing and interpreting actions determined by organisational priorities and procedures, so as to fit comfortably with their professional values and ethics (Sullivan, 2008). So, for example, in a risk-averse culture, care managers rely on bureaucratic procedure rather than professional knowledge (McDonald et al., 2007), justifying the application of, for example, restrictive eligibility criteria, with arguments about lack of resources and targeting of the most needy (Sullivan, 2008). The original rhetoric of tailored packages of care designed to meet individualised assessments of need has shifted to an emphasis on eligibility bands based on assessment of risk (DH, 2002b). Fuelling this tendency towards an administrative rather than professional culture of care management is the increasing use of temporary agency workers. Carey (2006, 2008) reports agency care managers as experiencing a lack of meaningful contact with service users as well as professional isolation, engaging instead in fragmented interventions and 'paper exercises'.

To understand how we have reached this position in the UK, it is necessary to examine the way in which care management was introduced. The immediate contradiction that jumps out is that although care management was built onto a social work culture rather than a home care culture (Welch, 1998), not only did the official guidance never address what the job of the social worker was intended to be (McDonald, 2006), but the new world of service delivery formally blurred professional roles and 'professionalised' new jobs. The 'old world' had been split between the established professions and care workers, who undertook more practically oriented tasks deemed to require neither expert knowledge nor the exercise of professional judgement. The new scenario resembled more of a job fair, with a world of 'workers', some of them with new labels, milling around newly configured tasks. Despite repeated arguments that the 'professional variant' of care management should be used only where it adds value (Welch, 1998) and that intensive care management should be reserved for a relatively few complex cases, with the majority being held within a care management system but not individually intensively care managed (Challis, 1994), most local authorities have continued with a 'one-size-fits-all' model. There is more to this than the important questions of screening and targeting. There is also the neglected issue of defining what the added value of the social work professional is, and demonstrating when, where and how it should be incorporated into the overall care management process.

The early literature on care management was preoccupied with the search for a model, in the course of which some opposing approaches were identified: administrative, caseworker, brokerage and social entrepreneur (Beardshaw and Towell, 1990; Biggs and Weinstein, 1991; Huxley, 1993; Challis, 1994). Ongoing work by the Personal Social Services Research Unit (PSSRU) has sought to develop a typology of the different care management arrangements that have developed across the UK and thereby to analyse whether particular models or features were more likely to result in desired outcomes for service users, such as the maintenance of quality of life and independence. This research has demonstrated that huge variation and inconsistency in care management arrangements exists across the UK, with inevitable negative implications for service users (Challis et al., 1998; Weiner et al., 2002). This confusion flies in the face of the government's 'modernisation' agenda, which prioritises person-centred care, standardised services and evidenced-based practice, linked to clearly demonstrable outcomes for the service user. Fragmented care remains a problem, despite the levers introduced to encourage interagency collaboration and initiatives such as 'one-stop shops' designed to provide integrated and wide-ranging services (Holloway and Lymbery, 2007).

Issues, dilemmas and potential at the front line

In summary, a number of tensions and dilemmas have been experienced by social workers and their managers in adult services in the implementation of care management, which appear to endure:

■ How to negotiate user choice and creative responses to need in a resource-constrained environment

■ How to maintain the therapeutic elements of the professional relationship in a service delivery culture of measurable outcomes, weighed down by bureaucratic procedure

■ How to provide continuity and attend to longer term processes in a system that appears to disrupt the dynamic interplay between assessment and intervention which social work has carefully nurtured.

There are no easy or complete answers to these questions. However, some of the research suggests that rather more lies in the power of the frontline care manager than most social workers appear to believe.

CASE EXAMPLE (cont'd)

Mrs Grant's case illustrates all three dilemmas. The medical opinion is that she will not regain her previous mobility and will need to use a wheelchair permanently. If she waits for a wheelchair to be provided, she will either have to go into supported accommodation temporarily or return home to a situation where she is highly dependent on the home care support and severely restricted in her activities outside carer visits. There is not much flexibility in the formal service provision systems, for example there is no negotiation of the wheelchair waiting list around priority criteria or avoidance of more costly alternative care. Even once provided with a wheelchair, Mrs Grant will have to wait 12 months for a ramp to be built to gain access to the house. The care provided in the rehabilitation unit is designated 'acute', with the requirement to transfer to another setting and different professionals at the end of a six-week period.

On the information currently collected by the health authority and the social services department, the only easily measurable outcomes at this point are the length of time Mrs Grant remains in the acute unit and whether she returns home or enters residential or nursing home care. For the social worker to negotiate with Mrs Grant around accepting her reduced capacity and managing the risks in her situation, she needs time to build a relationship and for Mrs Grant to adjust to her changed situation. The assessment, to be accurate and user-centred, needs to take account of Mrs Grant's personality, how she was functioning before the fall, the impact of the crisis hospital admission, her willingness to engage with the rehabilitation unit and her feelings about the future. Yet there is no one worker who will have developed this dynamic assessment throughout the intervention.

Despite the overall gloom that pervaded adult social work in the mid-1990s, some of the early research, which looked at the job care managers were doing at the micro-level, provided a counter to the picture of a deskilled, mechanistic response. For example,

Hardiker and Barker (1999: 421) claimed that social workers demonstrated 'skilled methods and proactive decision-making', adopting advocacy roles and identifying 'empowerment' as a method to enable service users to negotiate around limited choices. The case studies showed utilisation of 'a wider range of individualised, imaginative solutions' (p. 425). Similarly, the PSSRU's reporting of its wide-ranging 'Evaluating community care for elderly people' (ECCEP) research programme found that qualified social workers were responsible for the highest incidence of complex assessments and were the guardians of the holistic assessment. They were spending a higher proportion of their time in face-to-face contact with the service user or in contact with other agencies directly associated with the care package. Only one-fifth of the worker's time was being spent on administration and form-filling, even in the setting-up period. Care managers were undertaking direct work with service users and qualified social workers were more likely to provide counselling than other care managers. Moreover, the responses of the service users showed these 'social worker care managers' taking seriously the notion of user involvement and empowerment. For example, 87 per cent of the most 'dependent' category thought that their care manager understood their strengths as well as their problems. Sixty-nine per cent of all users felt that they could discuss alternatives, as equals, with their care manager (Bauld et al., 2000).

It is within these micro-level interactions that the glimmers of hope, as well as unrealised opportunities, to 'redeem' care management can be discovered. The point has repeatedly been made (for example Lymbery, 2004; Tanner, 2005) that social workers do have discretion in how they carry out policies, procedures and required tasks. In a study of the role of social work in hospital discharge to residential or nursing home care, Phillips and Waterson (2002) found that where the social workers prioritised involving and supporting the older person and their family in making choices, their input was appreciated and contributed significantly to humanising the process. However, there was evidence of a reluctance to challenge, or even get involved in, the initial decision to seek residential care – a process from which the older person themselves had often felt excluded – and too often failure to acknowledge the emotional dimensions of the experience for both the older person and their family. The recent introduction of individual budgets (IBs), aimed at enhancing users' choice and control, provides another example of potential in the social work role. In an evaluation of a pilot scheme, Rabjee et al. (2008) found that where service users could identify outcomes they wanted to achieve, IBs had great potential to enhance their quality of life. However, these people stated that they welcomed professional help in completing the self-assessment and felt that those who lacked informal support systems or had cognitive or intellectual impairments, as well as older people with some degree of confusion would be disadvantaged in this system. The researchers conclude that the development of assessment and resource allocation systems, which provide professional support for people with high or specialist needs, is essential. Tanner's (2005) study also highlighted the importance of skilled assessment in enabling service users to identify those factors that would contribute to their overall wellbeing. It appears to be down to social workers to nurture the holistic assessment and take responsibility for the integration of health and social care

(Ware et al., 2003). Despite government-led initiatives to expand the role of nurses as 'case managers', and evidence from the US of successful nurse care management programmes (Rosenman et al., 2006), the evidence appears to show that the involvement of healthcare staff in care management in the UK is limited both in scale and scope (Weiner et al., 2003).

A framework for good practice

Keeping the service user central

Repeatedly the message comes through that the only way to resist a bureaucracy-driven care management, which serves the interests of the service provider organisation, is for the social worker to maintain the central focus on the service user. It is important to acknowledge here that the initial direction of the community care reforms is fundamentally 'what people want'. My own research found people who were not service users and had no acquaintance with the care management system expressing the desire for a needs-led, multidisciplinary assessment, an individually tailored package of care and a flexible balance between formal services and informal support (Lloyd, 2000). Staying focused on the user when resources are tight can foster creativity because it requires us to think through with the potential service user what exactly the need is, and what the essential element(s) is to meet that need. However, Martin et al. (2004) argue from their research that the objective of cost containment has had a pervasive and overriding effect on the system and that social workers arranging individual care packages have adopted this same motivation. Overconsciousness of limited resources leads to a tendency to make a service-led assessment, not necessarily with any cost saving. Research into informal caring has long demonstrated that what carers actually want is often more low-key, cheaper alternatives than the sometimes underused schemes developed by service providers (for example Haffenden, 1991). It is salutary that the ECCEP study found care managers realising that what had seemed an inadequate care package to them initially had actually made a significant difference to people's lives.

Moreover, the value of undertaking a user-centred assessment of need, with the user respected and involved in the process, should not be underestimated. My own research demonstrated significant psychological benefits for carers of a community care assessment having been completed, independent of any ensuing service provision (Lloyd and Smith, 1998). Priestly (2000) points out that services which empower people to improve their own quality of life may have intrinsic value, even if this cannot be demonstrated through a measurable service outcome. This is not meant to cover up the inadequacies of service provision through dubious claims of therapeutic value. A user-centred process of assessment demands that it be part of an empowerment model of care management. This requires practitioners and managers to take risks in stimulating new responses and developing and reconfiguring existing services in response to locally defined user needs. It was my observation that those service managers and frontline practitioners who had got hold of this idea and were enthused by it were those who could see real possibilities to improve the quality of life of service users, despite struggling with the same resource problems as those who were negative about the 'reforms' (Lloyd and Smith, 1998). A recent study of micro-level commissioning concluded that care managers continue to be significantly hampered in their attempts to match care packages to assessed need by inadequate and unimaginative commissioning at service level (Ware et al., 2003). However, Foster et al. (2008) also found practitioner assessments continuing to focus on familiar social care services and outcomes despite the diverse range of potential outcomes identified by users.

An empowerment model also requires care managers to take seriously the resources of the service user/carer in understanding and managing their own situations (see Adams et al., 2009a, Ch. 19). The fact that these resources, even in the most resilient of people, can be undermined through lack of support or remain untapped through failure to access the system should lead the empowering care manager to see their task as identifying what is needed in this particular situation, in order to facilitate a working partnership that goes beyond the 'in principle' commitment to involve the service user. Sometimes it should lead us as professionals to take the even bolder step of resourcing service users as managers of their own care pathways (Holloway, 2007).

CASE EXAMPLE (cont'd)

Mrs Grant is articulate about her needs and able to express her clear priorities. Recognising that formal services are not going to be able to deliver what Mrs Grant needs in the time available, the social worker assists her with the self-assessment for an individualised budget. Mrs Grant makes arrangements to have a ramp built and orders an electric wheelchair. Mrs Grant is fully involved in individual assessment processes with the physiotherapist, occupational therapist and social worker and multidisciplinary planning meetings. Through these, Mrs Grant is able to see that her personal priorities of maintaining independence and mobility at home will only be achieved through attention to her excessive weight and compromising on accepting the pendant alarm for a trial period in order to reduce the risk arising from further falls. Importantly, the social worker advocates for Mrs Grant to stay in the acute unit while these arrangements are put in place rather than her having to move to another temporary unit.

Maintaining a holistic approach

This is not the first time that social work has faced a crisis of professional angst. Arguably, social work survived previous precarious moments because it managed to hold on to the 'whole person in total context' idea, despite the lure and challenge of psychotherapy, radical social work and community development. Yet it is that holistic approach that is most threatened by the culture of cost-effective task division and outcomes-focused accountability which has come to dominate the community care scenario. Cowen (1999: 101) argues that the global forces of marketisation, bureaucratisation and managerialism, combined with the loss of the public sector ethic, have 'served to downgrade the status of holistic models and ethical caring in social work practice'. A user-centred focus is, by definition, holistic. Holism is not concerned solely with the whole person, it is concerned with whole systems as well as wholeness in both persons and systems and the interactions between them. The simultaneous engagement with individuals, families, organisations and social structures is what should mark out social work as a profession. A holistic approach to the assessment and meeting of the needs of individuals requires a focus on the social structures that shape their lives and the mechanisms that impact on their experiences of services. Maintaining this holistic perspective and approach may seem to be the most impossible challenge of all, but, equally, holism – as a concept and practice – may hold the key to the way forward on some of the seemingly intractable issues in health and social care.

CASE EXAMPLE (cont'd)

Using a biographical approach to assessment, the social worker discovers that Mrs Grant used to be a clerical officer in the civil service and is keen to deal with services direct. She needs to regain some control over her life and is unlikely to respond well to the rehabilitation programme without this. The relationships she establishes with the different professionals, and their capacity to respond to her as a whole person interacting with the whole system, are crucial to the successful balancing of needs, resources, rights and risks.

Assuring quality

It is no accident that the emergence of 'quality talk' was simultaneous with the community care changes. Each of the intrinsic agendas of care management connects with the notion of quality and its definition and measurement. The original emphasis within 'service quality' developed as a preoccupation with easily quantifiable outputs and performance indicators based on such measures. Nocon and Qureshi (1996) comment that a repeated finding in community care studies is that senior managers tend to prefer quantitative information that can be aggregated and used in budgetary planning, whereas frontline professionals prefer qualitative outcomes that leave room for professional judgement and interpersonal processes. The emerging evaluation of care management surely leads us to the conclusion that we must integrate both. Differences in what is valued, by whom and by what indicators it is measured lie behind the division between 'service quality' and 'quality of life' approaches. Yet service outcomes may be one indicator of quality of life just as enhanced quality of life may be one service outcome. Both quality of life and service quality may contain aspects that are amenable to quantitative measurement, but their significance may be a subjective judgement. Thus, practitioners and managers seeking to deliver quality through care management can only do so by a determined attempt to integrate subjective and objective indicators in relation to quality of life, and by finding ways to identify and demonstrate outcomes that are not easily measurable but are equally significant.

CaSE EXaMPLE (cont'd)

Mrs Grant returns to her own home three months after her hospital admission and arrangements work well. The social worker feeds back to the service manager that without flexibility around the length of stay in the acute unit, the outcomes could have been very different. Recognising other cases where this has been so, the manager begins to collect data to inform the development of more flexible use of the different rehabilitation and support units.

Conclusion

The way in which social care for adults is delivered in the UK has been changed irreversibly by the introduction of care management. This is not peculiar to the UK – the health and social care systems of the developed world are shaped by common forces. However, the impact on social work does appear to be peculiar to the UK, arising from history and organisational context. Prevailing opinion is that 'traditional' social work is being squeezed out through time and resource constraints, its skills and values undermined by restrictive procedures, cumbersome bureaucracy and inflexible criteria. Nevertheless, the evidence from research also demonstrates that care managers and service managers are failing to utilise opportunities for a flexible, creative and empowering response to the needs of individuals and groups of service users. Where the care management process is infused with social work skills and values, there is evidence that this is what service users value.

It is a bold claim, but an arguable one, that social work will survive or fall according to its response to care management. The critical issues for social work practice and social care management that have been examined here are at the heart of the challenge of delivering health and social care in technologically advanced societies in the twenty-first century. Social work must have confidence in the contribution it has made to the understanding of individual and social problems in health and social care, and actively promote its holistic model of assessment and integrated response to need on the multiprofessional stage of the 'new world'. Undoubtedly, underfunding, restrictive policies and bureaucratic administration have contributed in no small measure to care management failing to fulfil its positive potential and having a negative impact on many aspects of social work. Ultimately, however, if the 'community care experiment' fails, it will be for none of these reasons per se, but because those professionals concerned with its delivery have failed to engage with the fundamental challenges for welfare services in the postmodern world.

For further discussion of assessment and planning, see Adams et al., 2009a, Chapters 16 and 17 respectively.

Cowen, H. (1999) *Community Care, Ideology and Social Policy*, London, Prentice Hall. Places discussion of the impact of the 1990s' policy developments on the health and social care professions in a political and global context.

Lymbery, M. (2005) *Social Work with Older People: Context, Policy and Practice*, London, Sage. Critique of care management and community care policy, including the government's 'modernisation' agenda, located within a detailed discussion of the history and contemporary issues in social work practice with older people.

McDonald, A. (2006) *Understanding Community Care*, 2nd edn, Basingstoke, Palgrave Macmillan. Clear and useful analysis of policy and practice targeted at the practitioner.

Means, R., Richards, S. and Smith, R. (2003) *Community Care: Policy and Practice*, 3rd edn, Basingstoke, Palgrave Macmillan. Good background to the community care reforms, with up-to-date commentary on evolving practice.

Raynes, N., Temple, B., Glenister, C. and Coulthard, L. (2001) *Quality at Home for Older People: Involving Service Users in Defining Home Care Specifications*, Bristol, Policy Press. Useful report on assuring quality in home care services through integration of service users views.

Mental health

This chapter offers some suggestions to mental health social workers about how to develop critical practice as a way of responding proactively to the challenge of delivering contemporary mental healthcare within a context of paradox and conflicting discourse.

Social work is only one contributing profession in the multidisciplinary mental health field that increasingly hinges on effective interprofessional working. For this reason, critical practice in mental health social work cannot be presented without reference to the multidisciplinary context that informs its delivery and to which it contributes. Critical practice in mental health social work must incorporate an emancipatory social change orientation (Healy, 2000), which ultimately involves workers in the difficult task of balancing safety and risk issues with the active involvement of service users. According to Ramon and Williams (2005: 15), this requires replacing a distanced, 'hands-off' with a more 'hands-on' approach that demonstrates emotional closeness to the service user and an interest in the everyday affairs that matter to them.

The challenge of writing this chapter is to present such an approach 'that engages critically and productively with what social work in mental health settings is rather than the received wisdom critical social science theory tells us it should be' (Healy, 2000: 77). As Hinselwood (1998: 25) claims, what is needed is not a 'simple "how to" manual' but an approach that encompasses the process of reflection in order to provide quality work in mental health that involves a 'human "being with"', rather than an operational "doing to"' individuals with mental health problems.

The modernisation agenda in mental health policy and practice has fundamentally altered the provision of mental healthcare (DH, 1999c, 2000c), replacing the bricks and mortar of the hospital setting with an ever-increasing complexity of community-based services glued together by paper-based systems for care planning, risk assessment and management (Bailey, 2009). As specialist mental health teams have evolved to provide services such as assertive community treatment, early intervention and crisis resolution (DH, 2001b), the challenge of multidisciplinary working has become increasingly onerous.

In the absence of a whole systems approach to the delivery of hospital and community mental health services, and with the introduction of the *New Ways of Working for Psychiatrists* initiative (DH et al., 2005), mental health practitioners struggle to be clear about the core skills and aptitudes they bring to their role and those that are common and shared with other multidisciplinary colleagues. According to Hinselwood (1998: 21), 'what has emerged in providing community care is that the distortions found in the old large institutions recur within the organisations of agencies in the community'. He cites some of these processes as staff demoralisation, stereotyped patients, scapegoating, a blame culture and schisms in the service.

Within this context, one possible approach to developing critical practice in mental health social work involves five stages and is helpful at several levels. In respect of individual practice, it potentially helps workers to feel more confident about exploring risky situations from the different perceptions of worker and service user and enables workers to be more confident about delineating the respective responsibilities for risk management. At the team level, it helps mental health social workers to be clear about their role within integrated or single line-managed teams and allows for the identification of the professional social work contribution within a multidisciplinary domain.

The approach requires practitioners to:

- *Examine the situations* they encounter with service users from the individual's perspective as distinct from their own
- *Weigh up the options for intervening*, including the value base underpinning practice and the practice context – theory, policy, power relations and legislation – together with their own previous experience
- *Make an informed judgement* that is acted upon
- *Reflect on the outcome* of their action/decision-making
- *Critically appraise* what they have learned.

The remainder of this chapter will explore this approach and apply it to a case example where inherent tensions lie between either adopting an empowering and enabling approach or resorting to controlling interventions. Through the case example, it is hoped to illustrate how the use of critical practice can redefine the power dynamics within the professional social work relationship, such that an intervention that has the potential to be coercive may actually involve the service user in working collaboratively with the practitioner to reach a shared responsibility for meeting care needs.

Exploring encounters with service users

Stickley (2006: 570) concludes that 'in no other arena in healthcare has there been the equivalent of what we now call the user/survivor movement in psychiatry'.

However, mixed views still exist about the extent to which this has been achieved that reflect scant evidence of it being translated into actual practice (Peck et al., 2002).

What we now know more about from a growing body of evidence is service users' satisfaction with and their views of services (Burns et al., 1993; Bindman et al., 1997; Faulkner, 1997, 2000; Leavey et al., 1997; Rogers et al., 2003), together with their personal perspectives about why and how some community programmes are effective (Rosenfield, 1992). They have provided first-hand evidence about what impacts upon their quality of life (Levitt et al., 1990; Ehlert and Griffiths, 1996; Leff et al., 1996a, 1996b; Trieman et al., 1999; Leff and Trieman, 2000) and their experiences of social support (Sullivan and Poertner, 1989). They have also shared their experiences of Mental Health Act assessments and coercion (Hoge et al., 1993; Quirk et al., 1999; Canvin et al., 2002), and discharge planning (Armitage and Kavanagh, 1998).

Through these studies, service users have described their 'lived' experiences of mental distress in their own terms, using a language that reinforces the concept of recovery (Polack, 1993; Carling, 1996). This is increasingly promoted through self-help approaches such as recovery groups and workbooks (see Leader, 1995; Coleman and Smith, 1997). Rather than focus on concepts such as 'cure' or being symptom free, the recovery approach encourages

> people to take stock and set new life paths [and it] provides a vision of moving from the despair of very changed circumstances on becoming a 'user' to hope. The hope is not about 'cure' but about leading a fulfilling life with mental health problems which are valued as part of experience. (Sayce, 2000: 132)

By exposing these different perceptions, critical practitioners can counter their complicity in the reproduction of oppressive conditions within the mental health system (Rojek et al., 1988; Sarri and Sarri, 1992), particularly in multidisciplinary contexts where a continued dominance of the medical model can result in a blinkered approach to care delivery, dismissing their subjective experience of mental distress and the meaning this has for them.

The process of engagement as a foundation for such relationship-building is probably by far the most important phase in reaching a negotiated perception of need. According to Perkins and Repper (1998a: 24), 'success will be measured by the quality of the relationship between mental health worker and client'. While they acknowledge the difficulties in defining what constitutes an 'effective relationship', they suggest that for people with severe and enduring mental health problems, 'it might best be judged in terms of the extent to which the person is facilitated in living the life they wish to lead and achieving their own goals' (Perkins and Repper, 1998a: 24).

However, acting as an individual agent of change can be an isolating experience for social workers within a multidisciplinary team (Carpenter et al., 2003), where role conflict and team identification have the potential to thwart emancipatory relationships with service users. Social workers need their professional affiliation with the General Social Care Council as a means of safeguarding standards and offering solidarity through professional identity and registration.

The focus on social work values that support working in partnership with service users and anti-discriminatory practice – as set out as the social work contribution to future mental health services (CSIP, 2005) – should encourage social workers to feel confident about using their power and authority to initiate consciousness-raising in other disciplines regarding the potential contribution that service users can make to their own care package and mental health services more generally.

Weighing options for intervention within the practice context

From 1 October 2008, the Mental Health Act 2007 revised the original 1983 Mental Health Act and widened the definition of medical treatment to include social work approaches. However, it also extended the traditional approved social work role to other professions, including nursing, occupational therapy and psychology.

Since then, an effective team approach hinges increasingly on all workers being clear about the unique contribution they offer as a result of their unidisciplinary training and professional affiliation, but also the skills, knowledge and philosophies they share with others. This respect for both uniqueness and diversity mirrors the approach outlined with service users in the previous section.

With the legislative changes comes an increasing focus on the biopsychosocial model for understanding the causative factors that contribute to and sustain mental distress (Watkins, 1997; Kingdon, 2000). This favoured framework is now recognised as promoting a more holistic, activist approach to care that reduces relapse and promotes individuals' coping strategies (Bailey, 2009) (Figure 29.1).

Perkins and Repper (1998a: 25) highlight the application of this model in practice:

> different people adopt different models for understanding what has happened to them ... organic constructions, psychological, social, religious or spiritual formulations. People have a right to define their own experiences for themselves and it is rarely helpful and more likely to be alienating for the clinician to insist that their understanding is correct.

For each individual, the respective elements of the model will therefore feature to a greater or lesser extent in terms of their specific understanding and experience but also in relation to effective interventions. As Perkins and Repper (1998b: 92) elaborate: 'If a person wants to be able to cook then an understanding of their neurotransmitters or intrapsychic processes may not be particularly useful.' The author agrees with Perkins and Repper's view (1998a) that because an individual understands their distress with particular emphasis on one or more aspects of the model, this does not preclude interventions that are based on different parts of the model. Indeed, if a holistic approach to mental healthcare is to be developed, a combination approach should be the rule rather than the exception.

By continually questioning how the respective elements of the biopsychosocial framework can feature to a greater or lesser extent in understanding an individual's mental distress, and how a combination of interventions from one or more disciplines may meet the care needs, the power bases of the disciplines themselves become intrinsically less valuable. Working collaboratively with service users to define their mental distress from their perspective and using their language – even if, for some individuals, medical terminology is their preferred frame of reference – optimises the chances of individuals taking responsibility for their mental health, using more effective coping and relapse prevention strategies than previously (Healy, 2000).

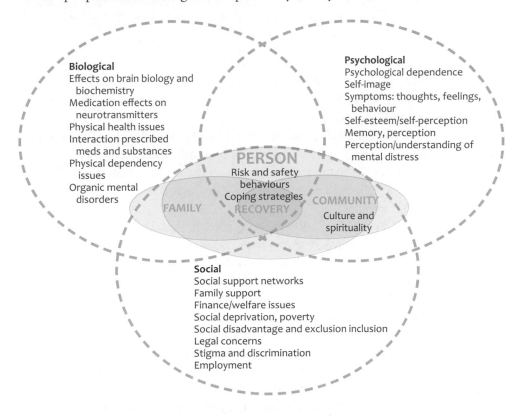

Figure 29.1 Inclusive biopsychosocial model of mental distress

Making informed judgements: reflection and critical appraisal

Faced with the dilemmas of interprofessional working and best practice guidance in respect of risk management (DH, 2007a), critical practice in mental health can only aid a process of questioning and self-questioning in the quest for an emancipatory approach – which recognises that working effectively with risk can only be achieved through a process of collaboration that involves service users and their carers as active participants.

As *Best Practice in Managing Risk* sets out (DH, 2007a: 11):

> Risk management should be conducted in a spirit of collaboration and based on a relationship between the service users and their carers that is as trusting as possible.

However, it does acknowledge that for some service users 'full engagement is sometimes not possible but the potential for it should always be considered' (DH, 2007a: 11).

One way of achieving the above is to ensure a balanced approach to risk assessment and management that includes positive risk-taking, negotiated and agreed between the service user and mental health professional. As Davis (1996: 114) explains:

> Risk taking … is an essential element of working with mental health service users to ensure autonomy, choice and social participation. It is a means of challenging the paternalism and overprotectiveness of mental health services.

This is echoed by Sayce (2000: 227), who supports 'a need to generate a more realistic debate about risk' as 'it is impossible to predict every crime'. However, it must be acknowledged that 'mental disturbance in any of us makes us emotionally and behaviourally unpredictable' (Foster, 1998: 85).

In the context of this debate, how can critical social work be assisted in the self-questioning process to rise to the challenge of working with risk? First, being clear about what is meant by 'risk assessment' is important as, in the author's view, this misleading term relates to only one element of a cyclical process, which, in the interests of the individual, needs to be ongoing.

The guidance (DH, 2007a) identifies the need for validated tools to assist the process but thankfully also recognises the importance of relationship-building, highlighted earlier, as integral to the making of informed judgements.

The guidance (DH, 2007a: 7) also identifies the need to draw on research-based knowledge of individual service users, their social context, and clinical judgement in the decision-making process. This reflects work done previously by B. Moore (1996) and Morgan (1999), which encourages the practitioner to critically review the information collected to highlight biases in how it is interpreted. This is necessary in order to identify more systematically which risks become apparent under what circumstances. When critical practice becomes more evidence based, it then becomes possible to design a risk management plan, as shown in Figure 29.2, which systematically delineates those risks that the service user has responsibility for managing and those that need to be managed by the multidisciplinary team. This approach embodies the collaborative efforts called for by the Department of Health in order to develop 'flexible strategies aimed at preventing any negative event from occurring or, if this is not possible, minimising the harm caused' (DH, 2007a: 13).

The importance of effective interprofessional communication has been highlighted as one of the most significant omissions in cases where mental health inquiries have been instigated (Reith, 1998). Thus such sharing of information is integral to collective decisions being taken, especially where it is unclear whether a risk-taking or risk minimisation approach is adopted. Also, by adopting a collaborative approach to risk work, critical practitioners are encouraged to involve their multidisciplinary team colleagues in the process of reflecting upon a course of action taken irrespective of the outcome.

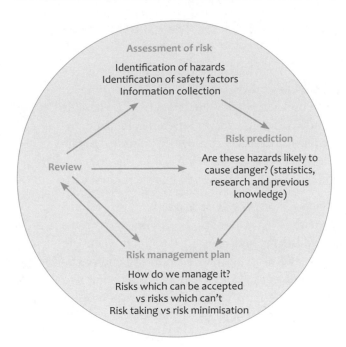

Figure 29.2 The process of risk assessment, planning and management showing the questions/issues to be considered at each stage

In an attempt to illustrate these issues together with those raised in the previous sections, the following case example is presented as an illustration of critical social work practice in mental health.

CASE EXAMPLE

Sally is a 25-year-old woman who has been experiencing difficulties with anorexia nervosa since her late teens. Despite three previous admissions to hospital – two as an informal patient and the latter under section 2 of the 1983 Mental Health Act – therapeutic intervention has been effective only in terms of weight gain. Social difficulties remain, as on discharge Sally has moved back to the family home where she lives with her younger sister aged 22 and her mother. Sally has identified her mother as the perpetrator of emotional and physical abuse spanning the past 13 years since her father left when she was 12 years old.

Sally contends that relationships within the family are fraught, with high levels of criticism, hostility and physical assaults from her mother, contrasted with an overprotectiveness that prevents Sally from holding down a job and restricts her finances and when she can see her friends. Sally's sister Ruth colludes with the mother's controlling behaviour as a way of sustaining her own role within the family, as the 'idealised daughter who can do no wrong', holding down a responsible job as a police officer, compared to Sally who is seen as a 'loser', intent on destroying herself with no hope of employment or independence.

An assessment of risk reveals at least two previous self-harm attempts motivated by Sally's despair connected to a need to get away from the home environment. One involved Sally taking an overdose of antidepressants prescribed by her GP, while the other, which had prompted the most recent referral to the community mental health team, involved her superficially cutting her wrists in a public toilet in the local park where she jogs several times each day. On this attempt, Sally was found by her sister who was routinely following her afternoon beat.

Both self-harm attempts are connected to periods of marked low self-esteem that stem from Sally's belief systems – 'I am unlovable', 'I must try to be a perfect daughter like my sister' and 'It's my fault that my father left' – and are triggered by rows with her mother following episodes of emotional and physical abuse. Sally's self-reports of the abuse are corroborated by a neighbour, Jan, who lives in the terraced house adjoining the family home and hears most of the arguments taking place. Sally's small social network includes Jan as an identified confidante and supporter, together with Clare, an old school friend who lives 10 miles away but visits in secret when Sally's mother is out at work.

Other risk factors include Sally's ritualised behaviour connected to her pursuit of weight loss, which is significant, but not life threatening. This involves eating little and taking excess exercise (jogging or swimming), together with an abuse of laxatives for purging and a problematic addiction to cough medicine to aid sleep. Until the overdose attempt with the antidepressants, Sally had maintained a good relationship with her GP. She is now frustrated that she has to visit the surgery weekly for a repeat prescription, feeling that this is an unnecessary infringement on her civil liberties. She also sees previous involvement of mental health professionals as coercive, due to the admission under section and a confrontational relationship with her consultant psychiatrist.

The temptation to wade into this situation and instigate another assessment under the revised mental health legislation as a means of minimising the risks by admission to hospital is great, but smacks of Hinselwood's 'doing to' approach, with little opportunity for reflection and consideration of alternatives. Also, Sally's previous experience of professional involvement suggests that pursuing this course of action would do little to foster a process of engagement and relationship-building, which, in the long term, might achieve greater success in promoting recovery rather than just weight gain. As the responsible approved mental health professional (AMHP), my preference was to pursue the latter option, provided that, through the process of engagement, I could identify and contain some of the apparent risks until I had a more appropriate opportunity to address them with Sally and the wider multidisciplinary team in a more proactive way.

Emancipatory encounters with service users need to commence on their terms, in order to demonstrate the dignity and respect of one human 'being with' another. Meeting with Sally at her request at Jan's house immediately communicated my desire to collaborate rather than control. However, as a qualified AMHP, I was faced with a dilemma at this point: whether to be up-front about this added dimension to my role and the associated powers it entails, thus risking the process of engagement, or, alternatively, reserving the discussion until the engagement process was further underway, which could then be jeopardised because I would be seen to have withheld vital information. It is worth pointing out that each individual service user will respond differently to whichever stage of disclosure is adopted – this is the kind of example where I, as a critical practitioner, needed to make a judgement as to when to take action and then reflect upon its outcome with the help of supervision.

In Sally's case, because of her previous encounters with professionals, I considered it necessary to be honest about my 'approved' status and explore the power relationship collaboratively, being clear that just as I could take a decision to pursue a formal Mental Health Act assessment, I could just as easily decide not to invoke my powers. Furthermore, it was necessary to indicate that I actually preferred to work with Sally without recourse to legislative measures, but that this required some joint effort to establish a collaborative relationship on which we might start to build some trust. Interestingly, Sally's response to my disclosure was to offer her own negotiating position for our relationship. While she was willing to give such collaboration a try, her provisos were that we did not have to involve her mother in our discussions at this stage, or spend session after session focusing on the past emotional and physical abuse, as she had found this kind of therapy of little use in terms of moving forward.

By engaging in an initial discussion that attempted to set some 'ground rules' for working together, we were able to move to an exploration of Sally's hopes and aspirations for the future, rather than focusing solely upon her eating disorder and self-harm attempts. Subsequent discussion revealed that Sally wished to leave home, live independently and have control over her own finances. She also expressed a wish to make contact again with her father whom she had written to in secret until she was 15 years old. Not surprisingly, a more in-depth discussion unearthed Sally's ambivalence about the costs required to achieve these goals, particularly her concerns that her mother would sabotage any attempt she made to leave the family home and the stress of managing financially and making the changes would exacerbate her eating disorder to a point where it would become out of control.

What became clear from discussing with Sally how the first steps towards this new 'life path' might be taken was that she had never been given the opportunity to reflect on her own understanding and interpretation of what had happened in her life over the years and how this had contributed to her mental distress and despair. Working in accordance with the biopsychosocial framework, I recognised Sally's need to understand:

- How the biological effects of her anorexia, including the associated use of laxatives and addiction to cough medicine, could contribute towards her mental health
- The interrelatedness of her belief systems with her self-harming behaviour
- How the social factors of unemployment and financial dependence on the benefit

system, coupled with domination and oppression within the family, featured in a complex presentation of interrelated need, such that previous strategies to extricate herself from this web were unsurprisingly ineffective.

In order to address the above, the contributions from the GP and consultant psychiatrist were important, not only in helping Sally and myself understand the biological contributions to Sally's presentation, but also in modelling for Sally that one professional group does not have a monopoly on explaining mental distress and that she too has an element of choice in deciding how she interprets her own experience.

So, in order to facilitate the first steps towards the new life path that Sally had identified, I needed to work collaboratively with her, together with other multidisciplinary colleagues and members of Sally's social network, to begin to provide the support necessary for her to move into independent living. While the care programme approach (CPA) (DH, 1995c) would provide the vehicle for such collaboration, the timing of CPA meetings and their focus on Sally's needs rather than on interprofessional rivalry were paramount. For this to be achieved, I had to undertake some 'behind-the-scenes' work, with Sally's permission, prior to a full meeting being convened.

As the care coordinator responsible for implementing Sally's care plan, my subsequent interventions with her included:

- Accompanying Sally to the housing department to complete an application for supported accommodation – 'being with' as opposed to 'doing to'
- Individual meetings with the GP and consultant to update them of the social work involvement on housing and finance issues, and also to highlight the need for effective medical treatment as part of a holistic approach – role clarification in the interests of interprofessional working
- Joint discussions with GP and consultant to agree a collaborative approach to risk management, taking on board Sally's aspirations – generating a more realistic debate about risk and guarding against it being left to an isolated practitioner
- Meetings with Sally together with Jan and Clare to explore the social support available and to explain the CPA as a framework for care planning in preparation for a CPA meeting in which they would feel more able to participate – encouraging collaborative decision-making
- Continuing individual sessions with Sally to foster the engagement process and monitor the risk issues as part of the care plan, with the opportunity to reflect on the ongoing work and issues arising in regular supervision sessions – providing a flexible yet systematic response
- Individual/joint sessions with Sally's mother and/or sister to explore family dynamics in more detail, facilitate Sally's move to independent living and promote ongoing support from close family members – sharing of information and making informed judgements.

All the above demonstrate how the use of professional power together with self-questioning and reflection can be used constructively to pursue an emancipatory approach, bearing testimony to the contribution that critical mental health social workers can make to 'the development of a perspective which empowers service users rather than labelling them as sick' (Braye and Varley, 1992: 46). Depending on the nature of the relationship established with individual services users and multidisciplinary colleagues, the behind-the-scenes work will be more or less necessary and there will be situations where collaborative joint meetings with service users involve possible rights from the outset. Supervision is an obvious and important vehicle to allow the critical practitioner the opportunity to reflect on how they might 'stage-manage' interprofessional working in order to promote optimum involvement for people like Sally.

Conclusion

Contemporary critical practice in mental health social work is shaped by a policy agenda that on the one hand promotes the involvement of service users but on the other considers the importance of public safety. Thus critical practitioners in mental health are forced to explore the situations they encounter with service users in the context of shifting power relations and the conflicting paradoxes apparent in the legislative and policy context. Only by working collaboratively with both service users and professional colleagues can critical mental health social workers rise to the challenge of making informed judgements that are proactive and underpinned by a bedrock of service user-oriented values. Through the process of collaboration together with supervision, reflective social work practitioners can engage in a process of ongoing reflection and professional development that serves to highlight the contribution of critical social work practice to contemporary mental healthcare.

For further discussion of mental capacity, see Chapter 7, and for rights in mental health work, see Adams et al., 2009c, Chapter 8.

LiNked reADinGs

fuRther ReadinG

Bailey, D. (2009) *Interdisciplinary Working in Mental Health*, Basingstoke, Palgrave Macmillan. In-depth look at current mental health issues from an interdisciplinary perspective.

DH (Department of Health) (2007) *Best Practice in Managing Risk: Principles and Evidence for Best Practice in the Assessment and Management of Risk to Self and Others in Mental Health Services*, London, DH. The most up-to-date policy guidance in managing risk in mental health practice.

Foster, A. and Roberts, V.Z. (eds) (1998) *Managing Mental Health in the Community: Chaos and Containment*, London, Routledge. A more theoretical book from a psychoanalytical perspective on current working in mental health, including a useful chapter on risk.

Healy, K. (2000) *Social Work Practices: Contemporary Perspectives on Change*, London, Sage. Useful analysis of more general critical social work practice.

Ramon. S. and Williams. J.E. (2005) *Mental Health at the Crossroads: The Promise of the Psychosocial Approach*, Aldershot, Ashgate. Useful book summarising contemporary psychosocial approaches to mental health from an international perspective.

30 Physical disability

Chapter overview

This chapter argues that if social workers are to play a positive role in the provision of welfare for disabled people, they will have to develop positive attitudes towards impairment in order not to cause further disablement.

To develop a critical practice, social workers working with disabled people should start by asking the question: Do disabled people need social work? On the one hand, this may be an administrative question – the organisation of welfare has traditionally required disabled people to access services via social workers, although the blurring of occupational boundaries with others and the move towards direct payments and individual budgets is reducing the reliance on social workers. However, more importantly, social workers ought to question the value of their involvement by asking the question in terms of whether disabled people benefit from or are disadvantaged by social work intervention.

Disability and social work

Since the 1960s, disabled people have consistently criticised the organisation of welfare services and, more importantly, have questioned whether the provision of welfare, as opposed to access to the mainstream social and economic worlds, is an appropriate response to people who are physically impaired. In this sense, social welfare and social workers are seen as contributing to the construction of a disabling society rather than being part of the solution. The social model of disability distinguishes between impairment and disability, the former referring to some form of physical loss, while the latter is taken as the disadvantages, restrictions and oppression that occur as a result of social responses to impairment. This model leads to an argument that, by its very nature, social work assumes that disabled people need to be 'cared for' and, as such, views them as unable to be in control of their own lives. If disabled people were full citizens of a society, there would be no need for a welfare system to offer care services as a substitute. Therefore, the receipt of care services through a welfare system is viewed as second best and any attempt to try and perpetuate it is seen as counter to the goals of citizenship.

To some extent, policy and the legal framework in the UK – the Disability Discrimination Act 1995, the Equality Act 2006 and the associated duty on public bodies to promote disability equality – have developed in the light of campaigns, with the disability movement in the forefront, for the rights of disabled people.

However, many social workers' practice is based on a belief in the collective provision of welfare – their aim is to deliver services in a non-stigmatising manner. With some awareness of the academic and political debates about disability and disablism, many social workers would consider their own position to be supportive of the disability movement. They aim to help disabled people to empower themselves and gain access to services that would meet their personal and social care needs. They aim to counter the oppression and discrimination that disabled people experience by encouraging self-assessment of need and the use of individual budgets – in so doing, many social workers consciously try to ensure that their practice is not disabling. Different social workers may take different approaches to these tasks, ranging from the politicisation of specific issues to personal counselling, but their aim is one of actively trying to help disabled people.

But, while social workers may use the term 'care' to signify positive attitudes and actions, it has been experienced by many on the receiving end as meaning some form of control or custody. Social workers may see welfare as an indicator of a mature society, but their clients often see it as no less than a form of apartheid, in that it singles out certain groups of people as having to be dependent. As part of the disability industry, social workers may well understand these arguments, but they may tend to temper them with the cultural reality faced daily in local authority social service departments – that welfare is a necessary and positive activity. The challenge is that while social workers may well try to make it positive, why should people with physical impairments be singled out to receive it?

Challenging practice

In the rest of this chapter, I use five case examples to explore different aspects of practice with people with physical impairments. It is clear that some people's impairments are severe and will benefit from additional resources. However, the test for social workers is how to ensure people have access to these without being stigmatised or, literally, being disabled in the process.

CASE EXAMPLE

Stephen had recently become paraplegic following a road accident. After a period in a spinal injuries unit, he had returned home to resume his life. Stephen's father was an influential local businessman and the family were quite affluent. They had good access to medical advice and were well informed of the consequences of the accident. When the accident occurred, they were shocked, saddened and distraught, and so the social services manager wanted to ensure that all the help his department might be able to offer would be available. However, by the time Stephen had returned from hospital, much of what could be done to make his previous life accessible to him had already happened. Because of the influence and efforts of his family, he was returning to a life in which he would be accepted rather than rejected, and in which his right to opportunity was ensured.

The social worker visited to establish what, if anything, would be required in the coming weeks. Stephen's father asked her what it was that she could do for him. This was an open question on one level, but it was also a challenge. The hospital and GP had referred the family to the social services department and they all expected them to need and benefit from their assistance. Over the years, they had invested in a range of institutional provisions for younger disabled people, in the belief that this was the way in which they should provide care. The social worker described the father's question as asking her if she represented a part of society that might treat his son as dependent. The consciousness-raising that had occurred over the past months was thorough and as a family they were fully capable of ensuring that Stephen was not disadvantaged. Clearly, there was no role for social work with this family at this time, as they had no need of the services to which social workers act as gatekeepers and they had the capacity to deal with the changes that had occurred as a result of the accident. The social worker closed the case.

CASE EXAMPLE

This contrasts with Philip, a disabled man in his late teens who was resident in a local authority home. The home had some influence with a local housing association and at a case conference, the staff were discussing how to help Philip to leave and live independently. Apart from being unemployed and homeless, he was not dependent on any other person and it seemed clear that what he needed was suitable accommodation. However, the senior manager who chaired these conferences made the observation that Philip had never appeared to have grieved his 'loss' through his physical impairment and its consequences in terms of being unemployed, and that until he had done so, he would be at risk if living independently. Therefore she was not willing to permit the social worker or staff in the home to recommend, to the housing association, rehousing Philip. Philip remained in the home a further year until he left to live in a flat he found for himself.

Philip's story illustrates the power that social services can have in restricting people when they expect them to conform to certain theoretical processes of adjustment. In Stephen's case, social services may have thought this to be true and the social worker was able to act in an empowering way by closing the case, but for Philip, his dependence in terms of his homelessness meant that he was unable to exercise the same choices.

So, while it may often be the case that disabled people do not need social workers to get involved with how they might live with their impairments, they can also experience considerable social inequalities. While those people with the financial freedom to provide for their own needs may be able to avoid state intervention in their lives, this is not the case for those who need the local authority to pay for services. For Philip, the price of being dependent was that the state assumed the right to involve itself forcefully and unhelpfully in his life. A common example of this intrusion is the control that many local authorities impose on the use of direct payments. However, there are times when the authority invested in social workers by the state can be useful, as the next case example shows.

CASE EXAMPLE

David was involved in a motorcycle accident that resulted in severe brain damage. Following the accident, he was unconscious for several weeks and this necessitated several months of medical rehabilitation in hospital, after which he was considered ready to be discharged. This meant that he was functioning well enough to go to a specialist rehabilitation centre, but not that he had the ability to live at home without being quite dependent on others. As this was a time of war, the best head injury rehabilitation centres were too busy to take civilian patients. The only opportunity for David was to go to a social services day centre. Within a few weeks, the staff at this centre decided that he was too disoriented to be productive and insisted that he leave. After a few weeks, he was found a place in a sports rehabilitation centre, but again, within one week, his disorientation resulted in him being rejected. Reports were sent by all involved to a rehabilitation centre that specialised in head injuries in the hope that they would now consider helping him, but they responded by saying that all they could do was recommend long-term nursing care.

In the meantime, David was living at home with his elderly parents and attending the physiotherapy department of the firm that had employed him. He was making steady progress in relearning a range of activities with the help of the physiotherapist, while the social worker supported his parents in learning to live with him. However, they were faced with a lack of any hope that he might get the specialist help he needed to make greater progress, which made the social worker look at the situation from a different perspective. He began to examine what help would actually be provided by these specialist centres and discovered that it would consist of sessions with various therapists. None of the services that would be offered within the rehabilitation centre would be different to those that could be offered locally, except that they would be coordinated. What the social worker then did was to talk to the therapists in the local community services and arrange for them to come together to form a rehabilitation team. While each person might have had a defined area of practice, what they achieved was a means of working together that was effective for David.

This example demonstrates the potential for social workers to affect the institutionalised processes of treatment, which was in turn useful to David. The services were inflexible and condemning of his potential for an autonomous life. The dominant social attitudes permitted people in positions of power to reject him and suggest that some form of incarceration in a nursing home was the best he could hope for. It was only by confronting the power of those organisations that the social worker was able to examine their actions and provide the services that would help this individual. This was made possible by the skills that social work brought to the problem because it was concerned with both his adaptation to the social world and the social world's adaptation to him. Most of the practical help he needed came from other sources, but these professions work to particular functional responsibilities and would not find it easy to confront their own organisational control. The power relations of the rehabilitation industry were a major part of the problem and the social worker played an important role in understanding and challenging these.

Despite policies based on the assumption that all disabled people need support and care, social services are generally provided for those people without the ability to survive or progress, particularly those who live in poverty. This raises some pertinent points regarding the initial question – do disabled people need social work? In an unjust society, poverty is more likely to hit particular groups of people, and disabled people are one such group. Therefore, it is important to recognise why people need social work assistance and not simply claim this as being an individual problem, directly attributable to their impairment. In effect, part of the social process of being disabled is to be economically disadvantaged, so it is dishonest to say that people with impairments need social workers per se, rather than disabled people may need some form of help to fight the oppression they are experiencing. The question remains, however, as to whether social work is or can be the right sort of help. There is clearly a legitimacy in the argument that social welfare and social work can contribute to the disablement of people with impairments, but it is also true that many people, both with and without impairments, need and benefit from the help that social work can provide. So how can this paradox be explained?

The argument that social work is part of the problem, in that it perpetuates the dependency of disabled people, is being made at a political level. This is the same argument that might be made against unemployment benefit as an insufficient substitute for employment, and, as a political analysis, it is sound. However, society cannot be examined from that perspective alone. As Thompson (2006) has argued, discrimination occurs within a complex interaction of the structural, cultural and personal levels of our social world. In this sense, we can begin to explain why it is that many people, both disabled and non-disabled, might subscribe to the view that people need to adjust to their disabilities. We are influenced by the cultural realities that we have grown up with, part of which is the construction of disability as a state of dependency and a personal problem. No matter how much we argue at a political or structural level that this is wrong, it will not change unless we also address the cultural influences on the personal.

While structural change will undoubtedly affect our cultural realities in the long term, in the immediate present we need some other means of dealing with the problems that individuals are experiencing. It is at this personal level that social work can help and be part of the solution. While the political arguments are made and before the changes they seek have occurred, there are individuals who will find that the only alternatives on offer are a life in institutions or inadequate, custodial care in the community. It is these individuals who social workers may be able to assist. What must be remembered, however, is that these levels are involved in a complex interaction and therefore social work practice at the personal level will also have its influence on the cultural and structural levels. What is needed is an understanding of the whole that will lead to models of practice at a personal level that are consistent with and supportive of the change being sought elsewhere. An example of this was a piece of work undertaken by a social work student while on placement with a social services department.

CASE EXAMPLE

The student was asked to deal with a referral from the mother of a 19-year-old man with spina bifida. On leaving 'special' school at 17, Michael had spent some time at home and had attended the local day centre to provide respite for his mother; the pattern of care throughout his life had been determined by the assumption that he was a 'burden' on his mother who was his 'carer'. He was also sent to a residential centre to learn the skills of independent living. This had largely concentrated on functional abilities and at the end of his stay, he returned home. Like many teenagers, he continued to rely on his mother who, worried that this could be a lifelong dependency, had requested that he be readmitted to the day centre. The expectation of social services was that this would be treated as a reasonable request and Michael would be offered a place, hence it was allocated to a student to learn how to carry out the administrative process of a routine task.

On first visiting the family, the student discovered that Michael did not wish to attend the day centre and he felt quite happy remaining at home while his mother was out at work. On the other hand, his mother reported having to provide a range of help to Michael during the day and considered that he would be at risk if he was left alone. The assessment was made more complex by the fact that some of the activities for which Michael was dependent on his mother were not things that he was incapable of doing for himself, but things for which, as a teenager, he chose to rely on her. The dilemma for the student was whether to help the mother or to accept Michael's right to refuse to be sent to the day centre.

The student initially attempted to get the authority to use the cost of daycare to purchase home support for Michael, but this was refused on budgetary grounds – this was prior to April 2004 when local authorities became obliged to provide direct payments. The advice from the agency was to 'counsel' Michael towards accepting the day centre placement in order to give his mother a break. This would have been perfectly acceptable for passing a social work degree and would be theorised as intervention in a situation of conflict in which both parties could not have exactly what they wanted. However, the student felt this would have made her part of the problem in relation to the structural aims of equal citizenship for disabled people.

Thus she approached the problem from a different perspective. She felt that it was necessary to help Michael to understand the politics of his predicament, so she did engage in counselling Michael, not in order to get him to accept the placement, but to help him become aware of the ways in which he was being denied his dependency as a teenager. The aim of this was that it would help him to adopt a strategy with which he would have a chance of succeeding, because he would be better informed about the true nature of what was happening. The student also took him to meet people from a nearby coalition of disabled people so that the politicisation could advance beyond that which could be offered by an able-bodied social worker.

This illustrates how it is possible to contribute at an individual level in a manner that is consistent with challenging the cultural and structural expectations of disabled people, and provides a sound basis for the way in which personal problems can be re-examined from a different perspective. However, Michael was receptive to the notion of developing a positive identity and this is not true for everyone.

CASE EXAMPLE

John was 50 years old when he was diagnosed with multiple sclerosis. The diagnosis was devastating for him and he viewed it as the end of life. He gave up work and his relationships with friends and family began to deteriorate. He regarded other people's acceptance of his disability as pity. He left his wife and returned to live with his mother. His physical condition was deteriorating rapidly and he soon began to use a wheelchair and could no longer manage

to live in his mother's small cottage. He requested that social services place
him in a residential home. He had already spent two weeks in a nursing home
and the staff complained that he seemed to find the sight of other disabled
people repugnant.

Following a conventional approach to assessment, John's behaviour would be examined in relation to his failure to adjust psychologically towards accepting his debilitating illness. There would be little questioning of the view that the multiple sclerosis would cause him to have to abandon positive roles and, while being a disabled person would be seen as undoubtedly a negative experience, he would be expected to have the emotional capacity to cope with it. Any failure to do so would be treated as a lack of ability on his part. He would be labelled as a problem because he was failing to conform to the goals of whatever rehabilitation had been planned. The focus of any intervention would be on getting John to behave in ways that would be acceptable to the services that he might need to receive.

I want to suggest another way of viewing John and his response to this illness. Throughout his life, John, like most other people, has been subjected to a cultural education and socialisation that has caused him to believe that disability is a negative state. This is not just a passive piece of information that he held in his mind, but a belief so strong that he had consistently thought of disabled people as lesser beings, or part of another world. In short, he was a disablist person. Therefore, when he was diagnosed as having an illness that would result in him becoming increasingly impaired, he was only able to view this as the start of a negative phase of his life. While clearly he was subjected to a range of stigmatising stereotypes, the predominant ones were already in place within his own mind and he was in effect his own oppressor. John's identity as an able-bodied person was of such importance to him that when it was threatened, it resulted in a range of self-damaging reactions.

Within this way of thinking, a number of questions arise as to how John might be helped. First, if he has been and continues to be influenced by a personal tragedy model of disability, then some form of consciousness-raising aimed at countering this, and providing him with an alternative way of understanding impairment and disability, may be of some value. However, can this be achieved through contact with a social worker, when the probability is that she will be able-bodied and, regardless of this, likely to be representing an organisation that is embedded in an individual model approach to disability issues (Oliver and Sapey, 2006)?

As John has retained his identity as an able-bodied person, it is possible that he may find it easier to relate to an able-bodied social worker, albeit in order to strengthen his conviction that impairment is a problem. This is important, because if a social worker, whether disabled or able-bodied, is going to even begin helping in this situation, they are going to have to ensure that they do not reinforce these beliefs. There are various ways of doing this according to the style and approach to practice of the individual, but one thing that is important here is the recognition and understanding that disability can be a universal experience.

While many people are already disabled, those who are not could be at some point in the future, which makes disability somewhat different to other issues of oppression such as gender or race. Indeed, John represented precisely that – an able-bodied person who had become disabled – and while he undoubtedly faced many problems because of that, his first and perhaps most significant difficulty is his prior failure to acknowledge disabled people as part of the same society as himself. The problem therefore lies not only in the negative identity that John perceives disability has brought to him, but also with the strong able-bodied identity he had prior to this.

Although individual social workers can be prepared for working in ways that do not reinforce the stigma that disabled people will experience, they also need to be able to provide people like John with some form of positive role models, and they need to consider how they do this while representing organisations that have traditionally been responsible for the large-scale segregation of disabled people. The problem here arises out of the ways in which social work agencies, in both the statutory and independent sectors, have developed their relationships with disabled people by treating them as 'other'. Finkelstein (1991) argues that such organisations have been practising an administrative model of disability in which social workers simply administer cures and care to disabled people who have already been deemed to be socially dead. But the process can be institutionalised in other ways. Social workers work in organisational structures that devalue direct work with clients. The rewards in terms of salary are in an inverse relationship to such contact, in that those jobs which have least direct contact pay most. In order to have a career in social work in the conventional sense of moving up the hierarchy and salary scale, social workers have to actively seek posts with reduced or no contact with their clients. If direct work is devalued, so too are clients.

Individual social workers can resist such a culture, although it does make it personally difficult for them within their employment. However, even if social workers individually are able to resist pressures to conform to their agencies' view of disabled people, they may still have difficulty in presenting themselves to their clients in such a way. Social services departments will have some form of popular reputation and this will contribute to the way the social worker is perceived from the outset of their working relationship, so it is important to try and establish a more personal basis for working together. This is not personal in the sense of being non-professional, but in terms of being symbolically separate from an oppressive organisation. The aim is to present oneself to John as someone whose identity is not determined by disablism, but by the idea that impairment can be part of a universal experience. Whether the social worker is disabled or not, this provides the potential of a positive role model.

Conclusion

All the examples discussed here are of men and there may therefore be other issues that should be considered in relation to disabled women; nevertheless, I am proposing that there is a possibility of positive social work practice with disabled people. Central to this is the recognition that the primary reason for that involvement is not the individual's impairment, but the ways in which society perceives people with impairments. This is made difficult by the structure of social welfare agencies and the focus of social policy, in which disabled people are identified, defined and made separate from the rest of society. The task for the social worker will involve overcoming the structural, institutional, cultural, professional and personal barriers that contribute to the problem. However, none of this can be achieved effectively if social workers themselves hold on to an identity that devalues difference and impairment. Social work is an interpersonal activity and it cannot take place effectively if one person in the working relationship believes they are superior to the other.

For further discussion of relevant aspects of care planning and adult services, see Adams et al., 2009a, Chapters 17 and 23.

www.disabilitystudies.net Contains the archives of the international disability studies conferences that have been held at Lancaster University since 2003.

www.leeds.ac.uk/disability-studies/archiveuk/ Holds an archive of disability studies materials, many of which are no longer in print.

www.disability-archive.leeds.ac.uk/ The Disability Archive at the University of Leeds contains hundreds of books, articles and papers that make up a history of disability studies in the UK.

www.lancs.ac.uk/cedr/ The Centre for Disability Research contains the archive of papers presented at each of the biennial disability studies conferences hosted by Lancaster University.

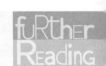

Morris, J. (1993) *Independent Lives: Community Care and Disabled People*, Basingstoke, Macmillan – now Palgrave Macmillan. This study of disabled people's experience of receiving care remains timely and relevant and contains many important messages, both positive and negative, for anyone involved in organising support services for disabled people.

Oliver, M. and Sapey, B. (2006) *Social Work with Disabled People*, 3rd edn, Basingstoke, Palgrave Macmillan. Key textbook, updated to include the major policy changes, which examines the relationship between the social model of disability and social work policies and practices.

Thomas, C. (2007) *Sociologies of Disability and Illness: Contested Ideas in Disability Studies and Medical Sociology*, Basingstoke, Palgrave Macmillan. Provides an accessible and comprehensive account of the main ways in which disability has been theorised with disability studies and medical sociology.

31 Learning disability

Chapter overview

This chapter examines the meaning of learning disability, recognising the barriers to reaching a specific definition. It discusses three dominant models or approaches to learning disability: the medico-psychological model; normalisation; and a rights and citizenship perspective. Finally, it looks at the implications of this last model for critical practice in social work.

Constructing difference

CASE EXAMPLE

Jones, B., male, 18, profound mental handicap due to unspecified brain damage at birth, mental age of 3 years 10 months, poor motor control due to mild cerebral palsy on left side, no verbal or other forms of communication, frequent episodes of aggressive behaviour towards staff and other residents, incontinent and lacking basic daily living skills. Requires a 2:1 staffing ratio to control behaviour.

Barry is a lively young man of 18 who has lived with a learning disability since birth. He is a bit unsteady on his feet but manages to get around without aides or assistance. He does not speak nor has he had the opportunity to learn other formal means of communication. He communicates his likes and dislikes clearly through his facial expressions and behaviour and those who know him well have no difficulty interpreting what he is communicating. After being admitted to hospital due to the lack of community support systems, Barry has occasionally lashed out at staff. This invariably would occur after visits home and was usually directed at unfamiliar staff who are trying to rush him through one of his routines. Barry was moved out of the long-stay hospital into a specialist behaviour group home, where he lives with four other men who are also labelled as having challenging behaviour. Barry needs support to go to the toilet at regular intervals. At his family home, he enjoys helping washing the dishes or the car, going for long drives, listening to rock music, and has his own drum set, which he uses regularly at home but has no access to at the group home. Family reports no difficulties while on his visits and activities.

So which one is the real Barry Jones? Well, both of them; at least they are as real as any of us get. They represent two different constructions of who Barry is. How he is constructed, though, has serious implications, not only for how we may perceive Barry and how we social workers might respond, but, more critically, what kind of life Barry has the opportunity to live. While we are all socially constructed to some degree, people with a learning disability have been more vulnerable than most individuals or groups to negative, stigmatising and exclusionary constructions, which, as in Barry's case, sometimes lead us to miss the person in favour of the labels and consequently to see what Barry might be trying to tell us, for example why is his behaviour so radically different with the family than in the group home?

A simple look at the labels used to describe learning disability illustrates the power of the negative construction to shape attitudes: idiot, moron, imbecile, retard, defective, mentally handicapped and so on. These are all terms that rightfully jar our contemporary sensibilities, but which all began their modern usage as 'scientific' terms or categories, but have been transformed into popular terms of derision in the English language. Such is the power of the construct that whatever term is used, it almost inevitably takes on an oppressive, derisory meaning. The power of any label to oppress is recognised by a group of people who have a learning disability, who chose 'People First' as the name of their movement, inherently recognising how their humanity has been suppressed by this plethora of labels.

A key aspect of critical practice – in this and most other areas of social work – is the ability to deconstruct imposed identities, to understand the power of various constructions and labels to oppress or emancipate, and to find the person beneath these constructions. As social workers, we are both subject to, and part of, this process of identity construction. If we accept uncritically Barry number one, we are likely simply to reinforce the oppressive and stigmatising identity that the description implies. We may recommend support options that will themselves reinforce the spoiled identity described – a self-fulfilling prophesy. Or we may ask ourselves: How did this person come to be reduced to this litany of negative identity features? Who is the person behind this construction? How can we help Barry to overcome identity number one and discover and build on a self-determined identity? This is not an easy challenge, as it requires both the skills and knowledge to deconstruct identities that are often mired in scientific complexity and the will to challenge systems, structures and professions that profit from the spoiling of Barry's identity.

In this chapter, we will look first at what we mean by 'learning disability' and the difficulty in arriving at any specific definition. We will then look at the dominant models or approaches to learning disability: the medico-psychological model; normalisation; and a rights and citizenship perspective. The first two have been, and continue to be, widely used perspectives and we will briefly consider each and how one might respond in practice using these models. The third model, that of rights and citizenship, has only recently emerged and we will concentrate on this model and what it implies for critical practice in social work.

Defining learning disability

The simple task of naming the category of people we currently refer to as having a 'learning disability' has often led to acrimonious debate and a large dose of political correctness. In the UK, 'learning difficulty or disability' are the current 'correct' terms, while in the US, the use of 'people first language' is de rigueur. Intellectual disability, developmental disability and older forms such as mentally handicapped, defective or retarded can all still be found in the literature and in practice. The reality is of course that there is no such thing as a neutral term, nor is any term perceived to be 'correct' today likely to remain so. Language is power and so will always reflect the shifting sands of power dialectics.

While the seemingly simple task of naming has proven complex, identifying exactly who we are talking about within whatever label we choose is equally complex and can have severe ramifications for those who are included or excluded. Over the years, the category has expanded and contracted, depending more on who was doing the categorising and why, than on any essential truth or scientific 'fact'. During the early part of the twentieth century, when the eugenics movement was at its height and intelligence tests were first being developed, the category expanded rapidly. Goddard's (1866–1957) rather poor interpretations of Binet's test created a situation where extreme numbers of persons were classified as 'mentally defective'. Goddard wrote:

> For many generations we have recognised and pitied the idiot. Of late we have recognised a higher type of defective, the moron, and have discovered he is a burden ... a menace to society and civilization, that he is responsible in large measure, for many, if not all, our social problems. (quoted in Abbott and Sapsford, 1987: 25)

Intelligence tests rely heavily on normative assumptions about what constitutes average or 'normal' functioning, with little regard to social or cultural factors. The arbitrary nature of determining what constitutes 'normal' can be seen in the fact that when the American Association on Mental Deficiency reclassified its IQ levels, 'thousands of people were cured of mental handicaps overnight' (Blatt, quoted in Bogdan and Taylor, 1982).

So, the question of 'what is learning disability?' is neither simple nor without dangers. Being included in the definition has, at different times, meant a total loss of rights, being subject to sterilisation, incarceration and, in some cases, killed. On the other side, being excluded may mean a lack of access to services or support. Therefore, the critical social worker must be aware of not only what the various definitions are but also, more critically, the implications for the person involved.

In general, at one end of the spectrum, we find definitions with an exclusive or predominant emphasis on the biological facts, the presence of a specific impairment such as Down's syndrome. The main problem with this type of definition is its exclusive focus on learning disability as a 'disease', an individual pathology, with little or no reference to the practical or social consequences that may be vastly different, given the severity or the individual and the social context. A more specific problem is the magnitude of possibilities and range of degrees that may be present in a given case. Most learning disabilities cannot be attributed to a specific biological factor. Down's syndrome represents the largest single identified 'cause' and yet includes only 10 per cent of the entire putative 'class'. This does not even begin to tell us about the degree or severity of the impairment.

Other definitions have focused on various forms of intelligence or adaptive behaviour tests, which purport to measure either intelligence or behavioural attributes or deficits. As noted above, these definitions rely heavily on normative assumptions about what constitutes average functioning or adaptive behaviour. They also tend to ignore the 'person' behind the behaviours or IQ levels and engender stereotypical responses and attitudes. Saying someone has a mental age of 13 gives the impression that they act like a 13-year-old or can only do things that a 13-year-old can. In fact, this tells us very little about who the person is or what they want and are capable of.

These types of definition generally are underpinned by what Oliver (1990) has termed the 'personal tragedy theory of disability' (see Chapter 30), where disability is seen exclusively as an individual, disease-based problem, thus encouraging a focus on the elimination of the impairment and a predominantly biopsychological approach to policy and practice. This tendency is increasing with the rapid growth of genetic testing and research, which cannot provide any 'cure' but has resulted in high rates of selective abortion based on the presence of Down's syndrome or other genetic impairments. If you were working from this model, you might recommend for Barry more psychological or psychiatric intervention and continued control.

Alternatively, a 'social model' of disability has begun to emerge, spurred on largely by the work of people with disabilities themselves and focusing not on the individual with a disability as the problem, but on social arrangements that 'construct disabilities'. The central idea is that through processes such as labelling, segregation, stigmatisation, lack of access and a denial of citizenship, we have constructed the disability. The model does not deny the presence of an impairment, but rather argues that any disability associated with that impairment is a consequence of social arrangements noted above.

Related to this type of approach is the World Health Organisation's *International Classification of Functioning, Disability and Health* (ICF), which tries to integrate both the 'impairment' and the social aspects of disability, its context and impact on participation, shifting the focus from cause to impact:

The ICF 'mainstreams' the experience of disability and recognises it as a universal human experience ... ICF takes into account the social aspects of disability and does not see disability only as 'medical' or 'biological' dysfunction. (www.who.int/classifications/icf/en/)

At the end of the day, the critical social worker must remember that definitions, of whatever type, are simply social constructs that help us to understand a general phenomenon, but tell us little about the person behind the label. But, the critical social worker must also remember that definitions are powerful tools that can be used for good or ill, can dictate our response and the response of others, and can mean access to services or denial of rights. A rose by any other name does not always smell as sweet.

Medical, psychological and normalisation approaches

The medical or psychological approaches discussed above engendered certain types of response, such as special school and classes, behavioural interventions, medical control, a focus on prevention and institutional or specialist provision. The eugenic fears reflected in Goddard's comments engendered a response of control, regulation and exclusion that still haunts our current system of services and policy, although now the most explicit eugenic focus is on prenatal detection and elimination. The medical and psychological approaches are still common in practice today, particularly in cases where people are thought to have either 'challenging behaviour', a dual diagnosis of mental health and learning disability, autism spectrum disorder or complex physical needs. Whether some or all of the practices associated with these approaches are justified is a question beyond the scope of this chapter, but one you may want to keep in the back of your mind as we look at other approaches that are more relevant to social work practice.

'Normalisation' – or as it has been renamed, 'social role valorisation' – was the dominant approach to learning disability from the 1970s through to the 1990s and is still common in practice today. The most influential version was developed by Wolfensberger, who described it as:

> The utilisation of culturally valued means in order to establish and/or maintain personal behaviours, experiences and characteristics that are culturally normative and valued. (quoted in O'Brien, 1981: 1)

Normalisation is based on social role theory and, as the name implies, is concerned with reversing negative roles and images and developing and enhancing more positive social roles for people with a learning disability. As such, normalisation is concerned with issues such as dress, the normal rhythms to people's day, the locations and company in which people spend their time and the things people spend their time doing. For example, normalisation advocates against large groupings of devalued people, segregated provision that reinforces their role as different, labelling and stigmatisation. In short, normalisation is concerned with ensuring that people with a learning disability fulfil roles that are both valued and non-stigmatising (see Brown and Smith, 1992, for further details on normalisation).

While the above brief review hardly does justice to what is a complex theory, you can see how this might influence practice, for example by ensuring that people have the opportunity to participate in meaningful activities, rather than spending their days in large day centres enduring endless, usually pointless training that only reinforces their differences. In short, it means ensuring that our interventions enhance people's positive roles in our community and minimise the occurrence of devalued or stigmatising activities and roles. Normalisation can also be a useful means of evaluating current or proposed services or interventions. In brief, we can ask ourselves: 'Does this activity encourage a positive identity or reinforce a negative image?'

In recent years, normalisation has come in for criticism from a number of directions (for example Brown and Smith, 1992; Oliver, 1999), but most of these can be summed up in two related questions: 'Does normalisation simply reinforce existing ideas about normality and what is culturally accepted?' 'Does normalisation simply encourage the appearance of normality without really giving the individual true choice and empowerment?' In the former case, concerns centre around reinforcing societal prejudices about race, gender, sexuality, class and so on. In order for people not to be further stigmatised, are they encouraged to accept roles that may be oppressive either to themselves or others? In the second case, does normalisation encourage people simply to 'pass' rather than challenging their oppressors and embracing and celebrating their own identity? Space precludes a full treatment of these issues, but we can look at what has evolved as a 'next step', that is, the rights, citizenship and self-determination movement.

Rights, citizenship and self-determination

The concepts of rights, citizenship and self-determination are increasingly seen as central to a new approach to learning disability. The UK learning disability strategy, of which the English White Paper (DH, 2001c) illustrates one leading edge, is based on four related principles: rights, independence, choice, and inclusion. The magnitude of this challenge can, however, be seen when one considers the historical exclusion – specifically from a rights-bearing status – of people with a learning disability. John Locke (1632–1704), a central figure in modern liberal political thought, was clear on this point in his *Two Treatises of Government* (1924: 145):

> But if through defects that may happen out of the ordinary course of Nature, any one comes not to such a degree of reason wherein he might be supposed capable of knowing the law ... he is never capable of being a free man ... So lunatics and idiots are never set free from the government of their parents.

This exclusion – not just politically but morally – has been taken even further by many leading moral and political philosophers who question the very humanness of people with a learning disability. Ryle notes that 'specifically human behavior' is that 'which is unachieved by animals, idiots and infants', and Quinton, discussing the centrality of rationality in humanness, notes that 'defective human beings who look and are physically constructed like men ... are only marginally or by a sort of prudent and humane courtesy fully human beings' (both quoted in Goodey, 1992: 28). In light of this, rights, citizenship and self-determination may seem a strange basis for an approach to learning disability. On the other hand, it may be that we are finally attacking the real root of their oppression and exclusion.

Rights in Western democratic states are grounded in the idea of autonomy or self-determination, that is, the ability to choose how to live one's own life, either on our own or, as is the case with most of us, in collaboration with others with whom we choose to live and work. Self-determination is not a new term, having long been considered the core value of the social work profession. It is also a core value in Western liberal democratic societies. This connection is useful in helping us to understand what self-determination means, and does not mean, for practice and policy. We will return to this question shortly, but first, we look at the concept of self-determination.

Put simply, it is choosing for oneself what one does or does not want to do, be or value. A slightly more complex definition of the related term 'autonomy' is the capacity to formulate and pursue plans and purposes that are self-determined (Stainton, 1994). This highlights a couple of key features that will help us to see what this means for practice. First, we are concerned here with capacity, not outcome. In other words, our goal is not to ensure that people achieve some specific outcome we think is valid, but that they have the capacity to determine what they would like to do and an equal chance of achieving their goal as anyone else. Notice that we are concerned with equal opportunity, not outcome. In service terms, this means that we will focus more on supporting choice-making through our planning systems and other supports such as advocacy, rather than deciding what programme or service is best for a person.

Second, we are concerned not only that people are able to decide something for themselves, but also with their ability to act on their choices. Telling someone they are free to decide to go to college, but not providing the means for them to do so is no choice at all. We are not looking at special rights here, but simply ensuring that people with a learning disability are not inhibited by discriminatory practices and have an equal chance to benefit from college as anyone else. So our goals in practice are to ensure that people have the means to make their choices, whether this entails support staff, benefits, or simply knowledge and skills.

The idea of equality requires some clarification here. If 'equal' implies simply 'getting the same as everyone else', in essence this means we are ignoring difference that may require either a different way of doing things or additional support. This problem, sometimes called the 'difference dilemma', refers to the problem that what people require in order to achieve equal citizenship differs with each individual. In other words, 'equal treatment' does not equate with 'equal citizenship', since different people require different types of treatment to achieve the same basic capacity for participation. For example, a person who is paraplegic requires different means to achieve basic mobility than does a fully ambulant person. They are not getting 'more' mobility, they simply require something different to achieve the same mobility as everyone else.

While the example above may be relatively easy, dealing with this dilemma becomes more acute as the nature and complexity of needs increases. This complexity makes it impossible to establish general universal provisions that will satisfy all needs. The challenge then for social work and policy is not to find better services, but to create a structure in which individuals can articulate their demands directly and which allows the state to adjudicate and meet legitimate claims. In essence, this is what the role of the local authority social worker is in a rights-based system, helping the person to articulate their needs and determining if these are needs that a person has a right to have met. If so, the social worker becomes the catalyst for making sure that they are met and monitoring any changes in the person's needs.

At heart, the struggle to recognise and respect the autonomy, citizenship and rights of people with a learning disability is a political struggle. It is not primarily a psychological concept concerned with changing the individual, but a political one concerned with changing the relationship between the individual, the state and society. On one level, this means focusing on obtaining basic legal equality and securing equality of rights. However, legal equality and rights are only one step towards equal citizenship. On a more structural level, social policy must begin to allow for individually determined choices about how, when and where support is provided. This is why policy developments in the UK such as direct funding, individual budgets and access to advocacy, which allow the individual to choose how their needs are to be met, are so critical to building self-determination and equal citizenship.

To go one stage further into the complexities of this, we can look at the situation in England, where *Valuing People* (DH, 2001c), the first White Paper for 30 years on learning disability, is based on promoting the rights, inclusion, choices and opportunities for independence of disabled people as citizens. Shakespeare (2006: 139) points out that for a person whose impairments are significant, the goal of autonomy – implying a significant level of services to support them – may be more realistic than aiming for independence. It is necessary to accept that the way forward is complex. He proposes a personalised approach, with a matrix of different types of service available, such as direct payments, home care and residential care, interwoven with the different components of care – such as companionship, flexibility, privacy and risk (Shakespeare, 2006: 149).

Such approaches provide the means for the individual citizen to emerge, participate and grow as a citizen rather than being a part of some excluded putative class. These types of change to the context of practice are critical if social workers are to be given the scope to truly recognise and support the rights and citizenship of people with a learning disability (see Stainton, 2007). The critical practitioner must be able to recognise where structural barriers exist and work to overcome them within their own communities and agencies.

On the level of practice, social workers' key roles as assessors and case managers are critical in determining if people are to be supported to be autonomous, rights-bearing citizens, or if they are to continue to be oppressed. From this perspective, critical practice requires a much sharper focus on the individual, both in terms of our planning and assessment systems and in determining needs and how they are best met. Planning and assessment systems such as person-centred planning (Sanderson, 1997) are useful tools in helping us to do this and help to break us out of existing ways of working with people.

In many ways, from a rights and citizenship perspective, critical practice is simply what has always been good practice in social work:

- making the user the centre of the assessment process

- acting as a facilitator to help people to determine for themselves what they need and want, and not deciding for them
- ensuring that they are supported to make decisions both with information and independent advocacy and advice – particularly important for people with more severe learning disabilities who may not be able to articulate formally their wants and needs.

The critical social worker is not an 'expert' on learning disability, but a skilled professional able to support people to determine and act on what they want and need in order to be the person they want to be. In the past, we predetermined the outcomes for people by labelling them and then assigning them to services; a day centre, a group home, a special school. A rights-based approach means that we must reject any preconceived notions of what some illusory category of 'people with a learning disability' needs, and focus on the individual as an individual, who happens to require some support because they have a learning disability. What a person wants and needs are questions that must be addressed to the specific individual, not to a label or category.

Conclusion

So to return to Barry, our goal is to see past the labels, diagnoses and so on and see the person, to find ways of helping Barry to express what he needs and wants and support him in achieving this, even if it may not be what 'we' think is 'best for him'. The critical practitioner needs to be aware of the often subtle ways in which Barry's identity has been distorted and the ways and means of helping him to reclaim his autonomy, rights and citizenship.

I have tried to outline what is required if we take the autonomy, rights and citizenship of people with a learning disability seriously:

- a foundation in rights and legal equality
- a social policy structure that supports and enhances individual autonomy and participation
- practice that truly focuses on the person and who they are and what they want.

As was noted, at heart, this perspective is a political concept that is also concerned with eliminating the oppression experienced by people with a learning disability. Is not the social work response then too individualistic to bring about this change? First, as was noted, a social worker has an ethical obligation to work towards broader structural changes that counter oppressive structures and practices. But in terms of practice with specific individuals, it is founded on the belief that only empowered individuals can form the collective force necessary to bring about full citizenship for people with learning disabilities. As Noel (1994) notes: 'Even though emancipation begins and ends with the individual, he or she has only collective means of ensuring its progress.' Critical practitioners must not only commit themselves to these goals, but also arm themselves with the knowledge and tools to identify means of oppression and support people to take their rightful place as full and equal citizens.

For further discussion of working with service users and carers, see Adams et al., 2009a, Chapter 15, and for rights approaches in mental health, see Adams et al., 2009c, Chapter 8. For a more general discussion of rights and citizenship, see Chapter 4.

Atkinson, D. (1999) *Advocacy: A Review*, Brighton, Pavilion. Excellent review of the literature on advocacy.

Bigby, C., Fyffe, C. and Ozanne, E. (eds) (2007) *Planning and Support for People with Intellectual Disabilities: Issues for Case Managers and other Professionals*, London, Jessica Kingsley. Provides an up-to-date look at a range of critical issues for practitioners in the learning disability field from working with families, working in a rights-based context and supporting people with complex needs.

Flynn, R. and Lemay, R. (eds) (1999) *A Quarter Century of Normalization and Social Role Valorization: Evolution and Impact*, Ottawa, University of Ottawa Press. Brings together a range of experts on normalisation from around the world and provides a good overview of the current state of practice and some of the main critiques.

Malin, N. (ed.) (1996) *Services for People with Learning Disabilities*, London, Routledge. Although slightly dated on services, remains the best overview of the history, definition and range of services for people with a learning disability.

Ramcharan, P., Roberts, G., Grant, G. and Borland, J. (eds) (1997) *Empowerment in Everyday Life: Learning Disability*, London, Jessica Kingsley. Excellent volume containing chapters on self-advocacy, families, legal aspects and citizenship and empowerment.

32 Older people

Chapter overview

This chapter addresses some key critical debates and dilemmas in social work practice with older people. It discusses the role of critical practice in the development of positive social work practice with older people and proposes an agenda for change and development which incorporates the key messages of critical practice.

CASE EXAMPLE

Mr Khalif is a divorced man in his late sixties, who lives alone on the outskirts of a large market town. He is from Somalia and came to England over 20 years ago. He has one son who lives and works in London. They maintain contact but Hussein is only able to visit his father every few months. Mr Khalif's health has deteriorated over the past six months. He was diagnosed with diabetes and high blood pressure over two years ago, but the GP and specialist nurse have indicated that Mr Khalif does not engage with treatment and does not follow an appropriate diet. Mr Khalif's eyesight has deteriorated markedly (diabetic retinopathy) and recently, he has had one toe and part of a second amputated. Unfortunately, the neuropathy in his toes has not abated and the clinic has indicated that Mr Khalif needs further surgery. He has refused to undergo surgery and has been told that the implications of this are that he risks his life. Mr Khalif often appears disoriented but is apparently very clear about his wish to be 'left alone' by healthcare professionals. Mr Khalif has a reputation among healthcare staff for being aggressive, uncooperative and 'stubborn'.

Mr Khalif has fallen several times following surgery. Until fairly recently, he has taken a taxi to the local café every day for lunch. His son Hussein visited his father and has contacted the office to make a referral (with

Mr Khalif's permission), as he is concerned that his father is not managing well at home. According to the referral, Mr Khalif has nothing to eat in the house, is struggling to care for himself and is resistant and reluctant to let any healthcare workers into the house. The referral is allocated to Yvonne, a duty social worker.

There are dilemmas and challenges as well as opportunities in developing the knowledge, skills and values important in social work practice with older people. The social work practice arena with older people is not a straightforward one.

Policy dilemmas

Resources and restrictions

The national eligibility criteria, *Fair Access to Care Services* (DH, 2002b), is intended to provide a framework to ensure equality of access to people who may need social services support and intervention. However, the imperative to manage finite resources means that social services agencies are, at the time of writing and to a large extent, only able to respond to needs assessed as being within 'critical' or 'substantial' areas of need (CSCI, 2008). These levels of need focus on the presence of indicators such as acute and severe risk to the service user.

Despite the current policy emphasis on promoting independence, the eligibility criteria, insecurities around the privatisation of care services, and the implementation of procedural rules of assessment are also likely to have a negative effect on older people's access to services and the options that are available to them (Lymbery, 2005).

Diverse needs of older people

Historically, policy has not adequately reflected the diversity of ageing and the range of physical, emotional and psychological transitions that older people face. The provision of care for older people has tended to rely on a sequential range of services, such as home care and daycare, and, once the person has reached a sufficiently complex level of need, residential or nursing care. Preventive services and strategies continue to be heavily emphasised in policy but remain largely underdeveloped or unavailable. As social work continues to move away from the one-size-fits-all approach to intervention and care planning, it is clear that crucial dilemmas remain in terms of how creative and innovative social work with older people can be achieved in the context of increasing managerialist workloads coupled with the lack of adequate preventive services.

Partnership and collaborative working

Partnership and collaborative working are key elements of developing critical practice in working with older people. This commitment is reflected in the proliferation over the past five years of policy documents relevant to older people, which unerringly point towards partnership and collaborative working as being the way forward in integrating health and social care to provide a seamless service (DH, 2005, 2007b, 2007c).

The realities of developing and maintaining effective collaboration between health and social care is harder to achieve than the rhetoric of policy would imply. Tensions and uncertainties exist between health and social care at all levels – from executive and strategic planning right down to the front line and the point of delivery, where one could argue it is most evident and tangible. Such tensions can in part be attributed to the lack of clarity and definition of the roles and functions of health and social care at government level (Lewis, 2001) and the historic differences in power and culture. Also implicated is the lack of an appropriate role for social work in the context of partnership working that has yet to be robustly defined (Lymbery, 2005).

Single assessment process

The single assessment process (SAP) for health and social care is a central tenet of recent policy to promote a person-centred, interagency approach to the assessment of the health and social care needs of older people (DH, 2001d). The SAP places a requirement on key agencies at the local level to develop and establish shared assessment tools and processes to prevent unnecessary delays in accessing services and avoid duplication (Powell et al., 2007).

The SAP sits within a broader context, where, as in all areas of public policy, the principle of modernisation is being mooted as a means of improving service delivery, challenging established professional boundaries, and focusing on outcomes for the service user (Holloway, 2007). Significant barriers remain, however, to the SAP asserting a tangible influence on the delivery of health and social care services. Barriers include the absence of clear agency protocols and processes for referral between agencies and dealing with anticipated issues at practitioner level, leading to a general confusion and the differently perceived professional status of health and social care (McDonald et al., 2007).

Mental Capacity Act 2005

The Mental Capacity Act 2005 (MCA) provides a statutory framework for people who lack capacity to make decisions for themselves. It also ensures that the individual remains at the centre of the decision-making process by placing particular responsibilities on those who are assessing the person's capacity. Under the MCA, a person's capacity can be assessed by anyone who is directly concerned with their care or welfare at the time the decision needs to be made. More complex decisions are deemed to require a higher degree of capacity, an area which will usually necessitate professional health and/or social care input. If there is reasonable belief that the person does not have the capacity to make the decision concerned, any decision made for, or any act done to, the person lacking capacity must be done in their 'best interests' (DH/Welsh Office,1999; Mental Capacity Act 2005).

The implementation of the MCA has brought significant challenges and, arguably, opportunities for social work with older people to not only further protect the rights and choices of older people who may lack capacity, but also to further assert the professional status of social work with older people and gain a clear voice in multi-agency and collaborative processes of assessment. The challenges have been in the form of the heightened insecurities experienced by individual practitioners and managers as to the level and validity of knowledge required to make a defensible professional judgement. It is perhaps inevitable that such insecurities exist, given the deprofessionalisation of social work with older people and is symptomatic of the 'fallout' of the NHS and Community Care Act 1991, which was to reduce working with older people to a primarily technical exercise of 'managing the problem' of ageing (Phillips et al., 2006) and promote social work as a purely bureaucratic role.

Practice and professional dilemmas

The managerial process of assessment

Another side effect of the managerialisation of social work with older people has been the tendency to view assessment as a means of determining eligibility to obtain resources rather than acquiring an understanding of the individual and their needs. Lloyd and Smith (1998) further argues that at the level of individual professional social work relationships, assessments of need are dominated by procedural and resource considerations, which have often prevented the articulation of the service user's own perceptions and assertion of self.

Proving eligibility can prevent an important focus on an older person's biography, exemplified through, for example, the person's strengths, abilities and lifelong continuities as well as transitional experiences that may be harnessed to cope with present challenges. How can social workers use their skills in assessment processes that are driven by the organisational imperative to prove eligibility? Research has demonstrated the impact on practice of increasingly proceduralised practice (Gorman and Postle, 2003) and a reduction in relevant knowledge and skills in favour of a focus on 'resource finding' (McDonald et al., 2007: 7). There are few studies of the value that older people place on social work services. However, one such study by Manthorpe et al. (2007: 9) found that negative evaluations focused on practice that endorsed the skills associated with an administrative model:

> Negative statements about social workers included references to unhelpful attitudes, guarding the council's money and rationing services, and being too slow to respond to requests for help or to undertake social care assessments, or in some cases, not responding at all.

Lymbery (2005: 178) has argued that practitioners can maintain a positive commitment to practice within a managerialist framework without compromising professional methods and skills by focusing on traditional social work values and skills that utilise a whole systems approach to the individual in their social world. Indeed, we argue that a critical practice highlights the importance of gerontological social workers possessing an appropriate knowledge base that reflects the complexities of social work practice in general, and practice with older people in particular. The kinds of skills that social workers are trained to have, such as the development of social understandings of complex situations, the ability to work with systems, drawing on eclectic theories and models to inform practice, and the importance of developing positive and participatory relationships with older people, are all critical elements of social work practice and should be retained.

The concept of risk and older people

A focus on risk has become a central concern in the current context of social work practice and often involves defining and constructing older people as being 'at risk'. Alongside this definition, terms such as 'frail' and 'dependent' are often used to evidence the degree of risk (Phillips et al., 2006). It is argued that working in a climate of cost containment, risk has become central to defining eligibility as well as shaping the ways in which practitioners and organisations are expected to practise (for example Kemshall et al., 1997). As a result, defining an older person as being 'frail and at risk' can increase the likelihood of their gaining access to limited personal social services. Indeed, the presence of 'risk' may be used so frequently to define eligibility for resources that it is often treated as a relatively unproblematic concept. Arguably, the emphasis is on minimal intervention and a focus on what is required to secure safety, health and autonomy, rather than optimal interventions aimed at enhancing quality of life and promoting opportunities for positive citizenship (see, for example, Kemshall, 2002).

Assessments of older people and their levels of risk tend to dwell on defining risk as an individual problem, such as poor mobility, risk of falling in the home, unable to cook for oneself. Of course, it is essential that practitioners consider how an individual's context, behaviour and environment may create risks to that person and those around them. However, it is important that social workers consciously engage with a wider definition and understanding of risk. Structural factors, such as the consequences of age-based discrimination or poverty, are likely to result in significant risks for older people, which have little to do with their individual behaviour. One consequence of low income is fuel poverty, which results in as many as 50,000 additional deaths of older people occurring in the winter months in England and Wales (www.poverty.org.uk). Older people may also be at risk from the very interventions that are designed to 'protect' them from risk. One case in point is medication in care homes. As recently as 2006, the Commision for Social Care Inspection (CSCI, 2006) reported that half of all care homes in England, many of whom provide homes for older people, do not meet the minimum standards in the administration and management of medication. Clearly, issues such as receiving the wrong medication, taking medication that is inappropriately stored, or not having the benefit of regular medication reviews create serious risks for older men and women.

Ageist stereotypes

Routinised assessments may also serve to reinforce ageist stereotypes about older people and, perhaps in particular, older people who need to use social and healthcare services (see also Chapter 3). For example, a focus on individual dysfunction and problems can reinforce ideas about the inevitable dependency of older people. A failure to consider an older person in their biographical context can have the effect of separating older age from the rest of the life course and rendering the complexities and uniqueness of a person's life invisible. Finally, failing to consider strengths and abilities can imply that older people are helpless in the face of change.

Balancing carer and user needs

Social workers and care managers face the practice tensions of working with carers and older service users who may have very different views about their circumstances and aspirations for the future. For example, how should social workers respond to the difficulties that Hussein has in, on the one hand, caring about his father and, on the other, needing to return to London to work and care for his immediate family. Care and caregiving are understandably complex, contested in their definitions, and dynamic in the ways in which care can shift and change over time. There is a need for social work to develop practice insight into the ways in which roles may change, often dramatically, over a relatively short time period (Ray, 2000). There is a need too for practitioners to recognise and understand the ways in which carers and those people they care for bring meaning and understanding to their situations, informed by the meaning of those relationships (Parker, 1994; Nolan et al., 1996). The social work role should be focused on unpicking the complexity of these contexts and providing interventions that enhance and support service users and carers rather than providing services which, at best, can only substitute existing help or, at worst, be experienced as unhelpful.

Crisis, change and transition

Transition and change are part of all our lives. Often it is the continuities in our biography and life experience that provide us with a store of resources and skills from which we may be able to draw when faced with managing change and transition. Older people are likely to face numerous transitions. Positive transitions may include having more time through retirement, becoming a grandparent and taking on new roles and responsibilities. Other transitions such as the experience of long-term illness, becoming a carer or receiving formal care services are more likely to fall within the remit of social work attention. Social workers are faced with the goal of working positively with older people who are experiencing complex and frightening situations.

In this context, social workers' skills and values must incorporate the ability to work with positive assessment but must also have the skill to provide positive and skilful interventions. This is a difficult issue, as community care teams are increasingly driven towards short-term assessment and purchasing provision and there is not always a place where the short-term worker can refer an older person for longer term work. This is not a call for a return to long-term, open-ended 'casework'. But we do challenge the notion that every service user has needs that will inevitably be short term. A person with dementia, for example, may need time for a social worker to build a relationship with them. Difficulties with memory and communication, together with an appropriate concern about a 'stranger' intruding on a private life, may make it impossible for a social worker to engage in a short-term 'assessment relationship'.

Older people bereft of lifelong partners may need time and skilful help to cope with, and manage in the aftermath of, their bereavement. Older people, like anyone else through the life course, may experience difficulties with alcohol and drugs, have sexual difficulties, find it hard to talk with their partner, be in an abusive relationship or face terminal illness. These life challenges can be as disabling as chronic physical or mental illness and do not necessarily lend themselves to a procedural assessment followed by the provision of off-the-peg interventions. How should social workers and care managers respond appropriately when they are faced with service users with complex needs requiring intervention beyond the provision of care services? What theoretical and practice bases should inform the gerontological social work agenda?

The contribution of critical practice

Glaister (2008: 8) identifies the key components of critical practice as:

> open-minded, reflective approaches that take account of different perspectives, experiences and assumptions ... What is required is a capacity to handle uncertainty and change, as well as being able to operate in accordance with professional skills and knowledge. Practitioners must, in a sense, face both ways, drawing on a sound knowledge and evidence base on the one hand, but at the same time being continually aware of the discretionary and contextual basis of their practice.

Citing the work of Barnett (1997), Glaister (2007) frames three domains of critical practice – critical action, critical reflexivity and critical analysis. How might these domains assist social workers in developing their practice skills within uncertain organisational contexts? The case study in this chapter highlights some of the practice dilemmas that a social worker may typically face and the ways in which the skills of critical practice may assist in complex practice situations.

~~~~~~ CaSE EXaMPLE (cont'd) ~~~~~~

Yvonne faces uncertainty in terms of Mr Khalif's future and in relation to the impossibility of knowing with any certainty what she should do for the best to support him. For example, she has to live with the knowledge that Mr Khalif is in many ways at risk, but that while there are interventions that may alleviate the risk, she is unlikely to solve all the challenges that he faces. Yvonne has had to recognise and work with the realisation that other people may have different perspectives informed by different knowledge, skills and value frameworks. For example, a mandate to treat and cure may contribute to what, at first, may appear to be unsympathetic responses to Mr Khalif's deteriorating situation. Yvonne has also had to make use of her knowledge of social work theory, for example biographical assessment, continuity theory and systemic approaches, as well as information about physical conditions, for example diabetes, diabetic retinopathy and peripheral neuropathy, to assist and inform her understanding of Mr Khalif's experiences and possible interventions. Yvonne's practice will be informed by the need to balance the tension between autonomy and agency and others' views about what he should do. An essential part of this process must involve evaluating the outcomes of her interventions and reflecting on the process of her involvement with him.

Critical action

Critical action should be at the heart of social work practice with older people. It highlights the importance of tackling inequalities and disadvantage and working towards the empowerment of service users (Glaister, 2008). As we have seen, a critical debate rests on the erroneous assumption that ageing is appropriately positioned along a dimension of dependence and independence. There are now signs of a shift away from pathologising older people. The focus of a critical perspective is to challenge assumptions that many of the experiences commonly associated with ageing are driven by biological imperatives. Instead, it is argued, many key experiences generally associated with the experience of ageing are constructed, sustained and reinforced by policy, legislation and organisational procedures that create structural inequalities (for example Townsend, 2007).

It could be argued within a critical perspective, for example, that the assumption that the most appropriate form of care for an older person with physical or cognitive disabilities is in residential care, fuelled by limited resources to invest in support of older people, creates and reinforces the inequalities experienced by older service users. The assumption that people with dementia cannot participate in complex decisions about their lives can be reinforced by practices that display tunnel vision and do not make use of evidence that challenges these assertions (for example Allan, 2001).

Anti-discriminatory practice

The promotion of anti-discriminatory approaches to working with older people is at the heart of critical practice. A gerontological social work agenda should vigorously challenge the notion that such work is boring and amounts to little more than providing a limited range of off-the-peg services. As we have seen, such approaches do nothing to challenge the assumption that older people are an essentially homogeneous group with the same or similar needs (Bytheway, 2000). Age-based discrimination of this nature reinforces myths about ageing and perpetuates superficial explanations of complex situations, together with standardised service responses. As individual social workers, we have a professional duty to challenge society's views and assumptions about older people. For example, social workers should seek to recognise and value the diversity among the older people with whom they work. This includes obvious differences such as membership of diverse ethnic minority groups, cultural experiences and sexual orientation. It also includes recognition and value being placed on the uniqueness of individual lives and the importance of a person's identity. Focusing on a strengths perspective is also crucial in a practice context where it is all too easy to overfocus on the 'problems of age'. A strengths-based approach is characterised by a number of fundamental principles and values (Saleeby, 2002):

- a commitment to the belief that individuals, groups, families and communities have strengths
- trauma, change and illness may be injurious and difficult to endure, but they may also constitute sources of challenge and opportunity for growth and development
- practitioners' approaches should be underpinned by collaboration and facilitating opportunities for empowerment
- practitioners should avoid making assumptions about the upper limits of a person's or group's capacity to grow and change.

Empowerment

A commitment to critical action would also empower older service users. It is important to work with service users' own definition of the problems or challenges they face. If practitioners are genuinely able to engage with this process, it is a crucial step away from the danger of service-led assessment. Part of the assessment process must recognise the importance of understanding the skills, abilities and active attempts that older people use in order to manage the threats or changes in their situations (Ray, 2000). Social work with Mr Khalif should involve ensuring that he is able to express his concerns and preferences and that his wish not to have further treatment is properly acknowledged as a starting point in the relationship.

Empowerment beyond the assessment process involves the participation of the service user in deciding on interventions or plans to meet identified needs. Participation and empowerment are fraught with problems in a context of the restrictions on public expenditure. Clearly, there is a continued need for organisations to shoulder the responsibility of communicating clearly with user groups about the demands on finite resources and what can and cannot be achieved. Ideally, too, service users should be enabled to participate in planning community care and social services. At an individual level, it is likely that service users will fare better within a social services setting if they are armed with the appropriate information about what they can and cannot expect in the process. In Mr Khalif's case, for example, what interventions might ensure that Mr Khalif can remain safely at home, and promote his wellbeing and dignity, at what may be the end of his life. Bringing older people's voices to the forefront of practice can provide empowering experiences for the social worker and the older person, offering insights which will be of great value to practitioners in listening to, for example, marginalised groups of older women with dementia (for example Allan, 2001).

Biography and life course

Inherent in this approach is a recognition of the biography of an individual (Bornat, 1999). Older people may have lifelong continuities, which they wish to preserve. Understanding the importance of biographical continuity can challenge and prevent a social worker from, for example, constructing apparent intransigence as the 'stubbornness' that is bound to accompany old age.

A snapshot approach tells us little about the entrances and exits that older people experience in relation to a range of problems over the course of their lives, what would help them to balance or juggle different dilemmas, or assist them in care-giving or transitions to care. A life course approach can illustrate the way in which continuities are used to construct current identities and explain the ways in which individual older people employ strategies for managing change.

In addition, there is a clear need for social workers engaged in critical action to have the knowledge base to mobilise appropriate resources. This may mean helping an older person to access direct payments, access other community care services or helping a person's referral to other agencies or services, such as primary healthcare professionals. Clearly, not all older service users will be in a position to receive complex information, weigh up the costs and benefits of various courses of action, or decide independently on the best decision for them (Brown, 2000). There is a crucial social work role in advocating for the service user to ensure that they have access to the appropriate support or obtaining an advocate.

Critical analysis

Glaister (2008) highlights the importance of practitioners being able to evaluate the diverse knowledge, theories and policies relevant to practice. According to Glaister (2008: 12), it is inevitable that such analysis recognises the importance of 'multiple perspectives and an orientation of ongoing enquiry'.

Social work practice with older people is notable for its lack of demonstrable practice evaluations. This is in part caused by the slowness of the disciplines contributing to social gerontology to systematically develop theoretical frameworks. Sheldon and Macdonald (1999) argue that professional beliefs that are not based on evidence and debate stand in the way of developing reflective, evidence-based practice. What sorts of theory might usefully be applied to social work with older people? The answer is that it depends on the nature of the need or situation the social worker is facing.

CASE EXAMPLE (cont'd)

Consider, for example, Mr Khalif's situation – what kinds of theories and knowledge base might inform Yvonne's assessment, intervention and practice? The following are possible responses:

- loss – for example visual impairment circulatory disease
- continuity and management of change
- identity theories
- impact of diabetes
- legal frameworks – for example community care legislation and associated adult legislation, current national and local policy
- risk and risk management
- biographical and life course perspectives
- capacity and consent and appropriate legislative frameworks.

Given the complexity of the individual lives of older people and the diverse situations likely to be encountered, it follows that social work assessment and intervention must be informed by a diverse and appropriate theoretical knowledge base, which can be transformed into practice that can be evaluated.

Critical reflexivity

Glaister (2008: 12) defines critical reflexivity as:

> an aware, reflective and engaged self; the term 'reflexivity' implies that practitioners recognise their engagement with service-users and others in a process of negotiating understandings and interventions and are aware of the assumptions and values they bring to this process.

Developing reflective skills through reflecting on our own understanding of ageing is an important and often overlooked aspect of social work practice with older people. Working with older people sharpens our focus on our own ageing and our possible future selves. Although the ability to examine one's self is a central preoccupation in social work, reflecting on self-ageing can be challenging and can call into question our own stereotypes and negativities associated with old age. Examining one's biases is not a once and for all experience but needs attention throughout the social work process in order to understand the social worker's impact on the service user. Reflexivity is one way of analysing the power differential and diversity within the relationship. It is a way of understanding our role in the process. Yvonne is likely to have to confront her own assumptions and values about compliance with treatments and decisions to refuse treatment for life-threatening illness.

Conclusion

We have argued that one way of working positively in complex environments is to develop critical practice in the context of gerontological social work. Such a development should engage in a debate about what should properly and appropriately constitute social work with older people. Most importantly, it should acknowledge the importance of developing sound knowledge bases and theoretical frameworks to both underpin and evaluate practice. Such practice should engage in broad agendas on a number of levels. The agendas would reflect the diversity associated with the experience of ageing and should include an active commitment to developing theoretical and practical interventions based on evidence. We believe that there should be a clear distinction between social work and care management, in order to develop as a respected and legitimate activity in the twenty-first century.

For further discussion of ethical issues, mental capacity and consent, see Chapter 7, and for work with frail older people, see Adams et al., 2009c, Chapter 7.

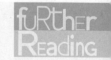

Lymbery, M. (2005) *Social Work with Older People; Context, Policy and Practice*, London, Sage. Discusses the current context in which social work practice takes place. Considers the role of interprofessional practice in some depth and offers ideas for the future development of social work with older people.

Phillips, J., Ray, M. and Marshall, M. (2006) *Social Work with Older People*, 3rd edn, Basingstoke, Palgrave Macmillan. Provides a useful introduction to social work practice with older people and considers the role of social work in key social work processes, for example assessment, care planning, monitoring and review.

Ray, M., Bernard, M. and Phillips, J. (2008) *Critical Issues in Social Work with Older People*, Basingstoke, Palgrave. Develops the ideas considered in this chapter and makes the case for a critical gerontological social work practice in key areas of social work practice with older people.

33

Care at the end of life and in bereavement

Chapter overview

This chapter sees dying and bereavement as matters of concern for workers in all areas of social care. Two factors are considered to be essential for critical practice: confidence about the practitioner's role, and the habit of reflectivity. Relevant concepts and models are outlined and several practice examples illustrate their application.

In line with the strategy for end-of-life care (DH, 2008), this chapter rests on the premise that dying and bereavement are clearly on the agenda for all workers in social care, whatever their area of practice. Despite the fact that social care workers have for many years worked with people who are dying or bereaved, many workers outside palliative care settings have seen this as ideally being work for specialists. If practitioners in mainstream social care are to be confident about their role, they need to be familiar with recent theoretical developments as well as sure that their managers will offer appropriate support and encouragement. This chapter outlines a number of relevant concepts and models, showing through the use of practice examples how these can be used as a basis for critical practice with people who are dying or bereaved in specialist and general settings.

Critical practice with people who are dying or bereaved

During 2008, the English government published an end-of-life care strategy (DH, 2008) promoting a widely accepted policy that is being adopted in many countries in the Western world. This shifts the focus on multiprofessional work with people who are dying and bereaved away from palliative care towards responding to end-of-life care needs wherever they arise. Palliative care deals primarily with people with an advanced life-threatening illness and focuses on medical and nursing practice concerned with symptom and particularly pain management. This is combined with psychological, social and spiritual care when personal and interpersonal issues arise for dying and bereaved people and their families. End-of-life care is a broader approach that extends the skills and knowledge of palliative care to the much greater number of people who approach the end of life increasingly frail and perhaps suffering from a number of debilitating medical conditions that are not life-threatening. Consequently, these people need help through non-specialised health and social care services, whose staff, including social workers and social care practitioners, need training and skills in responding to end-of-life issues. While this shift in strategy is to be welcomed, social work with people who are dying or bereaved is not, outside specialist settings, a unitary or defining area of work. For the mainstream worker, these aspects of experience may not be the main focus of involvement.

Moreover, dying and bereavement are very different events as, in any particular situation, they describe the situation of different actors, for whom the outcome of the crisis of death is totally different. In some instances, involvement may span the event of death, offering important benefits for service users who are bereaved. Nevertheless, it is still helpful to look separately at dying and bereavement if we are to understand both the experience of those concerned and the social work response to their situation.

Confidence about the social work contribution and reflective practice warrant some discussion at the outset. Parton and Marshall (1998: 245) sum up the paradox inherent within them:

> The contemporary challenge for social work is to take action, which demands that we have made up our mind, while being open minded.

In relation to work with people who are dying or bereaved, the issues that arise in relation to these two factors are different in specialist and mainstream settings.

Specialist social workers – usually working in palliative care settings – are in the forefront of thinking and writing about the social work contribution, particularly with people who are dying, but also in relation to bereavement (Sheldon, 1997; Monroe, 1998; Oliviere et al., 1998; Napier, 2003). In such settings, the issue is often the ways in which social work is defined in relation to the roles of other workers (Firth, 2003). 'Psychosocial palliative care' is a term used to refer to those areas of work that might previously have defined social work with dying or bereaved people, but are not exclusive to it. There are issues too in relation to the boundaries between the work done by specialist, hospice-based social workers and their social work colleagues in the community. Questions about the social work contribution may therefore centre less on *what* is the appropriate response –although this always has to be worked out afresh in any instance – and more on *who* is best placed to offer this care (often with attendant questions of funding).

Mainstream social workers are often unclear about the social work response to dying or bereavement that is desirable or possible in their situation. Some argue that 'real social work' (Lloyd, 1997) with people who are dying or bereaved needs more time than can be offered in the present climate of changes in social care. Concepts and understandings that apply in specialist palliative care settings have little relevance, some say, outside these protected environments. Along with Quinn (1998), I will refute this, arguing that current theoretical understandings do in fact form the basis for a strong remit for social workers in mainstream settings.

Reflective practice (Payne, 1998) is the other factor highlighted as essential for critical practice. Those who work with people facing death must be able to acknowledge and manage the strong feelings that this rouses in them. 'Our use of self is part of the service we offer to users and clients' (Lishman, 1998: 92). This cannot be sustained and developed without adequate training and supervision and – less often recognised – appropriate policies and structures (Currer, 2007). Managers have a key role in facilitating reflective practice on the part of workers meeting death and loss on a regular basis. Just as practitioners need to be able to hold their own emotions in balance, so their managers need to balance the pressures for measurable outcomes and 'results' against an awareness that process is as crucial as outcome and, in the last analysis, is part of it. Managers also need an understanding of the social work response to people who are dying or bereaved if they are to create policies and structures to facilitate it. It is in this respect that workers in specialist posts may be at an advantage, since the organisational culture is likely to be one where these aspects are recognised as important.

Two tasks face the confident and reflective critical practitioner. First, theoretical understandings and general ideas about the social work role have to be interpreted and probably adapted within a particular practice setting. Second, practices, policies and structures that undermine or threaten this response have to be challenged. This is an ongoing process and it occurs at many levels. It can involve 'stopping the action' for just five minutes to acknowledge someone's need to cry or say goodbye to a deceased relative. It can be about asking why there is no place for relatives to stay in a residential care setting if this enables them to be with a dying person, or asking who will accompany children from a residential unit to attend the funeral of a staff member. It can involve explaining to those pressing for an empty bed in hospital that informed choices about where an older person will live (and probably die) have an emotional component and cannot be made on the spot. It can involve putting in place (and monitoring) strict expectations in relation to the training and levels of supervision that private companies must offer if contracts for home care or other services are to be awarded. It may involve challenging national policies. While challenge is a factor that is particularly linked with social work (Ramon, 1997), this is actually no different to the response of any worker confident about their contribution to care; it is part of professional practice to seek to ensure the conditions that make it possible. As in other areas of social work, holding the service user at the centre is an essential starting point for such challenge (Monroe and Oliviere, 2003; Beresford et al., 2007).

Care at the end of life

Much of the theoretical work relating to dying is focused on those people who become aware, usually through the medical diagnosis of a terminal illness, that they are dying. Attention has been paid particularly to the emotional responses of individuals to this knowledge; the most influential of the frameworks being that outlined by Elisabeth Kübler-Ross (1970), who described an emotional progression from denial and anger through bargaining to depression and possible eventual acceptance. Subsequent authors (Corr, 1992; Buckman, 1998) have proposed alternative, more flexible frameworks (Sheldon, 1997).

Based in practice, this work has been enormously influential and has been strongly associated with the developing field of specialist palliative care, admission to which is also contingent on a terminal diagnosis. There can be a tendency, however, for frameworks to be rigidly applied in practice, rather than critically interpreted (Sheldon, 1997: 56). Other problems relate to the limits of these models. First, there is a focus on only a part of the experience of the dying person – a part referred to elsewhere as 'abandoning the future' (Currer, 2001). From the accounts of those who have written of their own dying (Moore, O., 1996; Picardie, 1998) and from research reports (Davies, 1995; Young and Cullen, 1996), we can see that 'managing the present' is also an important preoccupation. A part of this involves the renegotiation of social boundaries and managing issues of dependence and independence. This is apparent in the three scenarios below, where much of the focus of social care needs to be on practicalities that help the dying person and their carers to manage the present.

CASE EXAMPLE

Jane Truman is 10 years old and lives with her mother Sonia who has terminal cancer. A district nurse visits Sonia regularly. Sonia's current partner has refused to accept her illness and is rarely in the home, so Jane is, in effect, the main carer. The district nurse has asked a social worker from the hospice to visit Sonia and Jane. Sonia is worried about what will happen to Jane after her death, but this is a subject that Jane does not want to discuss.

CASE EXAMPLE

Lisa Jones has been severely disabled from birth and needs constant physical care. Her parents are aware that she is unlikely to live very long. Lisa's two sisters help with her care. The social worker from the local children's disability team has arranged for respite care to enable the family to have a holiday.

CASE EXAMPLE

Simon Shaw has AIDS. He is living at home with his partner. The social worker is arranging for a home carer to help the couple.

A second limitation of these models or frameworks relates to the issue of awareness of coming death. As Holloway (2007), Field (1996) and Seale et al. (1997) note, many people with long-term chronic conditions that result in death are never actually defined as 'dying'. In England and Wales, most deaths occur when people are over 75 years old (ONS, 1998). George and Sykes (1997) argue that the deaths of older people are often hard to predict. Siddell et al.'s study (1998) of residential care for older people makes it clear that deaths are frequent and not often accurately predicted in such settings. In such instances, we need a broader basis for the definition of dying, if theoretical understandings are to help the practitioner working with older people.

From a sociological perspective, Seale (1998: 149) defines dying as the severance of the social bond:

> Disruption of the social bond occurs as the body fails, self-identity becomes harder to hold together, and the normal expectations of human relations cannot be fulfilled.

This is a useful starting point for the social worker. Residents may decline the invitation to attend a funeral due to worries about their physical ability to sit through the service: the body is no longer reliable. In the following example, from a community setting, Violet Oliver's attempts to maintain 'respectability' in the eyes of neighbours, and the shame that can accompany failure to do so, will be familiar to many working with older people.

CASE EXAMPLE

Violet Oliver is a woman of 80, with a reputation for being immaculately dressed. Admitted to hospital following a fall, she is found to be badly undernourished. She is reluctant to agree to her neighbour's request for the keys to her home so that the neighbour can prepare for her return. The social worker sees her to make arrangements for her discharge.

For Violet, hospitalisation threatens to expose her attempts to preserve self-identity and to fulfil the 'normal expectations of human relations'. Seale's definition can also be applied to younger people with a terminal illness (Young and Cullen, 1996).

For those working with older people, understandings relating to dying have an application that is much broader than may be realised (Quinn, 1998). In relation to community care assessments, many social workers are acutely aware that service users (such as Violet Oliver) see the point of leaving their own home as a form of 'social death'. This concept has been defined as 'the cessation of the individual person as an active agent in others' lives' (Mulkay and Ernst, 1991: 178). Sweeting and Gilhooly (1997) have used the idea of 'social death' in their research into the experience of those caring at home for relatives with dementia. We could argue that the assessment of Violet's needs may result in a diagnosis of social death, should she be unable to return home, yet the pressure in many areas is to conduct such assessments in a routine way for the sake of speed.

Many people do of course spend their last years in some form of residential care. Let us consider just one of many situations that commonly arises.

CASE EXAMPLE

Maria Reed has been a resident in Green Meadows home for two years. She is 88 years old and has recently become confused, aggressive and disoriented. Her friend Grace, also a resident, has become increasingly withdrawn since Maria's deterioration. At present, the district nurse visits Maria at Green Meadows, but she is advising a move to a nursing home.

In this instance, the issue for staff caring for Maria concerns whether she will be able to die in the place that has become her home, a dilemma that relates to the separation of social and nursing care for older people. Siddell et al. (1998) report on national practice in this area, with recommendations for the wider application of good practice derived from experience in palliative care. The challenge for social care is to use insights from palliative care without reinforcing a stereotypical and potentially ageist association between old age and death.

Bereavement

While the dying person must abandon the future, the bereaved person must redefine it. The present is a struggle, maybe feeling unreal (Ironside, 1996; Currer, 2001). Social relationships are problematic and must be renegotiated. Anthropological studies see this as a time of transition (Littlewood, 1993). All social workers in ongoing contact with service users will be in touch with some experiencing bereavement, since this is a normal life event. Fear of 'opening up more than I can deal with' may lead to avoidance of the subject, in effect denying their grief (Currer, 2007). This is a reflection of general cultural uncertainties about how to respond to bereavement (Walter, 1994), and also of a context of change in social care, with the attendant devaluing of emotional work (Marsh and Triseliotis, 1996; Lishman, 1998; Quinn, 1998).

Until recently, there has been a dominant body of research with a focus on issues of emotional adjustment to the death of a significant person. Rooted in attachment theory (Bowlby, 1969, 1973, 1980), 'stages' of grieving have been described by Parkes (1996) and 'tasks of mourning' by Worden (1991). This body of research and knowledge has, with minor refinements, passed into the 'received wisdom' concerning bereavement, and been incorporated into advice leaflets in a range of spheres (for example Tebbutt, 1994; BODY, 1995; Help the Aged, 1996). Recent research has also focused on the experience of children who are bereaved (Silverman, 1996; Worden, 1996), and there are practice developments also in work with bereaved children (Hemmings, 1995; Smith and Pennells, 1995).

In the past decade, there has been what is described as a 'revolution' (Walter, 1997) in thinking about bereavement. Work by Stroebe and Schut (1999) and Walter (1996, 1999) extends the theoretical base in ways that have direct relevance for social care:

- The culture and gender blindness of earlier research and theory has been recognised (Stroebe, 1998; Stroebe and Schut, 1998).
- There has been sustained criticism – not least from bereaved people – of the notion that you 'get over' bereavement (Wortman and Silver, 1989), with exploration of what it means to 'move on'. Early ideas, rooted in Freud, of 'detachment' from the relationship with the person who has died have given way to ideas of 'relocation' (Walter, 1996).
- The focus of theoretical interest has shifted from looking at the experience of loss in a way that is passive – those emotions that are experienced, for example – to a more active focus on the ways in which people make sense of loss through meaning reconstruction (Neimeyer, 2001). This more positive focus is further developed in work that uses and applies the concept of 'resilience' (Monroe and Oliviere, 2007) in relation to both dying and bereavement.

Stroebe and Schut (1995, 1999) have proposed a dual process model of coping with bereavement, in which they suggest that the person who is bereaved is confronting two categories of stressor, the loss itself and the changes that result from it. There is, then, a dual orientation to loss and restoration, with oscillation between these two. A particular point of relevance for social care is that we are often associated with 'restoration': helping people with practical changes and adjustments that arise from bereavement. In some instances, these changes are forced, as for Jane in the example given above and for Tom and Imran Malik in the situations described below. In each case, involving different services, death has already or may in future precipitate a need for alternative (possibly residential) care.

CASE EXAMPLE

Tom is a child of mixed race who is in residential care following the breakdown of a placement in foster care. Eight years old, he was admitted to care after the suicide of his stepfather, when his mother became severely depressed and was admitted to hospital. His sister died at the age of two in an accident in the home.

CASE EXAMPLE

Imran Malik is 30 years old. He lives at home with his parents and his younger sister, helping in the family shop when he is not attending Wellton Resource Centre for adults with a learning disability, where he has a number of close friends. The sudden accidental death of both parents has led to a call to the department. Arrangements are being made for his sister's marriage, after which she will no longer live in the family home.

In such instances, opportunities to focus on the loss itself may be blocked. Conversely, where there is discrimination, attempts to focus on restoration may be particularly difficult (Currer, 2001: 104), and the person is thrust back into loss when they seek to take new steps. Therefore, understanding the social work task in terms of this model both validates our work and also highlights areas of particular vulnerability for some clients. Oscillation is the key, in Stroebe and Schut's model, to 'adaptive coping'. However, this rather prescriptive phrase is perhaps indicative of an overall question about even the more recent models. Work that considers bereavement in a broader social and cultural context, such as that of Walter (1994, 1999) and Holloway (2007), reminds us that responses to loss are negotiated rather than given, reflecting overall social understandings.

Responding to grief: the social work role in relation to bereavement and end-of-life care

Writing from the perspective of a specialist practitioner, Monroe (1998) identifies a number of features of social work in palliative care. Intervention will include giving information, helping communication and freeing up people's confidence to act, sometimes through helping with resources. Newburn (1993, 1996) gives feedback from those who have been in touch with social workers following the Hillsborough and other disasters. On the basis of such reports and interviews with practitioners from a wide range of social care settings, a number of features can be identified as central in social care work with people who are either dying or bereaved (Currer, 2001, 2007). Such features can offer a foundation for the confidence mentioned earlier. In all situations, the social work response is likely to combine emotional and practical support, recognising that these are inextricably linked.

In relation to work with people who are dying, dependability is crucial, facilitating efforts to 'manage the present'. This is clearly important for Lisa's family, as it is for all informal carers who have help with looking after someone in the community. Listening is also key. Such listening may be part of an assessment, and a means to the end of understanding what other services may be required, but it may also be enough in itself. This aspect of the work of home carers needs to be acknowledged, alongside their practical tasks. Encouraging and helping communication with others is an aspect of work that has clear links with the focus of social work on social relationships. It relates directly to the threat that can be posed to social relationships by increased dependency. For Sonia and Jane, this is a major issue. It also relates to the definition of dying as 'severance of the social bond' (Seale, 1998), and a time when human relationships become both more important and more difficult to sustain. Smith's (1976) existential analysis of bereavement proposes that even the apparently individual 'journey' of 'abandoning the future' can only be worked out in the context of social relationships with significant others. Finally, advocacy is seen, ideally, as a defining aspect of social work with those facing death.

Turning to consider bereavement, three features can be identified (Currer 2001).

First, there is the need to recognise and endorse the need to grieve. Another example illustrates this powerfully.

CASE EXAMPLE

A member of the emergency duty team is called to a house where a middle-aged woman has died in bed. Her mother, who is blind, is in the kitchen with a young police constable. The woman's body is about to be removed, and the social worker is asked to make arrangements for her mother's care. Although she has been informed of her daughter's death, the mother seems very confused.

For the emergency duty worker, it was essential to 'stop the action' and allow the mother time to be with her daughter before her body was removed. This involved challenge to those who wanted to 'get on' and avoid upsetting the mother. She did indeed burst into tears when she felt her daughter's face, but said later that she was enormously grateful that this opportunity for farewell had been created for her. Recognition of grief may be less dramatic. In the residential home referred to earlier, Grace's withdrawal in the face of Maria's decline suggests that her own distress needs to be recognised.

Practitioners also see a role as 'witness' – offering accompaniment to the grieving person, as well as support in relation to re-engagement. These two factors may be particularly important in relation to Jane's situation and influence the help that is offered. Sonia's primary carer is the district nurse; the social work role focuses on Jane. As a young carer, Jane is in need of immediate practical support. In the long term, there will be a need for alternative accommodation and care. Her emotional needs in the present and in the future include the need for someone to listen and be able to 'witness' to her current care of her mother as well as help her to remake her own life in the future. There is also a need to respect Jane's current reluctance to discuss her mother's death. It may be possible to identify a key worker who can offer long-term support to Jane, perhaps a young carers worker or a member of staff from a residential care setting. The task for this worker would not be 'grief counselling' either before or after her mother's death, but recognition of her current need for support and future need to grieve. If this person could meet Jane and Sonia together at home, they would be in a position to share memories of Sonia with Jane later, and in this way, they could fulfil the role of witness and give ongoing support at a pace that Jane can manage. This may involve support around the time of the funeral, and challenge to any well-meaning adults seeking to 'protect' Jane by limiting her involvement. Jane is likely to need both a well-informed advocate and accompaniment at this time.

Imran Malik and Tom also need accompaniment in their grief. Daycare and residential services are well placed to provide this, once workers recognise its importance. This is an active process involving appropriate acknowledgement of distress. In Pakistan, visits of condolence are customary following bereavement. Are staff at the centre aware of this? If Imran's friends wish to visit, how can this be facilitated? Is there an opportunity to explore with Imran his understanding of death and for him to talk about his parents? Rituals can easily be introduced in many settings, giving opportunities to remember, say goodbye and endorse the view that grief can be talked about. Tom has encountered multiple deaths in his short life. Is awareness of this a part of the brief for those working with him? A variety of resources have been developed to facilitate memory work with children (see Smith and Pennells, 1995). The critical practitioner is one who is aware of the range of resources available and seeks to adapt and use these within their own situation.

Conclusion

Despite strategy statements, it can be tempting to think that responding to the grief of people who are dying or bereaved is not possible for social workers except in specialist palliative care settings. Such a view is mistaken. In so far as dying and bereavement are everyday events, they arise in the course of social work practice in all areas. In many settings, we are ideally placed to respond appropriately – probably as members of a multidisciplinary team – given the necessary theoretical basis for intervention, and confidence concerning our part in care. It is part of the remit of those who work in specialist settings to encourage a wider awareness of good practice with people who are dying or bereaved (Oliviere et al., 1998; Monroe and Oliviere, 2003, 2007). To learn from this experience, interpret it realistically – adapting as necessary – and defend good practice vigorously in the context of mainstream practice are the challenges facing the critical practitioner in mainstream social care.

For further discussion of working with frail older people, see Adams et al., 2009c, Chapter 7, and for communication skills, see Adams et al., 2009a, Chapter 14.

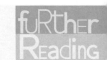

Currer, C. (2001) *Responding to Grief: Dying, Bereavement and Social Care*, Basingstoke, Palgrave – now Palgrave Macmillan. Written specifically for social care workers in mainstream settings, although it does also include reference to specialist work.

Currer, C. (2007) *Loss and Social Work*, Exeter, Learning Matters. Although having a broader focus than dying and bereavement, this introductory text focuses on issues for social workers.

Holloway, M. (2007) *Negotiating Death in Contemporary Health and Social Care*, Bristol, Policy Press. Combines a sociological overview with attention to developments in theory and practice issues for those in health and social care.

Monroe, B. and Oliviere, D. (eds) (2003) *Patient Participation in Palliative Care: A Voice for the Voiceless*, Oxford, Oxford University Press. Here the voice of the service user is central – a valuable collection of contributions from practitioners in palliative care.

Monroe, B. and Oliviere, D. (eds) (2007) *Resilience and Palliative Care: Achievement in Adversity*, Oxford, Oxford University Press. The international literature on resilience is outlined and applied to situations of dying and bereavement. Contributors include many leaders in the field.

Neimeyer, R. (ed.) (2001) *Meaning Reconstruction and the Experience of Loss*, Washington DC, American Psychological Association. Rather more theoretical papers exploring the ways in which people make meaning in situations of loss.

Concluding comment

In this book, we have scrutinised theories and approaches in social work. We have argued that it is important for social workers to try to reach an understanding of the complexities embedded within human relationships, the values on which they base practice, the approaches and methods that they try to use, and the specific settings in which they practise. It is impossible to practise without that alertness to the issues involved in these aspects of practice.

Also, we have explored what is involved in critically practising social work. Understanding, we say, has to be connected to action and the link between understanding and action is criticality. This is because action assumes a purpose, a direction in which we act. We call this direction 'agency'.

Agency and efficacy

Agency is the capacity of people to have an impact in their social environment, now and in the future; efficacy is the degree of self-belief that people have in their agency. These related concepts are examples of the way that social and psychological knowledge come together in social work. Agency is impact in social relationships, efficacy is psychological understanding about agency. Social workers need to work with the social and psychological aspects of a situation to achieve successful outcomes.

Both the practitioner and the service user have agency and use it in their activities, usually to meet their objectives and goals in maintaining or changing the world around them. Agency involves interaction between people as they negotiate their positions. As they are enabled to influence the world around them, users gain in efficacy; they become aware of and increase their belief in their agency. These two elements are interactive. They are able to stamp their own imprimatur (mark of ownership) on their relationship with practitioners and other people. Empowering practice therefore aims to increase people's agency, so that they can influence the world in directions that help them, and also their efficacy, because belief in their agency enables them to use it. If people do not believe they can influence the world, they are disempowered, because they are not aware of the impact they might have. Empowering social work practice must therefore help users socially and psychologically. It must help users to achieve their aims and relationships, and by so doing, help them to understand and believe in their capacity to do so in the future. One of the best ways of doing this is by practitioners being influenced by users within their practice relationships, by showing how users are helping practitioners to understand their problems and their story and by responding to what they learn from users. If practitioners are influenced by service users, they will in turn have greater influence with users because their relationship will be deeper. Being influenced does not mean that you lose power, it means that more agency is being achieved on both sides of a relationship; both are more empowered. It also recognises the interactive nature of social relationships, including those that are concerned with helping people.

Power differentials between users and practitioners often complicate interactions and disadvantage users, because they often have less formal power and resources to draw on in the negotiation than the practitioner does. It is important to remember, though, that they have better knowledge of their social situation, their story and the limitations in their lives than the practitioner. Therefore, the seeds of the help that practitioners offer to enable the service user to gain agency over the problems in their lives and efficacy in their capacity to do something about them are contained in the user's story. Empowering practice enables users to identify and use their power as they are helped to achieve their aims in life, and gain further power by understanding how their efficacy and control over their situation are increasing.

Social work cannot achieve this unless practitioners understand how inequalities in power and influence affect the social work relationship and also users' other relationships that are the focus of a social work intervention. For example, a practitioner helps a single parent to manage her income more effectively and to interact with her children to manage bad behaviour and improve their personal development. This increases the user's agency, because she can use her income and her interactions with her children to achieve her objectives more quickly or more successfully. She cannot be helped if the social worker does these things for her; for it to have an impact on her environment, she must understand how changes in her behaviour have their effect, so that she can incorporate them in the way she lives her life and adapt them for use in other situations. Through that understanding, her efficacy and sense of empowerment are augmented.

It is the same for a practitioner, and in particular a student practitioner. They may understand social work theories and possess knowledge about society, psychology and many other matters. However, experiencing having an impact using social work techniques and knowledge helps them to appreciate how ideas and knowledge influence social relationships, and realising that they have had an impact and how they achieved it gives them the efficacy to try it again and adapt it to use with other users in other situations. In social work, there is nothing so exciting as intervening in a situation, using skills and knowledge and realising that we have had a result.

When people say they have a purpose in a social relationship, they imply that the current position is not ideal, that they want to change it in some way; it may be a change in direction or a reduction in the pace of deterioration. This could be a small change, a minor correction of balance or stance, or a large change involving moving to a fresh position. Users coming or being referred for social work help may be aware of something being wrong without having a clear understanding of the issues they face. Without that understanding, they cannot be empowered to use their agency and improve their efficacy. Whatever the purpose, therefore, we need to understand what requires change so that we can help users to understand it and empower them to change our perceptions of it too. That is the reason for being critical in practice.

So, in Part 1 of this book, we have proposed that considering our values is essential to deciding on our critical approach. In Part 2, we have set out the main approaches on which we suggest critical practitioners are likely to draw. In Part 3, we have given illustrations of critical practice in some of the main areas of social work.

We regard it as axiomatic that, for adequate understanding, we must examine practice directly and not consider it at one remove. For this reason, authors of many of the chapters in this book have rooted their arguments in practice illustrations. Also, if critical practice is to be effective, we regard it as essential for our thinking and analysis to be examined minutely and systematically. This means devoting sufficient space to key areas and is reflected in our choice of topics in the foregoing chapters.

Critical practice and good practice: the example of diversity

We have reached the point where our argument that critical practice should be mainstream practice leads to the logical, if ideal, conclusion that all good practice should exemplify the aspects of values explored in Part 1 of this book.

An example is the area of diversity. Ideas of diversity are sometimes only used to update anti-discriminatory or anti-oppressive practice; in this meaning, they imply that we should value a variety of people in any community or workforce. It is a much broader term: it means the variety of different characteristics or features that form the identities of people in every aspect of life. To be concerned with diversity means having to think about how we deal with the impact of many different social identities on solidarity in our social relationships. For example, is a community damaged or strengthened by too much diversity? What is too much diversity? Does it mean there are too many different identities to promote collaboration? And is social work damaged and confused by its variety of theories and methods or is this a strength that leads to flexibility and opportunity?

We answer these questions with a positive view of diversity. Not only critical practice, but all good practice, should be exemplified by an understanding and celebration of diversities. This is reflected in the diversity of approaches to the different areas of practice illustrated in this book. We must celebrate and accept diversity if we are to promote inclusion. Citizens' rights can only be accepted if, whatever their other identities, their citizenship means that they are part of a shared community of interest. Anti-oppressive practice engages with this issue because it gives priority to solidarity over separate identities. The good practitioner is sensitive to attempts to attribute characteristics to people referring only to the social identity they acquire because of age, gender, race, geographical location and so on. Critical practice celebrates the range of identities in any community or social grouping, and thus regards it positively, but it extends further. Critical practitioners described throughout this book do not just acknowledge that diversity exists and do what is necessary, or just accept that they must behave correctly. Because critical practice involves careful attention to detail, diversities in the present situation need to be explored and understood and their implications for the people involved spelled out and acted upon. This is because, as we have argued, an understanding of the social situation in which we are helping is crucial to developing agency and efficacy; diverse understandings are just as important as other knowledge, skills and values.

Consequently, a critical practitioner is unable to polarise opinion about social groups, or stereotype people according to attributes of gender, role or ethnicity because such judgements will not survive critical analysis. They involve a form of essentialism, ascribing social behaviour to a particular essence of the individual, such as blackness or femaleness or disability. This results in a denial of diversity and difference, by assuming that all people who are socially constructed as black or old or disabled share the same experiences and aspirations.

But since, as with any successful practice, critical practice requires agency, this means acting in ways that value diversity, as well as awareness and analysis of it, even if we may feel challenged by it and its complexities. Action, therefore, can present more problems requiring further analysis and reflection. For example, we may seek to represent the diversity of the workforce by ensuring reasonably equal numbers of people of both sexes in promoted posts in the management team, having become aware through analysis that this represents a problem about a lack of diversity. Then, one or two appointments made by fair appointment processes lead to an imbalance of men, the traditional holders of power and management posts. Do we acquiesce? Do we accept a quota, which means that for individuals the appointment procedure may not be 'fair'? Do we take positive action and encourage and train women more actively? Do we look for hidden disincentives in the promoted posts? Or do we look for the incentives in practitioner posts, which leads us to accept that women might not want promoted posts of the present kind, and look for different ways to enable them to take up seniority and influence? That there are so many possibilities for action demonstrates how critical practice needs to apply to action as well as analysis.

We expect critical practitioners to be concerned to locate the practice in its broader historical, social and policy context. By doing so, we offer alternative possibilities for explanation and action. So, in the example given, power relations will emerge as embedded in social structures and human agency. If we celebrate rather than stereotype people, their identities appear to us as multidimensional and complex. As a result, a greater range of alternatives for action arises. How could our services involve a wider range of people from different minorities to give flexibility and responsiveness to our services? Ethnicity, of course, is only one aspect of this, other aspects being gender, age, class, school, neighbourhood, friends, the perceptions of family members and so on.

Critical practitioners are aware of the contradictions and dilemmas inherent in adopting a merely tolerant approach. It is necessary to move beyond the multicultural essentialism that stereotypes people as though their diversity, both culturally and ethnically, has only one meaning: 'lazy African-Caribbean youth, cohesive street gangs, supportive extended families, oppressed Muslim women'. The so-called lazy youth is not motivated by things that officials such as social workers talk to him about, but an approach based on diversity suggests that there will be things that motivate him and can carry him forward, and they must be found. The cohesive street gang can use its cohesiveness in mutual support and promote changes in both individual and gang behaviour, if it can be helped to do so. The supportive family may need to explore the violence hidden in many families and understand the paradox that supportiveness may also be exploitative for some family members. Also family members may benefit from understanding the value of giving and receiving affection, help and support. People without experience of Islam may gain from seeing the oppression which, for instance, in some Muslim families, permeates family relationships.

Critical practitioners recognise, like other good practitioners, that any understanding of difference is socially constructed and that oppression can be inherent in the way this happens, but diversity implies that such oppression is not a fixed or essentialised aspect of identity. A different understanding would construct the difference in different ways that are not oppressive; anti-oppressive practice seeks to validate those alternative constructions. Power is distributed in many social networks, and may be taken up and used even by people who are usually in less powerful positions. Social constructions may inhibit us from using such opportunities, but may also offer certainty and shared understanding that will help us to deal with social changes. After all, everyone – individually and collectively – is working across differences all the time. Also, it takes many different perspectives to construct, and experience, a difference. But we would expect critical practitioners to go further, for example into reconstructing individual and collective ideas and identities. Thus, critical practitioners may be unhappy about the way masculinity is constructed in the locality and may envisage reconstructing it so as to assert male partners' roles as carers for children, and older and disabled people in the household. Research evidence suggests that many men do take up caring roles successfully (Arber and Gilbert, 1989; Parker, 1993; Fisher, 1994), so among the possibilities for reconstructing understanding of this issue is raising awareness of models of equality that some men provide, celebrating their contribution and learning practicalities that can be passed on from the detail of their achievements. Critical practitioners attempt to achieve the reframing of qualities and activities associated with gender, on the basis that they are not attributes of gender but socially constructed cultural codes, valuable or disadvantageous in their own right as well as in their stereotypical identities. They do so by becoming aware of the detail of how people function in different ways, as they work with men who are caring within their families. This involves practitioners not only becoming aware of differences from a stereotype, but using their learning and understanding, gained through practice, to challenge the stereotype and empower others to overcome it. So, critical practitioners question dominant social constructions, resist or challenge oppressive constructions and seek hidden certainties in social constructions that inhibit people's self-empowerment. Critical ideas help them to identify stereotypes and diversities, but their practice involvements with and learning from carers and users enable them to put these ideas into action.

In this way, critical practice can be emancipatory practice, encouraging service users and carers also to reconstruct difference, thereby achieving the celebration of diversity and increasing their agency and efficacy. Thus, critical practice achieves the reconstruction of identities, valuing differences, and these differences, which have been marginal or oppressed, now become equally available to communities and individuals to contribute to the richness of their social relations. The critical practitioner working across difference may tackle the reconstruction, for example, of black women working with white men, or gay men and lesbian women working with heterosexuals.

Changing emphasis: from reflective to critical practice

Threaded through this book – Chapters 1, 7 and 21 – is our discussion of what critical practice entails. We would not dispute the claim of reflective practitioners to be critical. Just because we assert the need for developing critical practice built on reflection does not mean we are denying that other approaches to practice have a critical component. However, we argue that, for the critical practitioner, being critical is integral to the work and not something carried out incidentally or occasionally. Also, we have demonstrated in this book that shifting the territory of debates into practice has moved the centre of gravity of our discussion from 'being reflective' to 'being critical', because being critical involves action with a purpose as well as reflection, which assumes a neutrality of objective; we argue that social work's purpose is change sought by service users and their carers. We have illustrated how critical practice is experienced by, and feels to, the practitioner, as well as touching the knowledge and skill bases.

Constructing bridges

We can use the metaphor of bridges to emphasise how our critical practice can link diverse aspects, not destroying those that are vulnerable, not ignoring those that are marginal, but enabling them to interact with us and with each other. Critical practice may be a bridging activity, a means of reframing the different possibilities of our practice. Criticality can link alternative options. Being critical is powerful because it can enable us to exercise agency and reframe and treat equally a diversity of options, including those that are part of the status quo, and those that we otherwise might disregard as too problematic or risky. Critical practice offers bridges between the margins of possible practice and the centre. Through the medium of a diversity perspective, critical practice can bring the margins of our perceptions and experiences into the centre, the mainstream of our practice.

Critical practice also offers bridges between continuities and changes in the circumstances of our work, which enables us to transform our view of situations and act transformationally. Through criticality, we can make connections between the past, the present and the future, and achieve change. We conclude this chapter by considering what is involved in these key ideas of managing change and continuity, and critical practice as transformational. Inevitably, we engage with criticality as an unfinished agenda as we encounter the paradoxes and dilemmas of practice.

Managing change and continuity

Managing change is a difficult and complex process. People, both practitioners and service users, sometimes seek certainty. When this is so, ambiguous and constantly changing situations have to be managed in order to control and contain them. Anger and aggression must be calmed. Depression must be circumvented or overcome to permit progress. Without some form of order or view about a way forward, it would be impossible to act. Thus, control and containment may be valued features of social situations as well as oppressive elements. The failing is to value either control or a lack of it without a critical assessment of what people want and need in the situation. To value only control or only self-determination is to avoid being critical.

So it is with change and continuity. A problem with managing change is that people's fear of it often can leave them paralysed or disempowered. In those situations, a person with clearer ideas about what ought to be done may impose their views on another and reduce their potential to exercise agency or act in ways that take account of their own feelings and views. A problem with managing continuity is that frustration with it may lead them to seek change inappropriately. Sometimes, the answer to marital problems is to stay with it and work through them. This is often a tougher option than seeking change.

Reflecting on these alternatives and acting ethically, that is, in ways that do not abuse their formal power, is a critical stance that practitioners can adopt. To manage this tension, they need to be critical in action and critical of action.

Further practice development: tackling uncertainty, complexity and working across boundaries

In the third book in the trilogy (Adams et al., 2009c), we will be engaging with the tasks of practice development. We shall be working through the implications of the basis for critical practice established in this and the first book (Adams et al., 2009a). In the third book, we hope that you will feel a sense of excitement as you engage in the more challenging, imaginative and creative aspects of critical practice.

Bibliography

AASW (Australian Association of Social Workers) (1999) *Code of Ethics,* Canberra: AASW.

Abbott, P. and Sapsford, R. (1987) *Community Care for Mentally Handicapped Children,* Milton Keynes: Open University Press.

ACHSSW (Australian Council of Heads of Schools of Social Work) (2006) *We've Boundless Plans to Share: The First Report of the People's Inquiry into Detention,* Melbourne: ACHSSW.

Adams, R. (1990) *Self-help, Social Work and Empowerment,* London: Macmillan – now Palgrave Macmillan.

Adams, R. (1996) *Social Work and Empowerment,* Basingstoke: Macmillan – now Palgrave Macmillan.

Adams, R. (2002) 'Developing critical practice in social work', in R. Adams, L. Dominelli and M. Payne (eds) *Critical Practice in Social Work,* Basingstoke: Palgrave – now Palgrave Macmillan.

Adams, R. (2003) *Social Work and Empowerment,* 3rd edn, Basingstoke: Palgrave Macmillan.

Adams, R. (2008) *Empowerment, Participation and Social Work,* 4th edn, Basingstoke: Palgrave Macmillan.

Adams, R. and O'Sullivan, T. (1994) *Social Work With and Within Groups,* Birmingham: BASW Trading.

Adams, R., Dominell, L. and Payne, M. (2005a) 'Introduction', in R. Adams, L. Dominelli and M. Payne (eds) *Social Work Futures: Crossing Boundaries, Transforming Practice,* Basingstoke: Palgrave Macmillan.

Adams, R. Dominelli, L. and Payne, M. (2005b) 'Transformational social work', in R. Adams, L. Dominelli and M. Payne (eds) *Social Work Futures: Crossing Boundaries, Transforming Practice,* Basingstoke: Palgrave Macmillan.

Adams, R. Dominelli, L. and Payne, M. (2009a)

Social Work: Themes, Issues and Critical Debates, 3rd edn, Basingstoke: Palgrave Macmillan.

Adams, R. Dominelli, L. and Payne, M. (2009c) *Practising Social Work in a Complex World,* Basingstoke: Palgrave Macmillan.

Adorno, T. and Horkheimer, M. (1979) *The Dialectic of Enlightenment,* London: Verso.

ADSS (Association of Directors of Social Services) (2005) *Safeguarding Adults: A National Framework of Standards for Good Practice and Outcomes in Adult Protection Work,* London: ADSS.

Ahmad, B. (1990) *Black Perspectives in Social Work,* Birmingham: Venture.

Ahmed, S. (1986) 'Cultural racism in work with Asian women and girls', in S. Ahmed, J. Cheetham and J. Small (eds) *Social Work with Black Children and Their Families,* London: Batsford.

Ahmed, S. (2005) 'What is the evidence of early intervention, preventative services for black and minority ethnic group children and their families?', *Practice,* **17**(2): 89–102.

Ainsworth, M.D., Blehar, M.C., Walters, E. and Wall, S. (1978) *Patterns of Attachment: Psychological Study of the Strange Situation,* Hillsdale, NJ: Lawrence Erlbaum.

Aldgate J. and Tunstill J. (1995) *Section 17: The First 18 Months,* London: HMSO.

Allan J., Pease, B. and Briskman, L. (eds) (2003) *Critical Social Work: An Introduction to Theories and Practice,* Sydney: Allen & Unwin.

Allan, K. (2001) *Communication and Consultation: Exploring Ways for Staff to Involve People with Dementia in Developing Services,* York: Joseph Rowntree Foundation.

Allen, G. and Crow, G. (2000) *Families, Households and Society,* Basingstoke: Palgrave – now Palgrave Macmillan.

AMA (Association of Metropolitan Authorities) (1993) *Local Authorities and*

Community Development: A Strategic Opportunity for the 1990s, London: AMA.

Anderson, B. (1999) 'Youth crime and the politics of prevention', in B. Goldson (ed.) *Youth Justice: Contemporary Policy and Practice*, Aldershot: Ashgate.

Anwar, M. (1976) *Between Two Cultures*, London: CRC.

Anwar, M. (1998) *Between Two Cultures: A Study of Relationships between Generations in the Asian Community in Britain*, 2nd edn, London: Commission for Racial Equality.

Arber, S. and Gilbert, N. (1989) 'Men: the forgotten carers', *Sociology*, 23(1): 111–18.

Argyris, C. and Schön, D. (1974) *Theory in Practice: Increasing Professional Effectiveness*. San Francisco, CA: Jossey-Bass.

Armitage, S. and Kavanagh, K. (1998) 'Consumer-oriented outcomes in discharge planning: a pilot study', *Journal of Clinical Nursing*, 7(1): 67–74.

Arnup, K. (1997) *Lesbian Parenting: Living with Pride and Prejudice*, Charlottetown, PEI, Canada: Gynergy Books.

Askham, J., Henshaw, L. and Tarpey, M. (1993) 'Policies and perceptions of identity', in M. Evandrou and S. Arber (eds) *Ageing, Independence and the Life Course*, London: Jessica Kingsley.

Atkins, S. (2000) 'Developing underlying skills in the move towards reflective practice', in S. Burns and C. Bulman (2000) *Reflective Practice in Nursing: The Growth of the Professional Practitioner*, 2nd edn, Oxford: Blackwell Science.

Atkinson, D.R. and Hackett, G. (2004) *Counseling Diverse Populations*, 3rd edn, New York: McGraw-Hill.

Audit Commission (1996) *Misspent Youth*, London: Audit Commission.

Australian Broadcasting Commission (2005) 'Iranian refugee seeks compensation', on *AM*, 27/8/2005, www.abc.net.au/am/content/2005/s1447376.htm.

Ayre, P. (2001) 'Child protection and the media: lessons from the last three decades', *British Journal of Social Work*, 31(6): 887–901.

Badham, B. (ed.) (1989) '"Doing something with our lives when we're inside": self-directed groupwork in a youth custody centre', *Groupwork*, 2(1): 27–35.

Bagguley, P. (1991) *From Protest to Acquiescence? Political Movements of the Unemployed*, Basingstoke: Macmillan – now Palgrave Macmillan.

Bailey, D. (2009) *Interdisciplinary Working in Mental Health*, Basingstoke: Palgrave Macmillan.

Bailey, R. and Brake, M. (eds) (1975) *Radical Social Work and Practice*, London: Edward Arnold.

Baines, D. (2007) 'Anti-oppressive social work practice: fighting for space, fighting for change', in D. Baines (ed.) *Doing Anti-oppressive Practice: Building Transformative Politicized Social Work*, Halifax, Canada: Fernwood.

Bakhurst, D. and Sypnowich, C. (eds) (1995) *The Social Self*, London: Sage.

Balloch, S. (1997) 'Gender and occupational attainment in the social services', *Making a Difference: Women and Career Progression in Social Services*, Social Work Research Centre, Stirling University: NISW.

Balloch, S. and Taylor, M. (2001) *Partnership Working: Policy and Practice*, Bristol: Policy Press.

Balloch, S., Andrew, T., Ginn, J. et al. (1995) *Working in Social Services*, London: NISW.

Bamford, T. (1990) *The Future of Social Work*, Basingstoke: Macmillan – now Palgrave Macmillan.

Banks, S. (1995) *Ethics and Values in Social Work*, Basingstoke: Macmillan – now Palgrave Macmillan.

Banks, S. (1996) 'Youth work, informal education and professionalisation: the issues in the 1990s', *Youth and Policy*, 54: 13–25.

Banks, S. (1998) 'Professional ethics in social work – what future?', *British Journal of Social Work*, 28: 213–31.

Banks, S. (2001) *Ethics and Values in Social Work*, 2nd edn, Basingstoke: Palgrave – now Palgrave Macmillan.

Banks, S. (2004) *Ethics, Accountability and the Social Professions*, Basingstoke: Palgrave Macmillan.

Banks, S. (2006) *Ethics and Values in Social Work*, 3rd edn, Basingstoke: Palgrave Macmillan.

Banks, S. (2007) 'Becoming critical: developing the community practitioner', in H. Butcher, S. Banks, P. Henderson and J. Robertson (eds) *Critical Community Practice*, Bristol: Policy Press.

Bannister, A., Gordon, R. and Hendry, E. (eds) (1997) *Turning Points: A Resource Pack for Communicating with Children*, London: NSPCC.

Barber, J.G. (1991) *Beyond Casework*, Basingstoke: Macmillan – now Palgrave Macmillan.

Barclay, P.M. (ed.) (1982) *Social Workers: Their Role and Tasks*, London: Bedford Square Press.

Barker, R. and Roberts, H. (1993) 'The uses of the concept of power', in D. Morgan and L. Stanley (eds) *Debates in Sociology*, Manchester: Manchester University Press.

Barn, R. (1993) *Black Children in the Public Care System*, London: Batsford.

Barn, R. (2002) 'Race, ethnicity and child welfare', in B. Mason and M. Sawyer (eds) *Exploring the Unsaid*, London: Karnac.

Barn, R. (2007) '"Race, ethnicity and child welfare": a fine balancing act', *British Journal of Social Work*, **37**: 1425–34.

Barn, R. and Harman, V. (2006) 'A contested identity: an exploration of the competing social and political discourse concerning the identification and positioning of young people of inter-racial parentage', *British Journal of Social Work*, **36**: 1309–24.

Barn, R., Ladino, C. and Rogers, B. (2006) *Parenting in Multi-racial Britain*, London: NCH.

Barnoff, L. and Moffatt, K. (2007) 'Contradictory tensions in anti-oppression practice in feminist social services', *Afflilia: Journal of Women and Social Work*, **22**: 56–70.

Bartlett, H. (1970) *The Common Base of Social Work Practice*, Washington, DC: National Association of Social Workers.

BASW (British Association of Social Workers) (1979) *Clients are Fellow Citizens*, Birmingham: BASW.

BASW (British Association of Social Workers) (1996) *A Code of Ethics for Social Work*, Birmingham: BASW.

BASW (British Association of Social Workers) (2002) *The Code of Ethics for Social Work*, Birmingham: BASW.

Bateman, N. (2000) *Advocacy Skills for Health and Social Care Professionals*, London: Jessica Kingsley.

Batsleer, J. and Humphries, B. (eds) (2000) *Welfare, Exclusion and Political Agency*, London: Routledge.

Bauld, L., Chesterman, J., Davies, B. et al. (eds) (2000) *Caring for Older People: An Assessment of Community Care in the 1990s*, Aldershot: Ashgate.

Beardshaw, V. and Towell, D. (1990) *Assessment and Case Management: Implementation of 'Caring for People'*, Briefing Paper 10, London: King's Fund.

Bebbington, A. and Miles, J. (1989) 'The background of children who enter local authority care', *British Journal of Social Work*, **19**(5): 349–68.

Beck, A.T. (1976) *Cognitive Therapy and the Emotional Disorders*, New York: International Universities Press.

Beck, A.T. and Emery, G. (1985) *Anxiety Disorders and Phobias: A Cognitive Perspective*, New York: Basic Books.

Beck, U. (1992) *Risk Society: Towards a New Modernity*, London: Sage.

Belenky, M., Clinchy, B.M., Goldberger, N.R. and Tarule, J.M. (1997) *Women's Ways of Knowing: The Development of Self, Voice, and Mind*, 2nd edn, New York: Basic Books.

Bell, M. (2001) 'Promoting children's rights through the use of relationship', *Child and Family Social Work*, **7**(1): 1–12.

Beresford, P. and Trevillion, S. (1995) *Developing Skills for Community Care*, Aldershot: Arena.

Beresford, P., Adshead, L. and Croft, S. (2007) *Palliative Care, Social Work and Service Users*, London: Jessica Kingsley.

Berridge, D. (1997) *Foster Care: A Research Review*, London: TSO.

Berridge, D. and Brodie, I. (1998) *Children's Homes Revisited*, London: Jessica Kingsley.

Biehal, N., Clayden, J., Stein, M. and Wade, J. (1992) *Prepared for Living? A Survey of Young People Leaving the Care of Three Local Authorities*, London: National Children's Bureau.

Biestek, F. (1961) *The Casework Relationship*, London: Allen & Unwin.

Bigby, C., Fyffe, C. and Ozanne, E. (eds) (2007) *Planning and Support for People with Intellectual Disabilities: Issues for Case Managers and other Professionals*, London: Jessica Kingsley.

Biggs, S. and Weinstein, J. (1991) *Assessment, Case Management and Inspection in Community Care*, London: CCETSW.

Bilson, A. (2006) (ed.) *Evidence-based Practice in Social Work*, London: Whiting & Birch.

Bindman, J., Johnson, S., Wright, S. et al. (1997) 'Integration between primary and secondary services in the care of the severely mentally ill: patients' and general practitioners' views', *British Journal of Psychiatry*, **171**(8): 169–74.

Blakemore, K. and Boneham, M. (1994) *Age, Race and Ethnicity*, Buckingham: Open University Press.

Blaug, R. (1995) 'Distortion of the face to face: communicative reason and social work practice', *British Journal of Social Work*, **25**: 423–39.

Blom-Cooper, L. (1986) *A Child in Trust: The Report of the Panel of Inquiry into the Circumstances Surrounding the Death of Jasmine Beckford*, London: Borough of Brent.

Blyth, E. (1998) 'Donor assisted conception and donor offspring rights to genetic origins information', *International Journal of Children's Rights*, **6**: 237–53.

BODY (1995) *The Gift of Life* (2), Booklet available from the British Organ Donor Society, Balsham, Cambridgeshire CB1 6DL, 01223 893636.

Bogdan, R. and Taylor, S. (1982) *Inside Out: The Social Meaning of Mental Retardation*, Toronto, Canada: University of Toronto Press.

Bornat, J. (ed.) (1999) *Biographical Interviews: The Link Between Research and Practice*, London: Centre for Policy on Ageing.

Bottoms, A. (1995) *Intensive Community Supervision for Young Offenders: Outcomes, Process and Cost*, Cambridge: Institute of Criminology Publications.

Bottoms, A., Brown, P., McWilliams, B. et al. (1980) *Intermediate Treatment and Juvenile Justice*, London: HMSO.

Bourn, D.F. (1993) 'Over-chastisement, child non-compliance and parenting skills: a behavioural intervention by a family centre worker', *British Journal of Social Work*, **23**: 481–9.

Bowell, T. and Kemp, G. (2002) *Critical Thinking: A Concise Guide*. London: Routledge.

Bower, M. (2005) *Psychoanalytic Theory for Social Work Practice: Thinking Under Fire*, London: Routledge.

Bowes, E. (1998) *Away From Home*, London: Labos Housing Association/Lemos & Crane.

Bowlby, J. (1969) *Attachment and Loss*, vol. I: *Attachment*, London: Hogarth Press.

Bowlby, J. (1973) *Attachment and Loss*, vol. II: *Separation: Anxiety and Anger*, London: Hogarth Press.

Bowlby, J. (1979) *The Making and Breaking of Affectional Bonds*, London: Tavistock.

Bowlby, J. (1980) *Attachment and Loss*, vol. III: *Loss, Sadness and Depression*, London: Hogarth Press.

Bowlby, J. (1988) *A Secure Base: Clinical Applications of Attachment Theory*, London: Routledge.

Boylen, J. and Wyllie, J. (1999) 'Advocacy and child protection', in N. Parton and C. Wattam (eds) *Child Sexual Abuse: Responding to the Experiences of Children*, Chichester: Wiley.

Bracken, P. and Thomas, P. (2000) 'Ethics and self-injury', *Open Mind*, May/June.

Brammer, A. (2007) *Social Work Law*, 2nd edn, Harlow: Pearson.

Brandon, D. (1995) *Advocacy: Power to People with Disabilities*, Birmingham, Venture Press.

Braye, H. and Carr, H. (2008) *Law for Social Workers*, 10th edn, Oxford: Oxford University Press.

Braye, S. and Preston-Shoot, M. (1995) *Empowering Practice in Social Care*, Buckingham: Open University Press.

Braye, S. and Varley, M. (1992) 'Developing a mental health perspective in social work practice', *Social Work Education*, **11**(2): 41–59.

Brearley, J. (1995) *Counselling and Social Work*, Maidenhead: Open University Press.

Brechin, A. (2000) 'Introducing critical practice', in A. Brechin, H. Brown and M. Eby (eds) *Critical Practice in Health and Social Care*, London: Open University/Sage.

Breton M. (1994) 'On the meaning of empowerment and empowerment oriented social work practice', *Social Work with Groups*, **17**(3): 23–38.

Brewer, C. and Lait, J. (1980) *Can Social Work Survive?*, London: Temple Smith.

Briskman, L. (2003) 'Indigenous Australians: towards postcolonial social work', in J. Allan, B. Pease and L. Briskman (eds) *Critical Social Work: An Introduction to Theories and Practices*, Sydney: Allen & Unwin.

Briskman, L. and Fraser, H. (2002) 'Freedom first, then education', *The Age*, Melbourne, 7 August.

Briskman, L. and Goddard, C. (2007) 'Not in my name: the people's inquiry into immigration detention', in D. Lusher and N. Haslam (eds) *Yearning to Breathe Free*, Sydney: Federation Press.

Briskman, L. and Noble, C. (1999) 'Social work ethics: embracing diversity?', in B. Pease and J. Fook (eds) *Transforming Social Work Practice: Postmodern Critical Perspectives*, St Leonards: Allen & Unwin.

Brook, E. and Davis, A. (eds) (1985) *Women, the Family and Social Work*, London: Tavistock.

Brown, A. (1979) *Groupwork*, London: Heinemann.

Brown, A. (1986) *Groupwork*, 2nd edn, Aldershot: Gower.

Brown, A. (1992) *Groupwork*, 3rd edn, Aldershot: Ashgate.

Brown, A. (1994) 'Groupwork in Britain', in C. Hanvey and T. Philpot (eds) *Practising Social Work*, London: Routledge.

Brown, A. (1996) 'Groupwork into the future: some personal reflections', *Groupwork*, **9**(1): 80–96.

Brown, A. and Clough, R. (eds) (1989) *Groups and Groupings: Life and Work in Day and Residential Centres*, London: Tavistock/Routledge.

Brown, H. (2000) 'Challenges from service users', in A. Brechin, H. Brown, and M. Eby (eds) *Critical Practice in Health and Social Care*, London: Open University/Sage.

Brown, H. and Smith, H. (eds) (1992) *Normalisation: A Reader for the Nineties*, London: Routledge.

Brown, H.C. (1996) 'The knowledge base of social work', in A.A. Vass (ed.) *Social Work Competences: Core Knowledge, Values and Skills*, London: Sage.

Brown, H.C., Fry, E. and Howard, J. (2005) *Support Care: How Family Placement Can Keep Children and Families Together*, Lyme Regis: Russell House Publishing.

Brown, L. (2007) 'The adoption and implementation of a service innovation in a social work setting: a case study of family group conferencing in the UK', *Social Policy and Society*, **6**(3): 321–32.

Brown, P., Hadley, R. and White, K.J. (1982) 'A case for neighbourhood-based social work and social services', in P.M. Barclay (ed.) *Social*

Workers: Their Role and Tasks, London: Bedford Square Press.

Brownlee, I. (1998) 'New Labour – new penology? Punitive rhetoric and the limits of managerialism in criminal justice policy', *Journal of Law and Society*, **25**(3): 313–35.

Buckman, R. (1998) 'Communication in palliative care: a practical guide', in D. Doyle, G. Hanks and N. MacDonald (eds) *Oxford Textbook of Palliative Medicine*, 2nd edn, Oxford: Oxford University Press.

Bullock, R., Gooch, D. and Little, L. (1998) *Children Going Home: The Re-unification of Families*, Aldershot: Ashgate.

Bullock, R., Little, M. and Millham, S. (1993) *Going Home: The Return of Children Separated from their Families*, Dartington: Dartington Social Research Unit.

Bullock, R., Little, M. and Mount, K. (1999) *Research in Practice: Experiments in Development and Information Design*, Dartington: Dartington Social Research Unit.

Bulman, C. and Schutz, S. (eds) (2004) *Reflective Practice in Nursing*, 3rd edn, Oxford: Blackwell.

Bunyan, A. (1987) '"Help, I can't cope with my child": a behavioural approach to the treatment of a conduct disordered child within the natural home setting', *British Journal of Social Work*, **17**: 237–56.

Burfoot, A. (1990) 'The normalisation of a new reproductive technology', in M. McNeil, I. Varcoe and S. Yearley (eds) *The New Reproductive Technologies*, Basingstoke: Macmillan – now Palgrave Macmillan.

Burford, G. and Hudson, J. (eds) (2000) *New Directions in Community Centred Child and Family Practice*, New York: Aldine de Gruyter.

Burford, G., Morris, K. and Nixon P. (2007) Family Decision Making International Survey, unpublished.

Burke, P. and Cigno, K. (1996) *Support for Families: Helping Children with Learning Disabilities*, Aldershot, Avebury.

Burke, P. and Cigno, K. (2000) *Learning Disabilities in Children*, Oxford, Blackwell Science.

Burkitt, I. (1991) *Social Selves: Theories of the Formation of the Personality*, London: Sage.

Burns, D., Williams, C.C. and Windebank, J. (2004) *Community Self-help*, Basingstoke, Palgrave Macmillan.

Burns, T., Beadsmoore, A., Bhat, A. et al. (1993) 'A controlled trial of home-based acute psychiatric services: I, clinical and social outcome', *British Journal of Psychiatry*, **163**: 49–54.

Butler, M. (1990) *Gender Trouble: Feminism and the Subversion of Identity*, London: Routledge.

Butler, S. (1994) '"All I've got in my purse is mothballs!", The Social Action Women's Group', *Groupwork*, **7**(2): 163–79.

Butler, S. and Wintram, C. (1991) *Feminist Groupwork*, London: Sage.

Butler-Sloss, L. (1988) *Report of the Inquiry into Child Abuse in Cleveland*, London: HMSO.

Butt, J. (2006) *Are We There Yet?* Bristol: Policy Press.

Butt, J. and Box, C. (1998) *Family Centred: A Study of the Use of Family Centres by Black Families*, London: REU.

Buttny, R. (1993) *Social Accountability in Communication*, London: Sage.

Bytheway, W. (2000) 'Old age', in M. Davies and R. Barton (eds) *Blackwell Encyclopaedia of Social Work*, Oxford: Blackwell.

Cabinet Office (2000) *Adoption, Prime Minister's Review: A Performance and Innovation Unit Report*, London: TSO.

Caddick, B. (1991) 'Using groups in working with offenders: a survey of groupwork in the probation services of England and Wales', *Groupwork*, **4**(3): 197–216.

Calhoun, C. (1996) 'Social theory and the public sphere', in B. Turner (ed.) *The Blackwell Companion to Social Theory*, Oxford: Blackwell.

Cambridge, P. and Carnaby, S. (2006) *Personal and Intimate Care with People with Learning Disabilities*, London: Jessica Kingsley.

Cambridge, P., Beadle-Brown, J., Milne, A. et al. (2006) *Exploring the Incidence, Risk Factors, Nature and Monitoring of Adult Protection Alerts*, Canterbury, University of Kent: Tizard Centre.

Cameron, C. (2004) 'Social pedagogy and care: Danish and German practice in young people's residential care', *Journal of Social Work*, **4**(2): 133–51.

Campbell, J. and Pinkerton, J. (1997) 'Embracing change as opportunity: reflections on social work from a Northern Ireland perspective', in B. Lesnik (ed.) *Change in Social Work*, Aldershot: Ashgate.

Campbell, J.C. (ed.) (1995) *Assessing Dangerousness: Violence by Sex Offenders*, London: Sage.

Cannan, C. (1992) *Changing Families, Changing Welfare*, Hemel Hempstead: Harvester Wheatsheaf.

Cannan, C. (1994/95) 'Enterprise culture, professional socialisation and social work education in Britain', *Critical Social Policy*, **42**: 5–19.

Canvin, K., Bartlett A. and Pinfold, V. (2002) 'A "bittersweet pill to swallow": learning from mental health service users' responses to compulsory community care in England', *Health and Social Care in the Community*, **10**(5): 361–9.

Carey, M. (2006) '"Selling social work by the pound?" The pros and cons of agency care management', *Practice*, **18**(1): 3–15.

Carey, M. (in press) 'The order of chaos: exploring agency care managers' construction of social order within fragmented worlds of state social work', *British Journal of Social Work*, Advance Access, Jan 27 2008, doi10.1093/bjsw/bcm143.

Carlen, P. (1989) 'Feminist jurisprudence – or women-wise penology?', *Probation Journal*, **36**(3).

Carlen, P. and Worrall, A. (eds) (1987) *Gender, Crime and Justice*, Buckingham: Open University Press.

Carling, P. (1996) *Return to the Community: Building Support Systems for People with Psychiatric Disabilities*, New York: Guilford.

Carniol, B. (2005) *Case Critical: Social Justice and Social Services in Canada*, 5th edn, Toronto: Between the Lines.

Carpenter, J., Schneider, J., Brandon, T. and Wooff, D. (2003) 'Working in multidisciplinary community mental health teams: the impact on social workers and health professionals of integrated mental healthcare', *British Journal of Social Work*, **33**: 1081–103.

Carr, S. (2004) *Has Service User Participation Made a Difference to Social Care Services?* Position Paper 3, London: Social Care Institute for Excellence.

Carter, R.T. (1991) 'Racial identity attitudes and psychological functioning', *Journal of Multicultural Counseling and Development*, **19**: 105–15.

Case, S. Clutton, S. and Haines, K. (2005) 'Extending entitlement: a Welsh policy for children', *Wales Journal of Law and Policy*, **4**(2): 187–202.

Cavanagh, K. and Cree, V.E. (eds) (1996) *Working with Men: Feminism and Social Work*, London: Routledge.

CCETSW (1991) *DipSW: Rules and Requirements for the Diploma in Social Work*, CCETSW Paper 30, 2nd edn, London: CCETSW.

Cemlyn, S. and Briskman, L. (2003) 'Asylum, children's rights and social work', *Child and Family Social Work*, **8**(3): 163–78.

Challis, D. (1994) *Implementing Caring for People: Care Management: Factors Influencing its Development in the Implementation of Community Care*, London: DH.

Challis, D., Darton, R. and Stewart, K. (eds) (1998) *Community Care, Secondary Health Care and Care Management*, Aldershot: Ashgate.

Chambon, A., Irving, A. and Epstein, C. (eds) (1999) *Reading Foucault for Social Work*, New York: Columbia University Press.

Chapillon, L. (1996) 'A behaviour management group for parents in a family centre', *Behavioural Social Work Review*, **17**: 22–30.

Chapman, T. and Hough, M. (1998) *Evidence-based Practice: a Guide to Effective Practice*, London: Home Office.

Chrisafis, A. (2007) 'French families motives for signing up with agency at centre of Chad abduction inquiry', *Guardian*, 1 November.

Christie, A. (2001) *Men and Social Work: Theories and Practices*, Basingstoke: Palgrave – now Palgrave Macmillan.

Christie, A. (2006) 'Negotiating the uncomfortable intersections between gender and professional identities to social work', *Critical Social Policy*, **26**(2): 390–411.

Cigno, K. (1988) 'Consumer views of a family centre drop-in', *British Journal of Social Work*, **18**: 361–75.

Cigno, K. (1993) 'Changing behaviour in a residential group setting for elderly people with learning difficulties', *British Journal of Social Work*, **23**: 629–42.

Cigno, K. (1998) 'Intervention in group care for older people', in K. Cigno and D. Bourn (eds) *Cognitive-behavioural Social Work in Practice*, Aldershot: Ashgate.

Cigno, K. and Bourn, D. (eds) (1998) *Cognitive-behavioural Social Work in Practice*, Aldershot: Ashgate.

Cigno, K. and Wilson, K. (1994) 'Effective strategies for working with children and families: issues in the provision of therapeutic help', *Practice*, **6**: 285–98.

Clark, C. (1996) 'Innovation, tradition and compromise: ethical issues in community care practice', in R. Adams (ed.) *Crisis in the Human Services: National and International Issues*. Selected Conference Papers, Kingston upon Hull: University of Lincolnshire and Humberside.

Clark, C. with Asquith, S. (1985) *Social Work and Social Philosophy*, London: Routledge & Kegan Paul.

Clark, C.L. (2000) *Social Work Ethics: Politics, Principles and Practice*, Basingstoke: Macmillan – now Palgrave Macmillan.

Clark, J. (1996) 'After social work', in N. Parton (ed.) *Social Theory, Social Change and Social Work*, London: Routledge.

Clarke, J., Cochrane, A. and McLaughlin, E. (eds) (1994) *Managing Social Policy*, London: Sage.

Clifford, D.J. (1994) 'Critical life histories: a key anti-oppressive research method', in B. Humphries and C. Truman (eds) *Rethinking Social Research*, Aldershot: Avebury.

Clifford, D.J. (1995) 'Methods in oral history and social work', *Journal of the Oral History Society*, **23**(2).

Clough, R. and Corbett, J. (eds) (2000) *Theories of Inclusive Education*, London: Paul Chapman.

Clough, R., Bullock, R. and Ward, A. (2006) *What Works in Residential Childcare: A Review of Research Evidence and the Practical Considerations*, London: National Centre for Excellence in Residential Child Care/National Children's Bureau.

Coates, R. (1981) 'Community-based services for juvenile delinquents: concept and implications for practice', *Journal of Social Issues*, **37**(3): 87–101.

Cochrane, A. (1993) 'Challenges from the centre', in J. Clarke (ed.) *A Crisis in Care? Challenges to Social Work*, London: Sage/Open University Press.

Cocker, C. and Allain, L. (2008) *Social Work and Looked After Children*, Exeter: Learning Matters.

Cohen, M. and Mullender, A. (eds) (2003) *Gender and Groupwork*, London: Routledge.

Cohen, S. (1975) '"It's all right for you to talk": political and sociological manifestos for social action', in R. Bailey and M. Brake (eds) *Radical Social Work*, London: Edward Arnold.

Coleman, R. and Smith, M. (1997) *Working with Voices: From Victim to Victor*, Gloucester: Handsall.

Coles, B. (1995) *Youth and Social Policy*, London: UCL Press.

Collins, B. (1986) 'Defining feminist social work', *Social Work*, May–June: 214–19.

Collins, S. (1990) *Alcohol, Social Work and Helping*, London: Routledge.

Commission on Social Justice (1994) *Social Justice: Strategies for National Renewal*, London: Vintage.

Compton, B. and Galaway, B. (1975) *Social Work Processes*, Homewood, IL: Dorsey Press.

Compton, B., Galaway, B. and Cournoyer, B. (2004) *Social Work Processes*, Pacific Grove, CA: Brooks/Cole.

Connell, R. (2006) 'Northern theory: the political geography of general social theory', *Theory and Society*, **35**(2): 237–64.

Connolly, M. and Ward, T. (2008) *Morals, Rights and Practice in the Human Services*, London: Jessica Kingsley.

Constantine, M.C., Richardson, T.Q., Benjamin, E.M. and Wilson, J.W. (1998) 'An overview of Black racial identity theories: limitations and considerations for future theoretical conceptualizations', *Applied and Preventive Psychology*, **7**: 95–9.

Coote, A. (ed.) (1992) *The Welfare of Citizens: Developing New Social Rights*, London: Rivers Oram.

Coppock, V. and Hopton, J. (2000) *Critical Perspectives on Mental Health*, London: Routledge.

Corby, B. (2005) *Child Abuse: Towards a Knowledge Base*, 3rd edn, Buckingham: Open University Press.

Cornwall Social Services (2008) 'Findings of a serious case review into the death of Steven Hoskin', www.db.cornwall.gov.uk/documents/download.aspx?doc=274337.

Corr, C. (1992) 'A task-based approach to coping with dying', *Omega*, **24**(2): 81–94.

Corrigan, P. and Leonard, P. (1978) *Social Work Practice Under Capitalism: A Marxist Approach*, London: Macmillan – now Palgrave Macmillan.

Coulshed, V. (1991) *Social Work Practice: An Introduction*, Basingstoke: Macmillan – now Palgrave Macmillan.

Coulshed, V. and Mullender, A. (2001) *Management in Social Work*, 2nd edn, Basingstoke: Palgrave – now Palgrave Macmillan.

Coulshed, V. and Orme, J. (2006) *Social Work Practice: An Introduction*, 4th edn, Basingstoke: Palgrave Macmillan.

Cowan, J. (1998) *On Becoming an Innovative University Teacher: Reflection in Action*, Buckingham: Society for Research into Higher Education/Open University Press.

Cowburn, M. and Modi, P. (1995) 'Justice in an unjust context: implications for working with adult male sex offenders', in D. Ward and M. Lacey (eds) *Probation: Working for Justice*, London: Whiting & Birch.

Cowen, H. (1999) *Community Care, Ideology and Social Policy*, London: Prentice Hall.

Craig, G. (ed.) (2005) *Not Water – Not Life: Hydration in the Dying*, Alsager: Fairway Folio.

Cree, V.E. and Macaulay, C. (eds) (2001) *Transfer of Learning in Professional and Vocational Education*, London: Routledge.

Crimmens, D. and Milligan, I. (2005) 'Residential child care: becoming a positive choice', in D. Crimmens and I. Milligan (eds) *Facing Forward: Residential Child Care in the 21st Century*, Lyme Regis: Russell House Publishing.

Crinall, K. (1999) 'Offending mothers: theorising in a feminist minefield', in B. Pease and J. Fook (eds) *Transforming Social Work Practice: Postmodern Critical Perspectives*, London: Routledge.

Crittenden, P.M. (2000) 'A dynamic maturational exploration of the meaning of security and adaptation', in P.M. Crittenden and A.H. Claussen (eds) *The Organization of Attachment Relationships: Maturation, Culture and Context*, Cambridge: Cambridge University Press.

Crittenden, P.M. and Claussen, A.H. (2000) *The Organization of Attachment Relationships: Maturation, Culture and Context*, Cambridge: Cambridge University Press.

Croft, S. and Beresford, P. (2000) 'Empowerment', in M. Davies and R. Barton (eds) *Blackwell Encyclopaedia of Social Work*, Oxford: Blackwell.

Cross, W.E. (1971) 'The negro to black conversion experience: towards the psychology of black liberation', *Black World*, **20**: 13–27.

Cross, W.E. (1980) 'Models of psychological nigrescence: a literature review', in R.L. Jones (ed.) *Black Psychology*, 2nd edn, New York: Harper & Row.

Cross, W.E. (1991) *Shades of Black: Diversity in African American Identity*, Philadelphia, PA: Temple University Press.

Cross, W.E. (2001) 'Encountering nigrescence', in J.G. Ponterotto, J.M. Casas, L.A. Suzuki and C.M. Alexander (eds) *Handbook of Multicultural Counseling*, 2nd edn, Thousand Oaks, CA: Sage.

Cross, W.E. and Vandiver, B.J. (2001) 'Nigresence theory and measurement: introducing the Cross Racial Identity Scale (CRIS)', in J.G. Ponterotto, J.M. Casas, L.A. Suzuki and C.M. Alexander (eds) *Handbook of Multicultural Counseling*, 2nd edn, Thousand Oaks, CA: Sage.

Cross, W.E., Parham, T. and Helms, J. (1998) 'Nigrescence revisited: theory and research', in R.L. Jones (ed.) *African American Identity Development*, Hampton, VA: Cobb & Henry.

Cross, W.E., Parham, T. and Helms, J.. (2004) 'The stages of black identity development: nigrescence models', in R.L. Jones (ed.) *Black Psychology*, 4th edn, Berkeley, CA: Cobb & Henry.

Crow, G. and Allen, G. (1994) *Community Life*, Hemel Hempstead: Harvester Wheatsheaf.

CSCI (Commission for Social Care Inspection) (2008) *The State of Social Care in England 2006/2007*, London: CSCI.

CSIP (Care Services Improvement Partnership) (2005) *The Social Work Contribution to Mental Health Services: The Future Direction*, London: NIMHE.

Cullen, C., Campbell, M., Connelly, D. et al. (1995) *Approaches to People with Challenging Behaviour*, learning pack, St Andrews: University of St Andrews.

Cumming, E. and Henry, W.E. (1961) *Growing Old: The Process of Disengagement*, New York: Basic Books.

Currer, C. (2001) *Responding to Grief: Dying, Bereavement and Social Care*, Basingstoke: Palgrave – now Palgrave Macmillan.

Currer, C. (2007) *Loss and Social Work*, Exeter: Learning Matters.

D'Ardenne, P. and Mahtani, A. (1999) *Transcultural Counselling in Action*, 2nd edn, London: Sage.

D'Cruz, H., Gillingham, P. and Melendez, S. (2007) 'Reflexivity, its meanings and relevance for social work: a critical review of the literature', *British Journal of Social Work*, **37**: 73–90.

Dalal, F. (1988) 'The racism of Jung', *Race and Class*, **29**(3): 1–22.

Dale, J. and Foster, P. (1986) *Feminists and State Welfare*, London: Routledge & Kegan Paul.

Dale, P., Davies, M., Morrison, T. and Waters, J. (1986) *Dangerous Families: Assessment and Treatment of Child Abuse*, London: Tavistock.

Dalley, G. (1988) *Ideologies of Caring*, Basingstoke: Macmillan – now Palgrave Macmillan.

Dalrymple, J. and Burke, B. (1995) *Anti-oppressive Practice, Social Care and the Law*, Buckingham: Open University Press.

Dalrymple, J. and Burke, B. (2006) *Anti-oppressive Practice: Social Care and the Law*, 2nd edn, Buckingham: Open University Press.

Daniel, B., Featherstone, B., Hooper, C. and Scourfield, J. (2005) 'Why gender matters for every child matters', *British Journal of Social Work*, **35**(8): 1343–57.

Dattalo, P. (1997) 'A typology of child protective services cases: design and implementation issues for SW administrators', *Administration in Social Work*, **21**(2): 55–75.

Davies, B. (1975) *The Use of Groups in Social Work Practice*, London: Routledge & Kegan Paul.

Davies, B., Gottsche, M. and Bansel, P. (2006) 'The rise and fall of the neo-liberal university', *European Journal of Education*, **41**(2): 305–19.

Davies, D. and Neal, C. (eds) (2004) *Pink Therapy: A Guide for Counsellors Working with Lesbian, Gay and Bisexual Clients*, 2nd edn, Maidenhead: Open University Press.

Davies, H.T.O., Nutley, S.M. and Smith, P.C. (eds) (2000) *What Works? Evidence-based Practice in Public Services*, London: Policy Press.

Davies, M. and Barton, R. (eds) (2000) *Blackwell Encyclopaedia of Social Work*, Oxford: Blackwell.

Davies, R. (1995) I Wanted a Pink Coffin, unpublished report of the HIV/AIDS User Consultation Exercise for Norfolk Social Services, by Norfolk County Council Social Services Department.

Davies, R. (ed.) (1998) *Stress in Social Work*, London: Jessica Kingsley.

Davis, A. (1996) 'Risk work and mental health', in H. Kemshall and J. Pritchard (eds) *Good Practice in Risk Assessment and Risk Management 1*, London: Jessica Kingsley.

DCA (Department for Constitutional Affairs) (2006) *Review of Care Proceedings in England and Wales*, London: DCA.

DCLG (Department for Communities and Local Government) (2006) *The Community Development Challenge*, London: DCLG.

De Jong, P. and Berg, I.K. (2007) *Interviewing for Solutions*, Pacific Grove, CA: Brooks Cole.

de Jonge, J.M., Schippers, G.M. and Schaap, P.D.R. (2005) 'The motivational interviewing skill code: reliability and a critical appraisal', *Behavioural and Cognitive Psychotherapy*, **33**: 285–98.

De Maria, W. (1997) 'Flapping on clipped wings: social work ethics in the age of activism', *Australian Social Work*, **50**(4): 3–19.

De Shazer, S. (1985) *Keys to Solutions in Brief Therapy*, New York: W.W. Norton.

De Shazer, S. (1988) *Clues: Investigating Solutions in Brief Therapy*, New York: W.W. Norton.

De Shazer, S. (1991) *Putting Difference to Work*, New York: W.W. Norton.

De Shazer, S. (1994) *Words were Originally Magic*, New York: W.W. Norton.

De Zulueta, F. (1999) 'Borderline personality disorder as seen from an attachment perspective: a review', *Criminal Behaviour and Mental Health*, **9**: 237–53.

Dean, H. (ed.) (2004) *The Ethics of Welfare: Human Rights, Dependency and Responsibility*, Bristol: Policy Press.

DfES (Department for Education and Skills) (2003) *Every Child Matters*, Green Paper. London: TSO.

DfES (Department for Education and Skills) (2004) *Every Child Matters: Change for Children*, www.everychildmatters.gov.uk.

DfES (Department for Education and Skills) (2006) *Working Together to Safeguard Children*, London: TSO.

DfES (Department for Education and Skills) (2007) *Care Matters: Time for Change*, White Paper, London: TSO.

DH (Department of Health) (1989a) *An Introduction to the Children Act 1989*, London: HMSO.

DH (Department of Health) (1989b) *Caring for People: Community Care in the Next Decade and Beyond*, Cm 849, London: HMSO.

DH (Department of Health) (1991) *Patterns and Outcomes in Child Placement: Messages from Current Research and Their Implications*, London: HMSO.

DH (Department of Health) (1995a) *Child Protection: Messages from Research*, London: HMSO.

DH (Department of Health) (1995b) *Looking After Children, Essential Information*, Parts 1 and 2, London: HMSO.

DH (Department of Health) (1995c) *The Care Programme Approach for People with a Mental Illness Referred to the Specialist Psychiatric Services*, London: HSMO.

DH (Department of Health) (1995d) *Looking After Children: Assessment and Action Schedules*, London: HMSO.

DH (Department of Health) (1998) *Quality Protects: Framework for Action and Objectives for Social Services for Children*, London: DH.

DH (Department of Health) (1999a) *Adoption Now: Messages from Research*, Chichester: Wiley.

DH (Department of Health) (1999b) *The Quality Protects Programme: Transforming Children's Services 2000/2001*, London: DH.

DH (Department of Health) (1999c) *Modernising Mental Health Services: Safe, Sound and Supportive*, London: HSMO.

DH (Department of Health) (2000a) *A Quality Strategy for Social Care*, London: HMSO.

DH (Department of Health) (2000b) *'No Secrets': Guidance on Developing and Implementing Multi-Agency Policies and Procedures to Protect Vulnerable Adults from Abuse*, London: HMSO.

DH (Department of Health) (2000c) *The NHS Plan: A Plan for Investment and a Plan for Reform*, Cm 4818-I, London: TSO.

DH (Department of Health) (2001a) *Adoption: National Adoption Standards for England*, London: TSO.

DH (Department of Health) (2001b) *The Mental Health Policy Initiative*, London: TSO.

DH (Department of Health) (2001b) *National Service Framework for Older People* LAC(2001) 12, London: The Stationery Office).

DH (Department of Health) (2001c) *The Mental Health Policy Implementation Guide*, London: DH.

DH (Department of Health) (2001c) *Valuing People: A New Strategy for Learning Disability for the 21st Century*, White Paper, Cm 5086, London: TSO.

DH (Department of Health) (2001d) *National Service Framework for Older People*, London: TSO.

DH (Department of Health) (2002a) *Fostering Services: National Minimum Standards: Fostering Services Regulations*, London: TSO.

DH (Department of Health) (2002b) *Fair Access to Care Services*, London, DH.

DH (Department of Health) (2003a) *Requirements for the Social Work Degree*, London: DH.

DH (Department of Health) (2003b) *Report of an Independent Inquiry into the Death of David 'Rocky' Bennett*, London: DH.

DH (Department of Health) (2005) *Independence, Well being and Choice*, London: DH.

DH (Department of Health) (2007a) *Best Practice in Managing Risk: Principles and Evidence for Best Practice in the Assessment and Management of Risk to Self and Others in Mental Health Services*, London: DH.

DH (Department of Health) (2007b) *Putting People First: A Shared Vision and Commitment* to the Transformation of Adult Social Care, London: DH.

DH (Department of Health) (2007c) The Single Assessment Process: Guidance and Resources, London: DH.

DH (Department of Health) (2008) End of Life Care Strategy: Promoting High Quality Care for all Adults at the End of Life, London: DH.

DH/DfEE/Home Office (Department of Health/ Department for Education and Employment/ Home Office) (2000) Framework for the Assessment of Children in Need and Their Families, London: TSO.

DH, NIMHE and Partners (2005) New Ways of Working for Psychiatrists: Enhancing Effective, Person-centred Services Through New Ways of Working in Multidisciplinary and Multi-agency Contexts, London: DH.

DH/SSI (Department of Health/Social Services Inspectorate) (1991) Care Management and Assessment: Summary of Practice Guidance, London: HMSO.

DH/Welsh Office (Department of Health/Welsh Office) (1999) Mental Health Act 1983: Code of Practice, London: TSO.

Dodson, M. (1997) Bringing Them Home, video, Sydney: HREOC.

Doel, M. (1994) 'Task-centred work', in C. Hanvey and T. Philpot (eds) Practising Social Work, London: Routledge.

Doel, M. (2006) Using Groupwork, Oxford: Routledge.

Doel, M. and Lawson, B. (1986) 'Open records: the client's right to partnership', British Journal of Social Work, 16(4): 407–30.

Doel, M. and Marsh, P. (1992) Task-centred Social Work, Aldershot: Ashgate.

Dominelli, L. (1986) 'The power of the powerless: prostitution and the reinforcement of submissive femininity', Sociological Review, (spring): 65–92.

Dominelli, L. (1988) Anti-racist Social Work, Basingstoke: Macmillan – now Palgrave Macmillan.

Dominelli, L. (1990) Women and Community Action, Birmingham: Venture.

Dominelli, L. (1994) Anti-racist Social Work Education, paper given at the 27th Congress of the International Association of Schools of Social Work, Amsterdam, July.

Dominelli, L. (1996) 'Deprofessionalising social work: anti-oppressive practice, competencies and postmodernism, British Journal of Social Work, 26: 153–75.

Dominelli, L. (2000) 'Empowerment: help or hindrance in professional relationships?', in D. Ford and P. Stepney (eds) Social Work Models,

Methods and Theories: A Framework for Practice, Lyme Regis: Russell House Publishing.

Dominelli, L. (2002a) Feminist Social Work Theory and Practice, Basingstoke: Palgrave Macmillan.

Dominelli, L. (2002b) '"Glassed-in": problematising women's reproductive rights under the new reproductive technologies', in R. Adams, L. Dominelli and M. Payne (eds) Critical Practice in Social Work, Basingstoke: Palgrave Macmillan.

Dominelli, L. (2002c) Anti-oppressive Social Work Theory and Practice, Basingstoke: Palgrave Macmillan.

Dominelli, L. (2004a) Social Work: Theory and Practice for a Changing Profession, Cambridge: Polity Press.

Dominelli, L. (2004b) 'Practising social work in a globalising world', in N.-T. Tan and A. Rowlands (eds) Social Work Around the World III, Berne: International Federation of Social Workers.

Dominelli, L. and Gollins, T. (1997) 'Men, power and caring relationships', Sociological Review, 45(3): 396–415.

Dominelli, L. and Hoogvelt, A. (1996) 'Globalisation and the technocratisation of social work', Critical Social Policy, 47(2): 45–62.

Dominelli, L. and McLeod, E. (1989) Feminist Social Work, Basingstoke, Macmillan – now Palgrave Macmillan.

Doolan, M. (2007) 'Duty calls: the response of law, policy and practice to participation rights in child welfare systems', Protecting Children, 22(1): 10–18.

Douglas, T. (1978) Basic Groupwork, London: Tavistock.

Douglas, T. (1983) Groups: Understanding People Gathered Together, London: Tavistock.

Douglas, T. (1986) Group Living: The Application of Group Dynamics in Residential Settings, London: Tavistock.

Douglas, T. (1993) A Theory of Groupwork Practice, Basingstoke: Macmillan – now Palgrave Macmillan.

Dow, J. (2007) 'NHS learning disability services: implications of the Cornwall report', Journal of Adult Protection, 9(4): 34–8.

Dowden, D. and Andrews, D.A. (2004) 'The importance of staff practice in delivering effective correctional treatment: a meta-analytical review of core correctional practice', International Journal of Offender Therapy and Comparative Criminology, 48(2): 203–14.

Dowie, J. (1999) 'Communication for better decisions: not about "risk"', Health, Risk and Society, 1(1): 41–53.

Drakeford, M. (1994) 'Groupwork for parents of young people in trouble', Groupwork, 7(3): 236–47.

Dryden, W., Charles-Edwards, D. and Woolfe, R. (eds) (1989) *Handbook of Counselling in Great Britain*, London: Routledge.

Durkheim, E. (1972) *Selected Writings*, ed. A. Giddens, Cambridge: Cambridge University Press.

Durrant, P. (1997) 'Mapping the future? A contribution from community social work in the community care field', in C. Cannan and C. Warren (eds) *Social Action with Children and Families*, London: Routledge.

Dwivedi, K.N. (1996) 'Introduction', in K.N. Dwivedi and V.P. Varma (eds) *Meeting the Needs of Ethnic Minority Children: A Handbook for Professionals*, London: Jessica Kingsley.

Dwivedi, K.N. and Varma, V.P. (eds) (2002) *Meeting the Needs of Ethnic Minority Children: Including Refugee, Black and Mixed Parentage Children: A Handbook for Professionals*, 2nd edn, London: Jessica Kingsley.

Eekelaar, J. (1986) 'The emergence of children's rights', *Oxford Journal of Legal Studies*, 6(2): 177–82.

Egan, G. (1998) *The Skilled Helper*, 6th edn, Pacific Grove, CA: Brooks/Cole.

Egan, G. (2004) *The Skilled Helper*, Pacific Grove, CA: Brooks/Cole.

Egan, G. (2006) *The Skilled Helper: A Problem Management and Opportunity Approach to Helping*, 8th edn, Pacific Grove, CA: Brooks/Cole.

Ehlert, K. and Griffiths, D. (1996) 'Quality of life: a matched group comparison of long stay individuals and day patients manifesting psychiatric disabilities', *Journal of Mental Health*, 5(1): 91–100.

England, H. (1986) *Social Work as Art: Making Sense for Good Practice*, London: Allen & Unwin.

Epstein, L. (1992) *Brief Treatment and a New Look at the Task-centered Approach*, New York: Macmillan.

Eraut, M. (1994) *Developing Professional Knowledge and Competence*, London: Falmer.

Erikson, H. (1964) 'Memorandum on identity and Negro youth', *Journal of Social Issues*, 20(4): 29–42.

Erikson, H. (1968) *Identity: Youth and Crisis*, London: Faber.

Fahlberg, V.I (1994) *A Child's Journey through Placement*, London: BAAF.

Fairbairn, G. (1985) 'Responsibility in social work', in D. Watson (ed.) *A Code of Ethics for Social Work: The Second Step*, London: Routledge & Kegan Paul.

Falloon, I., Laporta, M., Fadden, G. and Graham-Hole, V. (1993) *Managing Stress in Families: Cognitive and Behavioural Strategies for Enhancing Coping Skills*, London: Routledge.

Faulkner, A. (1997) *Knowing our own Minds: A Survey of How People in Emotional Distress Take Control of their Lives*, London: Mental Health Foundation.

Faulkner, A. (2000) *Strategies for Living: A Report of User-led Research into Peoples' Strategies for Living with Mental Distress: Summary Report*, London: Mental Health Foundation.

Faulkner, D. (1995) 'The Criminal Justice Act 1991: policy, legislation and practice', in D. Ward and M. Lacey (eds) *Probation: Working for Justice*, London: Whiting & Birch.

Fawcett, B., Featherstone, B. and Goddard, J. (2004) *Contemporary Child Care Policy and Practice*, Basingstoke: Palgrave Macmillan.

Fawcett, B., Featherstone, B., Fook, J. and Rossiter, A. (eds) (2000) *Practice and Research in Social Work: Postmodern Feminist Perspectives*, London: Routledge.

Featherstone, B. (2003) 'Taking fathers seriously', *British Journal of Social Work*, 33: 239–54.

Featherstone, B. (2004) *Family Life and Family Support*, Basingstoke, Palgrave Macmillan.

Featherstone, B. (2005) 'Feminist social work: past present and future', in S.F. Hick, J. Fook and R. Pozzuto (eds) *Social Work: A Critical Turn*, Toronto: Thompson.

Featherstone, B. and Fawcett, B. (1995) 'Power, difference and social work: an exploration', *Social Work Education*, 15(1): 3–19.

Featherstone, B. and Lancaster, E. (1997) 'Contemplating the unthinkable: men who sexually abuse children', *Critical Social Policy*, 17(4): 57–71.

Featherstone, M. (1988) 'In pursuit of the post modern: an introduction', *Theory, Culture and Society*, 5(2/3): 195–216.

Feeley, S. and Simon, J. (1992) 'The new penology: notes on the emerging strategy of corrections and its implications', *Criminology*, 30(4): 452–74.

Feltham, C. (1995) *What is Counselling?* London: Sage.

Feltham, C. and Dryden, W. (2004) *Dictionary of Counselling*, 2nd edn, London: Whurr.

Feltham, C. and Dryden, W. (2006) *Brief Counselling: A Practical Integrative Approach*, Maidenhead: Open University Press.

Fennell, G., Phillipson, C. and Evers, H. (1988) *The Sociology of Old Age*, Milton Keynes: Open University Press.

Ferguson, H. (2003) 'Outline of a critical best practice perspective on social work and social care', *British Journal of Social Work*, 33: 1005–24.

Ferguson, H. (2008) 'The theory and practice of critical best practice in social work', in K. Jones, B. Cooper and H. Ferguson (eds) *Best Practice in Social Work: Critical Perspectives*, Basingstoke: Palgrave Macmillan.

Ferguson, I. (2008) *Reclaiming Social Work: Challenging Neoliberalism and Promoting Social Justice*, London: Sage.

Ferguson, I. and Lavalette, M. (1999) 'Social work, postmodernism and Marxism', *European Journal of Social Work*, 2(1): 27–40.

Ferguson, I., Lavalette, M. and Mooney, G. (2002) *Rethinking Welfare: A Critical Perspective*, London: Sage.

Fernando, S. (1991) *Mental Health, Race and Culture*, London: Macmillan – now Palgrave Macmillan.

Fernando, S. (2002) *Mental Health, Race and Culture*, 2nd edn, Basingstoke: Palgrave Macmillan.

Field, D. (1996) 'Awareness of modern dying', *Mortality*, 1(3): 255–65.

Finch, J. and Groves, D. (eds) (1983) *A Labour of Love: Women, Work and Caring*, London: Routledge & Kegan Paul.

Finer, C. and Nellis, M. (eds) (1998) *Crime and Social Exclusion*, Oxford: Blackwell.

Finkelstein, V. (1991) 'Disability: an administrative challenge? (the health and welfare heritage)', in M. Oliver (ed.) *Social Work, Disabled People and Disabling Environments*, London: Jessica Kingsley.

Finlay, L. and Gough, B. (2003) *Reflexivity: A Practical Guide for Researchers in Health and Social Sciences*, Oxford: Blackwell.

Firestone, S. (1971) *The Dialectic of Sex*, London: Jonathan Cape.

Firth, P. (2003) 'Multiprofessional teamwork', in B. Monroe and D. Oliviere (eds) *Patient Participation in Palliative Care: A Voice for the Voiceless*, Oxford: Oxford University Press.

Fischer, J. (1974) 'Is casework effective? A review', *Social Work*, 1: 107–10.

Fischer, J. (1978) *Effective Casework Practice: An Eclectic Approach*, New York: McGraw-Hill.

Fisher, M. (1994) 'Man-made *care*: community *care* and older male *carers*', *British Journal of Social Work*, 24(6): 659–80.

FitzGerald, M. and Chapman, Y. (2000) 'Theories of reflection for learning', in S. Burns and C. Bulman (eds) *Reflective Practice in Nursing: The Growth of the Professional Practitioner*, 2nd edn, Oxford: Blackwell Science.

Flaskas, C. (1997) 'Reclaiming the idea of truth: some thoughts on theory in response to practice', *Journal of Family Therapy*, 1(1): 1–20.

Fleet, F. (2000) 'Counselling and contemporary social work', in P. Stepney and D. Ford (eds) *Social Work Models, Methods and Theories: A Framework for Practice*, Lyme Regis: Russell House Publishing.

Fleming, J. and Ward, D. (1996) 'The ethics of community health needs assessment: searching for a participant centred approach', in M. Parker (ed.) *Ethics and Community*, Preston: Centre for Professional Ethics, University of Central Lancashire.

Fletcher, A. (1999) *Genes are Us? Genetics and Disability: RADAR Survey*, London: RADAR.

Flood, M., Gardiner, J., Pease, B. and Pringle, K. (eds) (2007) *International Encyclopedia of Men and Masculinities*, Milton Park: Routledge.

Flynn, M. (2007) 'Unlearned lessons from the Healthcare Commission's investigation into the services for people with learning disabilities provided by Sutton and Merton Primary Care Trust', *Journal of Adult Protection*, 9(4): 21–6.

Fook, J. (2002) *Social Work: Critical Theory and Practice*, London: Sage.

Fook, J. and Askeland, G.A. (2006) 'The "critical" in critical reflection', in S. White, J. Fook and F. Gardner (eds) *Critical Reflection in Health and Social Care*, Maidenhead: Open University Press.

Fook, J. and Gardner, F. (2007) *Practising Critical Refection: A Resource Handbook*, Maidenhead: Open University Press.

Fook, J., Ryan, M. and Hawkins, L. (2000) *Professional Expertise: Practice, Theory and Education for Working in Uncertainty*, London, Whiting & Birch.

Foster, A. (1998) 'Thinking about risk', in A. Foster and V. Roberts (eds) *Managing Mental Health in the Community: Chaos and Containment*, London: Routledge.

Foster, M., Harris, J., Jackson, K. and Glendinning, C. (2008) 'Practitioners' documentation of assessment and care planning in social care: the opportunities for organisational learning', *British Journal of Social Work*, 38(3): 546–60.

Fostering Network (2003) *The Skills to Foster*, London: Fostering Network.

Freeman, I., Morrison, A., Lockhart, F. and Swanson, M. (1996) 'Consulting service users: the views of young people', in M. Hill and J. Aldgate (eds) *Child Welfare Services: Developments in Law, Policy, Practice and Research*, London: Jessica Kingsley.

Freire, P. (1972) *Pedagogy of the Oppressed*, Harmondsworth: Penguin.

Freud, S. ([1913]1950) *Totem and Taboo*, Harmondsworth: Penguin Freud Library 13.

Freud, S. (1915) 'Thoughts for the times on war and death', *Imago*, 4(1): 1–21, trans. J. Strachey in *The Standard Edition of the Complete Psychological Works of Sigmund Freud*, vol. 14, London: Hogarth Press.

Freud, S. (1930) 'Civilization and its discontents', in J. Strachey (ed.) trans. J. Rivière, *The Standard Edition of the Complete Works of Sigmund Freud*, vol. 21, London: Hogarth Press.

Frith, U. (1989) *Autism: Explaining the Enigma*, Oxford: Blackwell.

Frosh, S. (1987) *The Politics of Psychoanalysis*, London: Macmillan – now Palgrave Macmillan.

Gallagher, G. (2003) 'Refugee treatment the world's harshest: Ozdowski', *The Age*, 10 October.

Galper, J. (1975) *The Politics of Social Services*, Englewood Cliffs, NJ: Prentice Hall.

Gambe, D., Gomes, J., Kapur, V. et al. (1992) *Improving Practice with Children and Families*, Leeds: CCETSW.

Gambrill, E. (1983) *Casework: A Competency-based Approach*, Englewood Cliffs, NJ: Prentice Hall.

Gambrill, E. (1986) 'Social skills training with the elderly', in C. Hollin and P. Trower (eds) *Handbook of Social Skills Training*, vol. 1, Oxford: Pergamon.

Gambrill, E. (1997) *Social Work Practice: A Critical Thinkers' Guide*, New York: Oxford University Press.

Gardiner, H.W. (1994) 'Child development', in L.L. Adler and U.P. Gielen (eds) *Cross-cultural Topics in Psychology*, New York: Praeger.

Garrett, K. (1996) 'Missing', *Background Briefing*, Radio National Transcript, 11 Feb: 3.

Gendreau, P. and Andrews, D.A. (1990) 'Tertiary prevention: what the meta-analyses of the treatment programme literature tell us about 'what works', *Canadian Journal of Criminology*, 32: 173–84.

Gendreau, P. and Ross, R. (1987) 'Revisitation of rehabilitation: evidence from the 1980s', *Justice Quarterly*, 4: 349–406.

George, E., Iveson, C. and Ratner, H. (1990) *Problem to Solution: Brief Therapy with Individuals and Families*, London: Brief Therapy Press.

George, R. and Sykes, J. (1997) 'Beyond cancer?', in D. Clark, J. Hockey and S. Ahmedzai (eds) *New Themes in Palliative Care*, Buckingham: Open University Press.

George, V. and Wilding, P. (1994) *Welfare and Ideology*, Hemel Hempstead: Harvester Wheatsheaf.

Gergen, K. (1999) *An Invitation to Social Construction*, London: Sage.

Gerth, H.H. and Mills, C.W. (eds) (1948) *From Max Weber*, London: Routledge & Kegan Paul.

Geyer, R. (2003) 'Beyond the third way: the science of complexity and the politics of choice', *British Journal of Politics and International Relations*, 5: 237–57.

Ghuman, P.A. (2003) *Double Loyalties: South Asian Adolescents in the West*, Cardiff: University of Wales Press.

Giddens, A. (1987) *Social Theory and Modern Sociology*, Oxford: Blackwell.

Giddens, A. (1990) *The Consequences of Modernity*, Cambridge: Polity Press.

Giddens, A. (1991) *Modernity and Self Identity: Self and Society in the Late Modern Age*, Cambridge: Polity Press.

Giddens, A. (1998a) *The Third Way: The Renewal of Social Democracy*, Cambridge: Polity Press.

Giddens, A. (1998b) 'Risk society: the context of British politics', in J. Franklin (ed.) *The Politics of Risk Society*, Cambridge: Polity Press.

Gilles, V. (2005) 'Meeting parents' needs? Discourses of "support" and "inclusion" in family policy', *Critical Social Policy*, 25(1): 70–90.

Gilligan, C. (1993) *In a Different Voice*, 2nd edn, Cambridge, MA: Harvard University Press.

Gilligan, P. and Akhtar, S. (2005) 'Child sexual abuse amongst Asian communities: developing materials to raise awareness in Bradford', *Practice*, 17(4): 267–84.

Gilligan, P. and Akhtar, S. (2006) 'Cultural barriers to the disclosure of child sexual abuse in Asian communities: listening to what women say', *British Journal of Social Work*, 36(8): 1361–77.

Glaister, A. (2007) 'Introducing critical practice', in S. Fraser and S. Matthews (eds) *The Critical Practitioner in Social Work and Health Care*, London: Sage.

Goddard, C. and Briskman, L. (2004) 'By any measure, it's official child abuse', *Herald Sun*, 19 February: 17.

Goldson, B. (1999) *Youth Justice: Contemporary Policy and Practice*, Aldershot: Ashgate.

Goldson, B. (2000) *The New Youth Justice*, Lyme Regis: Russell House Publishing.

Goldson, B. and Muncie, J. (eds) (2006) *Youth Crime and Justice*, London, Sage.

Goodey, C.F. (1992) 'Mental disabilities and human values in Plato's Late Dialogues', *Archiv Für Geschichte Der Philosophie*, 74: 26–42.

Gorman, H. and Postle, K. (2003) *Transforming Community Care: A Distorted Vision?*, Birmingham: Venture Press.

Gorman, K. (2001) 'Cognitive behaviourism and the Holy Grail: the quest for a universal means of managing offender risk', *Probation Journal*, 48: 3–9.

Gorman, K., Gregory, M., Hayles, M. and Parton, N. (eds) (2006) *Constructive Work with Offenders*, London: Kessica Kingsley.

Gould, N. (1996) 'Using imagery in reflective learning', in N. Gould, and I. Taylor (eds) *Reflective Learning for Social Work*, Aldershot: Arena.

Graham, M. (2007) *Black Issues in Social Work*, Bristol: Policy Press.

Gray, M. and Webb, S. (2008a) 'Critical social work', in M. Gray and S. Webb (eds) *Social Work Theories and Methods*, London: Sage.

Gray, M. and Webb, S. (eds) (2008b) *Thinking About Social Work*, London: Sage.

Green, P. (2003) 'Feminist dilemmas in data analysis: researching the use of creative writing in women survivors of sexual abuse', *Qualitative Social Work*, **2**(1): 45–60.

Greenfield, P. and Cocking, R. (1994) 'Preface', in P. Greenfield and R. Cocking (eds) *Cross-cultural Roots of Minority Child Development*, Hillsdale, NJ: Lawrence Erlbaum.

Griffiths, R. (1988) *Community Care: Agenda for Action*, London: HMSO.

Grossman, K., Grossmann, K.E., Spangler, S. et al. (1985) 'Maternal sensitivity and newborn attachment orientation responses as related to quality of attachment in northern Germany', in I. Bretherton and E. Waters (eds) *Growing Points of Attachment Theory: Monographs of the Society of Research in Child Development*, **50**(1/2).

Gunaratnam, Y. (2003) *Researching Race and Ethnicity: Methods, Knowledge and Power*, London: Sage.

Habermas, J. (1984) *The Theory of Communicative Action: vol. 1 Reason and the Rationalisation of Society*, Cambridge: Polity Press.

Habermas, J. (1987) *The Theory of Communicative Action: vol. 2 The Critique of Functionalist Reason*, Cambridge: Polity Press.

Haebich, A. (1998) 'Grim facts we've known', *The Adelaide Review*, **173**: 8–9.

Haffenden, S. (1991) *Getting it Right for Carers: Setting Up Services for Carers: A Guide for Practitioners*, London: HMSO.

Hague, G., Mullender, A. and Aris, R. (2003) *Is Anyone Listening? Accountability and Women Survivors of Domestic Violence*, London: Routledge.

Haines, K. (1996) *Understanding Modern Juvenile Justice*, Aldershot: Avebury.

Haines, K. (1997) 'Young offenders and family support services: a European perspective', *International Journal of Child and Family Welfare*, **2**(1): 61–73.

Haines, K. (2000) 'Referral orders and the new youth justice', in B. Goldson (ed.) *The New Youth Justice*, Lyme Regis: Russell House Publishing.

Haines, K. and Drakeford, M. (1998) *Young People and Youth Justice*, Basingstoke: Macmillan – now Palgrave Macmillan.

Haines, K., Jones, R. and Isles, E. (1999) Promoting Positive Behaviour in Schools, report submitted to the Wales Office of Research and Development.

Hale, J. (1983) 'Feminism and social work practice', in B. Jordan and N. Parton (eds) *The Political Dimensions of Social Work*, Oxford: Blackwell.

Hall, C. (1997) *Social Work as Narratives: Storytelling and Persuasion in Professional Texts*, Aldershot: Ashgate.

Hall, C., Juhila K., Parton, N. and Pösö T. (eds) (2003) *Constructive Clienthood in Social Work and Human Services: Interaction, Identities and Practices*, London: Jessica Kingsley.

Halter, M., Brown, H. and Stone, J. (2007) *Sexual Boundary Violations by Health Employees: An Overview of the Published Empirical Literature*, London: Council for Healthcare Regulatory Excellence/DH.

Hanmer, J. and Maynard, M. (1987) *Women, Violence and Social Control*, London: Macmillan – now Palgrave Macmillan.

Hanmer, J. and Statham, D. (1988) *Women and Social Work: Towards a Woman-centred Practice*, London: Macmillan – now Palgrave Macmillan.

Harder, M. and Pringle, K. (eds) (1997) *Protecting Children in Europe Towards a New Millennium*, Aalborg University Press.

Hardiker, P. and Barker, M. (1999) 'Early steps in implementing the new community care: the role of social work practice', *Health and Social Care in the Community*, **7**(6): 417–26.

Harms, L. (2007) *Working with People: Communication Skills for Reflective Practice*, Melbourne: Oxford University Press.

Harris, R. (1997) 'Power', in M. Davies (ed.) *Blackwell Companion to Social Work*, Oxford: Blackwell.

Harrison, A., Wilson, M., Pine, C. et al. (1990) 'Family ecologies of ethnic minority children', *Child Development*, **61**: 347–62.

Hart, R. (1992) *Children's Participation from Tokenism to Citizenship*, Innocenti Essays, No. 4, Florence: UNICEF.

Hartley, J. and McKee, A. (2001) *The Indigenous Public Sphere: The Reporting and Recognition of Indigenous Issues in the Australian Media, 1994–1997*, New York: Oxford University Press.

Hassett, P. and Stevens, I. (2005) *Risk Management and Risk Assessment: A Training Pack*, Glasgow: SIRCC.

Hawkesworth, M.E. (1989) 'Knower, knowing, known: feminist theory and claims of truth', *Signs: Journal of Women in Culture and Society*, **14**(31): 533–57.

Healy, K. (2000) *Social Work Practices: Contemporary Perspectives on Change*, London: Sage.

Healy, K. (2005) *Social Work Theories in Context: Creating Frameworks for Practice*, Basingstoke: Palgrave Macmillan.

Healy, K. and Meagher, G. (2004) 'The reprofessionalization of social work: collaborative approaches for achieving professional recognition', *British Journal of Social Work*, **34**: 243–60.

Healy, L. (2001) *International Social Work*, Oxford: Oxford University Press.

Heap, K. (1985) *The Practice of Social Work with Groups*, London: Allen & Unwin.

Hearn, J. (1998) *The Violences of Men*, London: Sage.

Heelas, P., Lash, S. and Morris, P. (eds) (1996) *Detraditionalization: Critical Reflections on Authority and Identity*, Oxford: Blackwell.

Hek, R. (2006) *The Experiences and Needs of Refugee and Asylum Seeking Children in the UK*, London: DfES.

Help the Aged (1996) *Bereavement*, advice leaflet, 207–21 Pentonville Road, London N1 9UZ, 0207 278 1114.

Hemmings, P. (1995) 'Social work intervention with bereaved children', *Journal of Social Work Practice*, **9**(2): 109–30.

Herbert, M. (1987a) *Conduct Disorders of Childhood and Adolescence: A Social Learning Perspective*, 2nd edn, Chichester: Wiley.

Herbert, M. (1987b) *Behavioural Treatment of Children with Problems: A Practice Manual*, 2nd edn, London: Academic Press.

Herbert, M. and Harper-Dorton, K.V. (2002) *Working with Children, Adolescents and their Families*, 3rd edn, Oxford: BPS-Blackwell.

Heritage, J. (1983) 'Accounts in action', in G. Gilbert and P. Abell (eds) *Accounts and Action*, London: Gower.

Hester, M., Kelly, L. and Radford, J. (eds) (1996) *Women, Violence and Male Power*, Buckingham: Open University Press.

Hick, S. and Pozzuto, R. (2005) 'Introduction: towards "becoming" a critical social worker', in S. Hick, J. Fook and R. Pozzuto (eds) *Social Work: A Critical Turn*, Toronto: Thompson.

Hick, S., Fook, J. and Pozzuto, R. (eds) (2005) *Social Work: A Critical Turn*, Toronto: Thompson.

Hill Collins, P. (2000) *Black Feminist Thought: Knowledge, Consciousness, and the Politics of Empowerment*, 2nd edn, Routledge: London.

Hill, M. (2000) 'Social services and social security', in M. Hill (ed.) *Local Authority Social Services: An Introduction*, Oxford: Blackwell.

Hill, M. and Tisdall, K. (1997) *Children and Society*, New York: Longman.

Hill, S. (1999) *African American Children: Socialization and Development in Families*, Newport, CA: Sage.

Hinkson, M. (2007) 'Introduction: in the name of the child', in J. Altman and M. Hinkson (eds) *Coercive Reconciliation: Stabilise, Normalise, Exit Aboriginal Australia*, North Carlton: Arena.

Hinselwood, R.D. (1998) 'Creatures of each other: some historical considerations of responsibility and care, and some present undercurrents', in A. Foster and V. Roberts (eds) *Managing Mental Health in the Community: Chaos and Containment*, London: Routledge.

HM Government (2008) *Putting People First: A Shared Vision and Commitment to the Transformation of Adult Social Care*, London: TSO.

Hochschild, A.R. (1975) 'Disengagement theory: a critique and proposal', *American Sociological Review*, **40**: 553–69.

Hoge, S., Lidz, C., Mulvey, E. et al. (1993) 'Patients, family and staff perceptions of coercion in mental hospital admission: an exploratory study', *Behavioural Sciences and the Law*, **11**: 281–93.

Holdsworth, D. (1994) 'Accountability: the obligation to lay oneself open to criticism', in R. Chadwick (ed.) *Ethics and Professions*, Aldershot: Avebury.

Holland, S. (2000) 'The assessment relationship: interactions between social workers and parents in child protection assessments', *British Journal of Social Work*, **30**: 149–63.

Holland, S. and Scourfield, J. (2004) 'Liberty and respect in child protection', *British Journal of Social Work*, **34**(1): 21–36.

Hollin, C.R. and Trower, P. (eds) (1986) *Handbook of Social Skills Training*, vol. 1, Oxford: Pergamon.

Hollin, C.R., Epps, K.J. and Kendrick, A.J. (1995) *Managing Behavioural Treatment*, London: Routledge.

Hollis, F. (1972) *Casework: A Psychosocial Therapy*, 2nd edn, New York: Random House.

Holloway, M. (2007) *Negotiating Death in Contemporary Health and Social Care*, Bristol: Policy Press.

Holloway, M. and Lymbery, M. (2007) 'Editorial – caring for people: social work with adults in the next decade and beyond', *British Journal of Social Work*, **37**(3): 375–86.

Holman, B. (1983) *Resourceful Friends: Skills in Community Social Work*, London: Children's Society.

Holman, B. (1993) *A New Deal for Social Welfare*, Oxford: Lion Publishing.

Home Office (1997) *No More Excuses: A New Approach to Tackling Youth Crime in England and Wales*, White Paper, London: TSO.

Home Office (1999) *Supporting Families*, London: TSO.

Home Office (2000a) *What Works: First Report from the Joint Prison Probation Accreditation Panel*, www.homeoffice.gov.uk.

Home Office (2000b) *Report of the Policy Action Team 12: Young People*, London: HMSO.

Home Office (annual) *Criminal Statistics for England and Wales*, London: Home Office.

hooks, b. (1981) *Ain't I a Woman: Black Women and Feminism*, London: Pluto Press.

hooks, b. (1984a) 'Feminism: a movement to end sexist oppression', in A. Philips (ed.) *Feminism and Equality*, Oxford: Blackwell.

hooks, b. (1984b) *Feminist Theory: From Margin to Center*, Boston: South End Press.

hooks, b. (1989) *Talking Back: Thinking Feminist, Thinking Black*, Boston: South End Press.

hooks, b. (1991) *Yearning: Race, Gender and Cultural Politics*, London: Turnaround.

hooks, b. (1994) *Teaching to Transgress: Education as the Practice of Freedom*, Routledge: London.

Hope, M. and Chapman, T. (1998) *Evidence Based Practice: A Guide to Effective Practice*, London: Home Office.

Horkheimer, M. (1978) 'The authoritarian state', in A. Arato and E. Gebhardt (eds) *The Essential Frankfurt School Reader*, Oxford: Blackwell.

Hough, G. and Briskman, L. (2003) 'Responding to the changing socio-political context of practice', in J. Allan, B. Pease and L. Briskman (eds) *Critical Social Work: An Introduction to Theories and Practices*, Sydney: Allen & Unwin.

Houston, G. (1984) *The Red Book of Groups*, London: Rochester Foundation.

Howe, D. (1987) *An Introduction to Social Work Theory, Community Care Practice Handbook*, Aldershot: Arena.

Howe, D. (1993) *On Being a Client: Understanding the Process of Counselling and Psychotherapy*, London: Sage.

Howe, D. (1994) 'Modernity, postmodernity and social work', *British Journal of Social Work*, **24**(5): 513–32.

Howe, D. (1995) *Attachment Theory for Social Work Practice*, Basingstoke: Macmillan – now Palgrave Macmillan.

Howe, D. (1996) 'Relating theory to practice', in M. Davies (ed.) *Blackwell Companion to Social Work*, Oxford: Blackwell.

Howe, D. (2005) *Child Abuse and Neglect: Attachment, Development and Intervention*, Basingstoke: Palgrave Macmillan.

Howe, D. (2008) *The Emotionally Intelligent Social Worker*, Basingstoke: Palgrave Macmillan.

Howe, D., Brandon, M., Hinings, D. and Schofield, G. (1999) *Attachment Theory, Child Maltreatment and Family Support*, Basingstoke: Macmillan – now Palgrave Macmillan.

HREOC (Human Rights and Equal Opportunity Commission) (1997) *Bringing Them Home: Report of the National Inquiry into the Separa-tion of Aboriginal and Islander Children from their Families*, Sydney: HREOC.

Hudson, A. (1992) 'The child sex abuse "industry" and gender relations in social work', in M. Langan and L. Day (eds) *Women, Oppression and Social Work: Issues in Anti-discriminatory Practice*, London: Routledge.

Hudson, B.L. (1982) *Social Work with Psychiatric Patients*, London: Macmillan – now Palgrave Macmillan.

Hudson, B.L. and Macdonald, G. (1986) *Behavioural Social Work: An Introduction*, London: Macmillan – now Palgrave Macmillan.

Huggins, J. (1998) *Sister Girl: The Writings of an Aboriginal Activist and Historian*, Brisbane, University of Queensland Press.

Hugman, R. (1991) *Power in Caring Professions*, Basingstoke: Macmillan – now Palgrave Macmillan.

Humphreys, C., Akhtar, S. and Baldwin, N. (1999) 'Discrimination in child protection work: recurring themes in work with Asian families', *Child and Family Social Work*, **4**: 283–91.

Humphries, B. (ed.) (1996) *Critical Perspectives on Empowerment*, Birmingham: Venture.

Humphries, B. (2004) 'Refugees, asylum seekers and social work' in D. Hayes and B. Humphries (eds) *Social Work, Immigration and Asylum: Debates, Dilemmas and Ethical Issues for Social Work and Social Care Practice*, London: Jessica Kingsley.

Humphries, B. (2005) 'From margin to centre: shifting the emphasis of social work research', in R. Adams, L. Dominelli and M. Payne (eds) *Social Work Futures: Crossing Boundaries, Transforming Practice*, Basingstoke: Palgrave Macmillan.

Huxley, P. (1993) 'Case management and care management in community care', *British Journal of Social Work*, **23**: 365–81.

Ife, J. (1997) *Rethinking Social Work: Towards a Critical Practice*, Melbourne: Longman.

Ife, J. (2001) *Human Rights and Social Work: Towards Rights-based Practice*, Cambridge: Cambridge University Press.

IFSW (International Federation of Social Work) (2004) *Ethics in Social Work, Statement of Principles*, www.ifsw.org/en/p38000324.html.

Indigenous Social Justice Association (2003) 'Deaths in custody: an Aboriginal inquisition', *Djadi-Dugarang*, **5**(1): 1–32.

Inman, K. (1998) 'Generation eggs', *Community Care*, 26 November–2 December: 29.

Ironside, V. (1996) *You'll Get Over It: The Rage of Bereavement*, Harmondsworth: Penguin.

Iwaniec, D. (1995) *The Emotionally Abused and Neglected Child: Identification, Assessment and Intervention*, Chichester: Wiley.

Iwaniec, I., Herbert, M. and McNeish, A.S. (1985a) 'Assessment and treatment of failure-to-thrive children and their families: Part I. Psychosocial factors', *British Journal of Social Work*, **15**: 243–59.

Iwaniec, I., Herbert, M. and McNeish, A.S. (1985b) 'Social work with failure-to-thrive children and their families: Part II. Behavioural social work intervention', *British Journal of Social Work*, **15**: 375–98.

Ixer, G. (1999) 'There's no such thing as reflection', *British Journal of Social Work*, **29**(4): 523–37.

Jackson, M., Kolody, B. and Wood, J.L. (1982) 'To be old and black: the case for double jeopardy on income and health', in R.C. Manuel (ed.) *Minority Ageing*, Westport, CT: Greenwood Press.

Jackson, S. (1998) 'Looking after children: a new approach or just an exercise in form filling? A response to Knight and Caveney', *British Journal of Social Work*, **28**: 45–56.

Jackson, S. and Thomas, N. (1999) *On the Move Again? What Works in Creating Stability for Looked After Children*, Ilford: Barnardo's.

Jackson, S., Fisher, M., and Ward, H. (2000) 'Key concepts in looking after children: parenting, partnership, outcomes', in DoH, *A Child's World*, London: HMSO.

Jacobs, M. (2004) *Psychodynamic Counselling in Action*, 3rd edn, London: Sage.

Jacobson, A. and Richardson, B. (1987) 'Assault experiences of 100 psychiatric inpatients: evidence of the need for routine inquiry', *American Journal of Psychiatry*, **144**: 908–13.

James, A. (1994) *Managing to Care: Public Service and the Market*, London: Longman.

James, A. and James, A.L. (2004) *Constructing Childhood: Theory, Policy and Practice*, Basingstoke: Palgrave Macmillan.

James, A. and Prout, A. (eds) (1997) *Constructing and Reconstructing Childhood: Contemporary Issues in the Sociological Study of Childhood*, 2nd edn, London: Routledge.

James, S.M. and Busia, A.P. (eds) (1993) *Theorizing Black Feminisms: The Visionary Pragmatism of Black Women*, Routledge: London.

Jaspers, M. (2003) *Beginning Reflective Practice*, Cheltenham: Nelson Thornes.

Jehu, D. (1967) *Learning Theory and Social Work*, London: Routledge & Kegan Paul.

John Baptiste, A. (2001) 'Appropriateness of social work practice with communities of African origins', in L. Dominelli, W. Lorenz and H. Soydan (eds) *Beyond Racial Divides: Ethnicities in Social Work Practice*, Aldershot: Ashgate.

Johnstone, D. (2001) *An Introduction to Disability Studies*, 2nd edn, London: David Fulton.

Jokinen, A., Juhila, K. and Pösö, T. (eds) (1999) *Constructing Social Work Practices*, Aldershot: Ashgate.

Jones, A. and May, J. (1992) *Working in Human Service Organisations*, Melbourne: Longman.

Jones, A. and Waul, D. (2005) 'Residential care for black children', in D. Crimmens and I. Milligan (eds) *Facing Forward: Residential Child Care in the 21st Century*, Lyme Regis: Russell House Publishing.

Jones, C., Ferguson, I., Lavalette, M. and Penketh, L. (2004) *Social Work and Social Justice: A Manifesto for a New Engaged Practice*, Liverpool: University of Liverpool, www.liv.ac.uk/ssp/Social_Work_Manifesto.html.

Jones, K., Cooper, B. and Ferguson, H. (2008a) 'Concluding reflections on the nature and future of critical best practice', in K. Jones, B. Cooper and H. Ferguson (eds) *Best Practice in Social Work: Critical Perspectives*, Basingstoke: Palgrave Macmillan.

Jones, K., Cooper, B. and Ferguson, H. (eds) (2008b) *Best Practice in Social Work: Critical Perspectives*, Basingstoke: Palgrave Macmillan.

Jones, K., Cooper, B. and Ferguson, H. (2008c) 'Introducing critical best practice in social work', in K. Jones, B. Cooper, and H. Ferguson (eds) *Best Practice in Social Work: Critical Perspectives*, Basingstoke: Palgrave Macmillan.

Jones, M.A. (1985) *A Second Chance for Families: Five Years Later: A Follow Up Study of a Program to Prevent Foster Care*, New York: Child Welfare League of America.

Jones, R.L. (ed.) (2004) *Black Psychology*, 4th edn, Berkeley, CA: Cobb & Henry.

Jordan, B. (1990) *Social Work in an Unjust Society*, Hemel Hempstead: Harvester Wheatsheaf.

Jordan, B. (1997) 'Partnership with service users in child protection and family support', in N. Parton (ed.) *Child Protection and Family Support: Tensions, Contradictions and Possibilities*, London: Routledge.

Jordan, B. (2006) 'Well-being: the next revolution in children's services?', *Journal of Children's Services*, **1**: 41–50.

Jordan, B. with Jordan, C. (2000) *Social Work and the Third Way: Tough Love as Social Policy*, London: Sage.

Jordan, J. (1989) *Moving Towards Home: Political Essays*, London: Virago.

Jung, C. (1950) 'On the psychology of the Negro', in W. McGuire (ed.) *Collected Works of Carl Jung*, vol. 18, Princeton, NJ: Princeton University Press.

Katz, A.H. and Bender, E.I. (1976) *The Strength in Us: Self-help Groups in the Modern World*, New York: New Viewpoints/Franklin Watts.

Kelly, L., Regan, I. and Burton, S. (1991) *An Explor-atory Study of the Prevalence of Sexual Abuse in a Sample of 16–21 Year Olds*, London: Poly-technic of North London.

Kemshall, H. (2002) *Risk, Social Policy and Welfare*, Buckingham: Open University Press.

Kemshall, H., Parton, N., Walsh, M. and Waterson, J. (1997) 'Concepts of risk in relation to organi-sational structure and functioning within the personal social services and probation', *Social Policy and Administration*, **31**(3): 213–32.

Khan, P. and Dominelli, L. (2000) 'The impact of globalization on social work in the UK', *Euro-pean Journal of Social Work*, **3**(2): 95–108.

Kingdon, D. (2000) 'Schizophrenia and mood (affective) disorder', in D. Bailey (ed.) *At the Core of Mental Health Practice: Key Issues for Practitioners, Managers and Mental Health Trainers*, Brighton: Pavilion.

Kirby, P., Lanyon, C., Cronin, K. and Sinclair, R. (2003a) *Building a Culture of Participation: Involving Children and Young People in Policy, Service Planning, Delivery and Evaluation*, Research Report, London: DfES.

Kirby, P., Lanyon, C., Cronin, K. and Sinclair, R. (2003b) *Building a Culture of Participation: Involving Children and Young People in Policy, Service Planning, Delivery and Evaluation*, The Handbook, London: DfES.

Klein, R. (1989) *The Exploitation of Our Desire: Women's Experiences with In Vitro Fertilisation*, paper presented at the Women's Studies Summer Institute, Deakin University, Victoria, Australia.

Krueger, R. (1994) *Focus Groups: A Practical Guide for Applied Research*, Newbury Park, CA: Sage.

Krumer-Nevo, M. (2003) 'From a coalition of despair to a covenant of help in social work with families in distress', *European Journal of Social Work*, **6**(3): 273–82.

Kübler-Ross, E. (1970) *On Death and Dying*, London: Tavistock.

Kurland, R. and Salmon, R. (1993) 'Groupwork versus casework in a group', *Groupwork*, **6**(1): 5–16.

Laming, H. (2003) *Inquiry into the Death of Victo-ria Climbié*, London: TSO.

Langan, M. (2002) 'The legacy of radical social work', in R. Adams, L. Dominelli and M. Payne (eds) *Social Work: Themes, Issues and Critical Debates*, 2nd edn, Basingstoke: Palgrave Macmillan.

Langan, M. and Lee, P. (1989) 'Whatever happened to radical social work?', in M. Langan and P. Lee (eds) *Radical Social Work Today*, London: Unwin Hyman.

Law Commission (1997) *Who Decides? Making Decisions on Behalf of Mentally Incapacitated Adults*, London: HMSO.

Leadbetter, D. (2002) 'Anger Management', in M. Davies (ed.) *The Blackwell Companion to Social Work*, Oxford: Blackwell.

Leader, A. (1995) *Direct Power: A Resource Pack for People who Want to Develop Their own Care Plans and Support Networks*, London: Commu-nity Support Network/Brixton Community Sanctuary/Pavilion Publishing/MIND.

Leavey, G., King, M., Cole, E. et al. (1997) 'First-onset psychotic illness: patients' and relatives' satisfaction with services', *British Journal of Psychiatry*, **170**: 53–7.

Lee, J. (1994) *The Empowerment Approach to Social Work Practice*, New York: Columbia University Press.

Leff, J. and Trieman, N. (2000) 'Long-stay patients discharged from psychiatric hospitals: social and clinical outcomes after 5 years in the community', TAPS project 46, *British Journal of Psychiatry*, **176**: 217–23.

Leff, J., Dayson, D., Gooch, C. et al. (1996a) 'Quality of life of long-stay patients discharged from two psychiatric institutions', *Psychiatric Services*, **47**(1): 62–7.

Leff, J., Trieman, N. and Gooch, C. (1996b) 'TAPS project 33: prospective follow-up study of long-stay patients discharged from two psychiatric hospitals', *American Journal of Psychiatry*, **153**(10): 1318–24.

Leonard, P. (1984) *Personality and Ideology: Towards a Materialist Theory of the Individual*, London: Macmillan – now Palgrave Macmillan.

Leonard, P. (1995) 'Towards a paradigm for radical practice', in R. Bailey and M. Brake (eds) *Radical Social Work*, London: Edward Arnold.

Leonard, P. (1997) *Postmodern Welfare: Reconstruct-ing an Emancipatory Project*, London: Sage.

Levitt, A., Hogan, T. and Bucosky, C. (1990) 'Quality of life in chronically mentally ill patients in day treatment', *Psychological Medi-cine*, **20**: 703–10.

Levy, A. and Kahan, B. (1991) *The Pindown Experi-ence and the Protection of Children*, Stafford: Staffordshire County Council.

Lewis, J. (1996) 'The paradigm shift in the deliv-ery of public services and the crisis of professionalism', in R. Adams (ed.) *Crisis in the Human Services: National and Interna-tional Issues. Selected Conference Papers*, Kingston upon Hull: University of Lincoln-shire and Humberside.

Lewis, J. (2001) 'Older people and the health-social care boundary in the UK: half a century of hidden policy conflict', *Social Policy and Administration*, **35**(4): 343–59.

Lewis, J. and Glennerster, H. (1996) *Implementing the New Community Care*, Buckingham: Open University Press.

Lishman, J. (1998) 'Personal and professional development', in R. Adams, L. Dominelli and M. Payne (eds) *Social Work: Themes, Issues and Critical Debates,* Basingstoke: Macmillan – now Palgrave Macmillan.

Littlewood, J. (1993) 'The denial of death and rites of passage in contemporary societies', in Clark, D. (ed.) *The Sociology of Death,* Oxford: Blackwell.

Lloyd, L. (2004) 'Mortality and morality: ageing and the ethic of care', *Ageing and Society,* **24**: 235–56.

Lloyd, M. (1997) 'Dying and bereavement, spirituality and social work in a market economy of welfare', *British Journal of Social Work,* **27**: 175–90.

Lloyd, M. (2000) 'Where has all the care management gone? The challenge of Parkinson's disease to the health and social care interface', *British Journal of Social Work,* **30**: 737–54.

Lloyd, M. and Smith, M. (1998) *Assessment and Service Provision under the New Community Care Arrangements for People with Parkinson's Disease and their Carers,* Research Report No. 13, Manchester: University of Manchester.

Locke, J. (1924) *Two Treatises of Government,* London: J.M. Dent.

London to Edinburgh Weekend Return Group (1980) *In and Against the State,* London: Pluto.

Loney, M. (1983) *Community Against Government: The British Community Development Projects, 1968–1978: A Study of Government Incompetence,* London: Heinemann.

Long, C.G., Williams, M. and Hollin, C.R. (1998) 'Treating alcohol problems: a study of programme effectiveness and cost effectiveness according to length and delivery of treatment', *Addiction,* **93**(4): 561–71.

Looney, J. (1988) 'Ego development and black identity', *Journal of Black Psychology,* **15**(1): 41–56.

Lorde, A. (1984) *Sister Outsider,* New York: The Crossing Press.

Lukes, S. (2005) *Power: A Radical View,* 2nd edn, Basingstoke: Palgrave Macmillan.

Lundy, C. (2004) *Social Work and Social Justice: A Structural Approach to Practice,* Peterborough, ON: Broadview Press.

Lymbery, M. (2004) *Social Work Ideals and Practice Realities: An Introduction,* Basingstoke: Palgrave Macmillan.

Lymbery, M. (2005) *Social Work with Older People: Context, Policy and Practice,* London: Sage.

Lymbery, M. and Butler, S. (eds) (2004) *Social Work Ideals and Practice Realities,* Basingstoke: Palgrave Macmillan.

Lynn, R. and Pye, R. (1990) 'Anti-racist welfare education: pie in the sky?', in J. Petruchenia and R. Thorpe (eds) *Social Change and Social Welfare Practice,* Sydney: Hale & Iremonger.

Lyotard, J.F. (1984) *The Postmodern Condition: A Report on Knowledge,* Manchester: Manchester University Press.

McBeath, G. and Webb, S. (2005) 'Post critical social work analytics', in S. Hick, J. Fook and R. Pozzuto (eds) *Social Work: A Critical Turn,* Toronto: Thompson.

McBrian, J. and Felce, D. (1992) *Working with People who Have a Severe Learning Difficulty and Challenging Behaviour: A Practice Manual,* Clevedon: British Institute for Learning Disabilities.

McDonald, A., Postle, K. and Dawson, C. (2007) 'Barriers to retaining and using professional knowledge in local authority social work practice with adults in the UK', *British Journal of Social Work,* Advance Access, 25 April, doi:10.1093/bjsw/bcm042.

McDonald, C. (2006) *Challenging Social Work: The Context of Practice,* Basingstoke: Palgrave Macmillan.

Macdonald, G. (1994) 'Developing empirically-based practice in probation', *British Journal of Social Work,* **24**: 405–27.

Macdonald, G. (2001) *Effective Interventions for Child Abuse and Neglect,* Chichester: Wiley.

Macdonald, G., Sheldon, B. with Gillespie, J. (1992) 'Contemporary studies of the effectiveness of social work', *British Journal of Social Work,* **22**: 615–43.

McGlone, F., Park, A. and Smith, K. (1998) *Families and Kinship,* York: Joseph Rowntree Foundation.

McGrath, A. (1995) *Contested Ground: Australian Aborigines under the British Crown,* Sydney: Allen & Unwin.

McGuire, J. (ed.) (1995) *What Works: Reducing Reoffending: Guidelines from Research and Practice,* Chichester: Wiley.

McGuire, J. (2000) *Cognitive Behavioural Approaches: An Introduction to Theory and Research,* London: Home Office.

McLaughlin, E. and Muncie, J. (1994) 'Managing the criminal justice system', in J. Clarke, A. Cochrane and E. McLaughlin (eds) *Managing Social Policy,* London: Sage.

McLean, L. (1996) 'Forced removal of children: an Australian Holocaust', *The Age,* (28 May): 4.

McLeod, A. (2007) 'Whose agenda? Issues of power and relationship when listening to looked after children', *Child and Family Social Work,* **12**: 287–6.

McLeod, J. (2003) *An Introduction to Counselling,* 3rd edn, Maidenhead: Open University Press.

McLoughlin, J. and Pinkerton, J. (1996) 'Ethical dilemmas in practice: some thoughts on the Children (NI) Order', *Child Care in Practice,* **1**(4): 40–51.

McMurran, M. and Hollin, C.R. (1993) *Young Offenders and Alcohol-related Crime,* Chichester: Wiley.

McNamee, S. and Gergen, K. (eds) (1999) *Relational Responsibility: Resources for Sustainable Dialogue*, London: Sage.

McTaggart, R. (1999) 'Reflection on the purposes of research, action and scholarship: a case of cross-cultural participatory action research', *Systemic Practice and Action Research*, **12**(5): 493–511.

McWilliams, W. (1992) 'The rise and development of management thought in the English probation system', in R. Statham and P. Whitehead (eds) *Managing the Probation Service: Issues for the 1990s*, Harlow: Longman.

Maguire, N. (2006) 'Cognitive-behavioural therapy and homelessness: a case series pilot study', *Behavioural and Cognitive Psychotherapy*, **34**: 113–18.

Mama, A. (1995) *Beyond the Masks*, London: Routledge.

Mama, A. (1996) *The Hidden Struggle: Statutory and Voluntary Sector Responses to Violence against Black Women in the Home*, 2nd edn, London: Whiting & Birch.

Manthorpe, J., Moriarty, J., Rapaport, J. et al. (2007) '"There are wonderful social workers but it's a lottery": older people's views about social workers', *British Journal of Social Work*, advance access, 9 February, doi:10.1093.

Marchant, H. and Wearing, B. (eds) (1986) *Gender Reclaimed: Women in Social Work*, Sydney: Hale & Iremonger.

Marcuse, H. (1964) *One-dimensional Man*, London: Paladin.

Margolin, L. (1997) *Under the Cover of Kindness: The Invention of Social Work*, Charlottesville, VA: University Press of Virginia.

Marks, B., Settles, I.H., Cooke, D.Y. et al. (2004) 'African American racial identity: a review of contemporary models and measures', in R.L. Jones (ed.) *Black Psychology*, 4th edn, Berkeley, CA: Cobb & Henry.

Marsh P. (2008) 'Engaging children, young people and their families via family group conferences', in M. Calder (ed.) *The Carrot or the Stick? Toward Effective Practice with Involuntary Clients in Safeguarding Children Work*, Lyme Regis: Russell House Publishing.

Marsh, P. and Crow, G. (1998) *Family Group Conferences in Child Welfare*, Oxford: Blackwell.

Marsh, P. and Doel, M. (2006) *The Task-Centred Book*, London: Routledge/Community Care.

Marsh, P. and Fisher, M. (1992) *Good Intentions: Developing Partnership in Social Services*, York: Joseph Rowntree Foundation/Community Care.

Marsh, P. and Triseliotis, J. (1996) 'Social workers: their training and first year in work', in N. Connelly (ed.) *Training Social Services Staff: Evidence From New Research*, report of a conference, Research in Social Work Education No. 4, London: NISW.

Marston, G. (2003) *Temporary Protection Permanent Uncertainty: The Experience of Refugees Living on Temporary Protection Visas*, Melbourne: Centre for Applied Social Research, RMIT University.

Martin, G., Phelps, K. and Katbamna, S. (2004) 'Human motivation and professional practice: of knights, knaves and social workers', *Social Policy and Administration*, **38**(5): 470–87.

Martin, J. (2003) 'Historical development of critical social work practice', in J. Allan, B. Pease and L. Briskman (eds) *Critical Social Work: An Introduction to Theories and Practice*, Sydney: Allen & Unwin.

Martyn, H. (ed.) (2001) *Developing Reflective Practice: Making Sense of Social Work in a World of Change*, Bristol: Policy Press.

Marx, K. (1972) *Selected Writings*, ed. D. McClennan, Oxford: Oxford University Press.

Mason, J. and Fattore, T. (eds) (2005) *Children Taken Seriously: In Theory, Policy and Practice*, London: Jessica Kingsley.

Massey, D. (1995) 'Imagining the world', in D. Massey and J. Allen (eds) *Geographical Worlds*, Oxford: Oxford University Press.

Matahaere-Atariki, D., Bertanees, C. and Hoffman, L. (2001) 'Anti-oppressive practices in a colonial context', in M. Connolly (ed.) *New Zealand Social Work: Contexts and Practice*, Auckland: Oxford University Press.

Matthews, S., Harvey, A. and Trevithick, P. (2003) 'Surviving the swamp: using cbt in a social work setting', *Journal of Social Work Practice*, **17**: 177–85.

Mattinson, J. (1975) *The Reflection Process in Casework Supervision*, London: Institute of Marital Studies.

Maxime, J. (1986) 'Some psychological models of black self-concept', in S. Ahmed, J. Cheetham and J. Small (eds) *Social Work with Black Children and their Families*, London: Batsford.

Maxime, J. (1993) 'The therapeutic importance of racial identity in working with black children who hate', in V. Varma (ed.) *How and Why Children Hate*, London: Jessica Kingsley.

Mayer, J.E. and Timms, N. (1970) *The Client Speaks*, London: Routledge & Kegan Paul.

Mayo, M. (1994a) *Communities and Caring*, Basingstoke: Macmillan – now Palgrave Macmillan.

Mayo, M. (1994b) 'Community work', in C. Hanvey and T. Philpot (eds) *Practising Social Work*, London: Routledge.

Mayo, M. (2000) *Cultures, Communities, Identities: Cultural Strategies for Participation and Empowerment*, Basingstoke: Palgrave – now Palgrave Macmillan.

Mayoux, L. (2000) *Micro-finance and the Empowerment of Women: A Review of the Key Issues*, e paper, www.ilo.org/public/english/employment/finance/download/wpap23.pdf.

Mehlbye, J. and Walgrave, L. (1998) *Confronting Youth in Europe*, Copenhagen: AKF.

Meinert, R.G., Pardeck, J.T. and Murphy, J.W. (eds) (1998) *Postmodernism, Religion and the Future of Social Work*, New York: Haworth Press.

Mezirow, J. (1983) 'A critical theory of adult learning and education', in M. Tight (ed.) *Adult Learning and Education*, London: Croom Helm.

Millar, M. (2008) '"Anti-oppressiveness": critical comments on a discourse and its context', *British Journal of Social Work*, **38**(2): 362–75.

Miller, G. (1997) *Becoming Miracle Workers: Language and Meaning in Brief Therapy*, New York: Aldine de Gruyter.

Miller, L. (2006) *Counselling Skills for Social Work*, London: Sage.

Millett, K. (1972) *Sexual Politics*, London: Abacus.

Mills, M. (1999) 'Using the narrative in dementia care', in J. Bornat (ed.) *Biographical Interviews: The Link Between Research and Practice*, London: Centre for Policy on Ageing.

Milner, J. (2001) *Women and Social Work: Narrative Approaches*, Basingstoke: Palgrave – now Palgrave Macmillan.

Minajalku Aboriginal Corporation (1997) *Home Still Waiting*, Melbourne: Minajalku.

Ministry of Justice (2008) *The Public Law Outline*, London: Ministry of Justice.

Mirza, H.S. (1992) *Young, Female and Black*, London: Routledge.

Mirza, H.S (ed.) (1997) *Black British Feminism: A Reader*, Routledge: London.

Mitchell, J. (1974) *Feminism and Psychoanalysis*, London: Allen Lane.

Modood, T. (2007) *Multiculturalism: A Civic Idea*. Cambridge: Polity Press.

Monroe, B. (1998) 'Social work in palliative care', in D. Doyle, G. Hanks and N. MacDonald (eds) *The Oxford Textbook of Palliative Medicine*, 2nd edn, Oxford: Oxford University Press.

Monroe, B. and Oliviere, D. (eds) (2003) *Patient Participation in Palliative Care: A Voice for the Voiceless*, Oxford: Oxford University Press.

Monroe, B. and Oliviere, D. (eds) (2007) *Resilience and Palliative Care: Achievement in Adversity*, Oxford: Oxford University Press.

Moore, B. (1996) *Risk Assessment: A Practitioners' Guide to Predicting Harmful Behaviour*, London: Whiting & Birch.

Moore, O. (1996) *PWA: Looking AIDS in the Face*, London: Picador.

Moreau, M. (1979) 'A structural approach to social work practice', *Canadian Journal of Social Work Education*, **5**(1): 78–94.

Morgan, D. (1988) *Focus Groups as Qualitative Research*, London: Sage.

Morgan, S. (1999) *Assessing and Managing Risk: A Training Pack for Practitioners and Managers of Comprehensive Mental Health Services*, Brighton: Pavilion.

Morgans, D. (2007) 'Beyond practice and beyond theory?', in S.R. Smith (ed.) *Applying Theory to Policy and Practice: Issues for Critical Reflection*, Aldershot: Ashgate.

Morris, J. (1991) *Pride Against Prejudice: Transforming Attitudes to Disability*, London: Women's Press.

Morris, J. (1993) 'Feminism and disability', *Feminist Review*, **43**: 57–70.

Morris, J. (1996) 'Gender and disability', in J. Wain, V. Finkelstein, S. French and M. Oliver (eds) *Disabling Barriers: Enabling Environments*, London: Sage/Open University.

Morris, K. (2007) *An Evaluation of Camden FGC Service*, London: London Borough of Camden.

Morris, K. and Burford, G. (2006) 'Working with children's networks: building opportunities for change?', *Social Policy and Society*, **6**: 209–19.

Morris, K. and Shepherd, C. (2000) 'Quality social work with children and families', *Social Work*, **5**: 169–176.

Morris, K., Hughes, N., Clarke, H. et al. (2008) *Think Family: A Literature Review of Whole Family Approaches*, London: Social Exclusion Task Force/Cabinet Office.

Morrison, T. (1987) *Beloved*, London: Picador.

Morrow, V. (1998) *Understanding Families: Children's Perspectives*, London: National Children's Bureau.

Moss, P. and Petrie, P. (2002) *From Children's Services to Children's Spaces*, London: Routledge.

Mulkay, M. and Ernst, J. (1991) 'The changing profile of social death', *Archives of European Sociology*, **32**: 172–96.

Mullaly, B. (2002) *Challenging Oppression: A Critical Social Work Approach*, Toronto: Oxford University Press.

Mullaly, B. (2007) *The New Structural Social Work*, Don Mills, Ontario: Oxford University Press.

Mullender, A. (1996) *Rethinking Domestic Violence: The Social Work and Probation Response*, London: Routledge.

Mullender, A. and Ward, D. (1991) *Self-directed Groupwork: Users Take Action for Empowerment*, London: Whiting & Birch.

Muncie, J. (1999) *Youth and Crime: A Critical Introduction*, London: Sage.

Munro, E. (2002) *Effective Child Protection*, London: Sage.

Munro, E. (2004) 'The impact of audit on social work practice', *British Journal of Social Work*, 34(8): 1075–95.

Napier, L. (2003) 'Palliative care social work', in B. Monroe and D. Oliviere (eds) *Patient Participation in Palliative Care: A Voice for the Voiceless*, Oxford: Oxford University Press.

NAPO (National Association of Probation Officers) (1990) 'Working with women: an anti-sexist approach', in Probation Practice Committee (ed.) *Practice Guidelines*, London: NAPO.

NASW (National Association of Social Workers) (1996) *Code of Ethics*, Washington: NASW.

National Foster Care Association (1994) *Safe Caring*, London: National Foster Care Association.

National Foster Care Association UK Joint Working Party on Foster Care (1999a) *Code of Practice on the Recruitment, Assessment, Approval, Training, Management and Support of Foster Carers*, London: National Foster Care Association.

National Foster Care Association UK Joint Working Party on Foster Care (1999b) *UK National Standards for Foster Care*, London: National Foster Care Association.

National Offender Management Service (2006) *The NOMS Offender Management Model*, London: Home Office.

National Statistics (2008) www.statistics.gov.uk/cci/nugget.asp?id=167&Pos=1&ColRank=1&Rank=192.

National Urban League (1964) *Double Jeopardy: the Older Negro in America Today*, New York: National Urban League.

Neale-Hurston, Z. (1986) *Their Eyes were Watching God*, London: Virago.

Neimeyer, R. (ed) (2001) *Meaning Reconstruction and the Experience of Loss*, Washington, DC: American Psychological Association.

Nellis, M. (2000) 'Taking oppression seriously: a critique of managerialism in social work/probation', in I., Paylor, L. Froggett and J. Harris (eds) *Reclaiming Social Work: The Southport Papers*, vol. 2, Birmingham: Venture Press.

Newburn, T. (1993) *Disaster and After*, London: Jessica Kingsley.

Newburn, T. (1996) 'Some lessons from Hillsborough', in C. Mead (ed.) *Journeys of Discovery: Creative Learning from Disaster*, London: NISW.

Newman, T., Oakley, A. and Roberts, H. (1996) 'Weighing up the evidence', *Guardian*, 10 January: 9.

NISW (National Institute for Social Work) (1996) *Social Exclusion, Civil Society and Social Work*, Policy Briefings No. 18, London: NISW.

Nixon, S. (2000) 'Safe care, abuse and allegations of abuse in foster care', in G. Kelly and R. Gilligan (eds) *Issues in Foster Care: Policy, Practice and Research*, London: Jessica Kingsley.

Nocon, A. and Qureshi, H. (1996) *Outcomes of Community Care for Users and Carers: A Social Services Perspective*, Buckingham: Open University Press.

Noel, L. (1994) *Intolerance: A General Survey*, Montreal: McGill-Queen's.

Nolan, M., Grant, G. and Keady, J. (1996) *Understanding Family Care*, Buckingham: Open University Press.

Nutt, L. (2006) *The Lives of Foster Carers: Private Sacrifices, Public Restrictions*, London: Routledge.

O'Brien, J. (1981) *The Principle of Normalisation*, London: Campaign for Mental Health.

O'Hagan, K. (2001) *Cultural Competence in the Caring Professions*, London: Jessica Kingsley.

O'Hanlon, B. (1993) 'Possibility theory', in S. Gilligan and R. Price (eds) *Therapeutic Conversations*, New York: Norton.

O'Hanlon, B. and Beadle, S. (1994) *A Field Guide to Possibility Land*, Omaha, NE: Possibility Press.

O'Hanlon, B. and Weiner-Davis, M. (1989) *In Search of Solutions*, New York: Norton.

O'Keefe, M., Hills, A., Doyle, M. et al. (2007) *UK Study of Abuse and Neglect of Older People*, prevalence survey report, London: National Centre for Social Research.

O'Sullivan, T. (1999) *Decision Making in Social Work*, Basingstoke: Macmillan – now Palgrave Macmillan.

Oakley, A. (1999) 'People's ways of knowing: gender and methodology', in S. Hood, B. Mayal and S. Oliver (eds) *Critical Issues in Social Research: Power and Prejudice*, Buckingham: Open University Press.

Oldham, F. (2002) *Supporting and Enhancing Learning through the Use of Reflective Journals in an MBA Programme*, Edinburgh: Napier University Business School.

Oliver, J. and Hudson, B. (1998) 'Behavioural work, crisis intervention and the mental health call-out', in K. Cigno and D. Bourn (eds) *Cognitive-behavioural Social Work in Practice*, Aldershot: Ashgate.

Oliver, J., Huley, P. and Butler, A. (1989) *Mental Health Casework: Illuminations and Reflections*, Manchester: Manchester University Press.

Oliver, M. (1990) *The Politics of Disablement*, London: Macmillan – now Palgrave Macmillan.

Oliver, M.J. (1999) 'Capitalism, disability and ideology: a materialist critique of the normalization principle', in R.J. Flynn and R.A. Lemay (eds) *A Quarter Century of*

Normalization and Social Role Valorization: Evolution and Impact, Ottawa, ON: University of Ottawa Press.

Oliver, M. and Sapey, B. (2006) *Social Work with Disabled People*, 3rd edn, Basingstoke, Palgrave Macmillan.

Oliviere, D., Hargreaves, R. and Monroe, B. (1998) *Good Practices in Palliative Care*, Aldershot: Ashgate.

ONS (Office for National Statistics) (1998) *Mortality Statistics (Registrations), England and Wales*, London: ONS.

Orme, J. (1997) 'Research into practice', in G. McKenzie, J. Powell and R. Usher (eds) *Understanding Research: Perspectives on Methodology and Practice*, Hove: Falmer Press.

Orme, J. (2001) *Gender and Community Care: Social Work and Social Care Perspectives*, Basingstoke: Palgrave – now Palgrave Macmillan.

Orme, J. (2002) 'Social work: gender, care and justice', *British Journal of Social Work*, **32**: 799–814.

Orme, J. (2003) '"It's feminist because I say so!" Feminism, social work and critical practice', *Qualitative Social Work*, **2**(2): 131–53.

Orme, J., Dominelli, L. and Mullender, A. (2000) 'Working with violent men from a feminist social work perspective', *International Social Work*, **43**(1): 89–105.

Paisley, F. (1997) 'Assimilation: a protest as old as the policy', *The Australian*, 5 June.

Parham, T.A. (1989) 'Cycles of psychological nigrescence', *Counseling Psychologist*, **17**(2): 187–226.

Parham, T.A. and Helms, J. (1985) 'Relation of racial identity to self-actualization and affective states of black students', *Journal of Counseling Psychology*, **28**(3): 250–6.

Parker, G. (1993) *With this Body: Caring and Disability in Marriage*, Buckingham: Open University Press.

Parker, G. (1994) *Where Next for Research on Carers?*, Leicester: Leicester University.

Parker, G. and Clarke, H. (2002) 'Making the ends meet: do carers and disabled people have a common agenda?', *Policy and Politics*, **30**(3): 347–59.

Parkes, C.M. (1996) *Bereavement*, 3rd edn, London: Routledge.

Parmar, P. (1981) 'Young Asian women: a critique of the pathological approach', *Multi-racial Education*, **9**(3): 19–29.

Parton, N. (1991) *Governing the Family: Child Care, Child Protection and the State*, Basingstoke: Macmillan – now Palgrave Macmillan.

Parton, N. (1994) 'The nature of social work under conditions of (post)modernity', *Social Work and Social Sciences Review*, **5**(2): 93–112.

Parton, N. (1998a) 'Risk, advanced liberalism and child welfare: the need to rediscover uncertainty and ambiguity', *British Journal of Social Work*, **28**: 5–27.

Parton, N. (1998b) 'Advanced liberalism, (post)modernity and social work: some emerging social configurations', *Social Thought*, **18**(3): 71–88.

Parton, N. (2003) 'Rethinking professional practice: the contribution of social constructionism and the feminist "ethic of care"', *British Journal of Social Work*, **33**: 1–16.

Parton, N. (2005) *Safeguarding Children: Early Intervention and Surveillance in a Late Modern Society*, Basingstoke: Palgrave Macmillan.

Parton, N. and Marshall, W. (1998) 'Postmodernism and discourse approaches to social work', in R. Adams, L. Dominelli and M. Payne (eds) *Social Work: Themes, Issues and Critical Debates*, Basingstoke: Macmillan – now Palgrave Macmillan.

Parton, N. and O'Byrne, P. (2000) *Constructive Social Work: Towards a New Practice*, Basingstoke: Palgrave – now Palgrave Macmillan.

Patel, N. (1990) *A 'Race Against Time?' Social Services Provision to Black Elders*, London: Runnymede Trust.

Patel, N. (ed.) (2003) *Minority Elderly Care in Europe: Country Profiles*, Leeds: PRAIE.

Pawson, R., Boaz, A., Grayson, L. et al. (2003) *Types and Quality of Knowledge in Social Care*, London: SCIE.

Payne, M. (1991) *Modern Social Work Theory: A Critical Introduction*, Basingstoke: Macmillan – now Palgrave Macmillan.

Payne, M. (1992) 'Psychodynamic theory within the politics of social work theory', *Journal of Social Work Practice*, **6**(2): 141–9.

Payne, M. (1995) *Social Work and Community Care*, Basingstoke: Macmillan – now Palgrave Macmillan.

Payne, M. (1998) 'Social work theories and reflective practice', in R. Adams, L. Dominelli and M. Payne (eds) *Social Work: Themes, Issues and Critical Debates*, Basingstoke: Macmillan – now Palgrave Macmillan.

Payne, M. (2005) *Modern Social Work Theory*, 3rd edn, Basingstoke: Palgrave Macmillan.

Payne, M. and Askeland, G.A. (2008) *Globalisation and International Social Work: Postmodern Change and Challenge*, Aldershot: Ashgate.

Pearson, G. (1983) 'The Barclay Report and community social work: Samuel Smiles revisited?', *Critical Social Policy*, **2**: 73–86.

Pearson, G., Treseder, J. and Yelloly, M. (1988) *Social Work and the Legacy of Freud*, London: Macmillan – now Palgrave Macmillan.

Pearson, R.E. (1990) *Counselling and Social Support: Perspectives and Practice,* London: Sage.

Pease, B. (1987) Towards a Socialist Praxis in Social Work, unpublished MA thesis, Melbourne: La Trobe University,

Pease, B. (1990) 'Towards collaborative research on socialist theory and practice in social work', in J. Petrucenia and R. Thorpe (eds) *Social Change and Social Welfare Practice,* Sydney: Hale & Iremonger.

Pease, B. (1996) Reforming Men: Masculine Subjectivities and the Politics and Practices of Profeminism, unpublished PhD thesis, Melbourne: La Trobe University.

Pease, B. (2000) *Recreating Men: Postmodern Masculinity Politics,* London: Sage.

Pease, B. (2002) *Men and Gender Relations,* Melbourne: Tertiary Press.

Pease, B. (2003) 'Rethinking the relationship between the self and society', in J. Allan, B. Pease and L. Briskman (eds) *Critical Social Work: An Introduction to Theories and Practice,* Sydney: Allen & Unwin.

Pease, B. (2006) 'Encouraging critical reflections on privilege in social work and the human services', *Practice Reflexions,* **1**(1): 15–26.

Pease, B. (2007) 'Critical social work theory meets evidence-based practice in Australia: towards critical knowledge-informed practice in social work', in K. Yokota (ed.) *Emancipatory Social Work,* Kyoto: Sekai Shisou-sya.

Pease, B. and Camilleri, P. (2001) *Working with Men in the Human Services,* London: Allen & Unwin.

Pease, B. and Fook, J. (eds) (1999) *Transforming Social Work Practice: Postmodern Critical Perspectives,* Sydney: Allen & Unwin.

Pease, B. and Pringle, K. (eds) (2001) *A Man's World? Changing Men's Practices in a Globalised World,* London: Zed Books.

Pease, B., Allan, J. and Briskman, L. (2003) 'Introducing critical theories of social work', in J. Allan, B. Pease and L. Briskman (eds) *Critical Social Work: An Introduction to Theories and Practices,* Crows Nest, NSW: Allen & Unwin.

Peck, E., Gulliver, P. and Towel, D. (2002) 'Information, consultation or control: user involvement in mental health services at the turn of the century', *Journal of Mental Health,* **11**(4): 441–51.

Penna, S. and O'Brien, M. (1996) 'Postmodernism and social policy: a small step forwards?', *Journal of Social Policy,* **25**(1): 39–61.

Perkins, R. and Repper, J. (1998a) 'Principles of working with people who experience mental health problems', in C. Brooker and J. Repper

(eds) *Serious Mental Health Problems in the Community: Policy, Practice and Research,* London: Baillière Tindall.

Perkins, R. and Repper, J. (1998b) *Dilemmas in Community Mental Health Practice: Choice or Control,* Oxford: Radcliffe Medical Press.

Perlman, H.H. (1957) *Social Casework: a Problem-solving Process,* Chicago: University of Chicago Press.

Perry, B. (2001) *In the Name of Hate: Understanding Hate Crimes,* New York: Routledge.

Peters, A. (1986) 'Main currents in criminological law theory', in J. van Dijk, C. Haffmans, F. Ruter et al. (eds) *Criminal Law in Action,* Arnheim: Gouda Quint.

Peters, M.F. (1985) 'Racial socialization of young black children', in H. McAdoo and J. McAdoo (eds) *Black Children: Social, Educational and Parental Environments,* Newbury Park, CA: Sage.

Phillips, J. (2001) *Groupwork in Social Care: Planning and Setting Up Groups,* London: Jessica Kingsley.

Phillips, J. and Waterson, J. (2002) 'Care management and social work: a case study of the role of social work in hospital discharge to residential and nursing home care', *European Journal of Social Work,* **5**(2): 171–86.

Phillips, J., Ray, M. and Marshall, M. (2006) *Social Work with Older People,* 3rd edn, Basingstoke: Palgrave Macmillan.

Phillipson, J. (1991) *Practising Equality: Women, Men and Social Work,* London: CCETSW.

Phinney, J. (1990) 'Ethnic identity in adolescents and adults: review of research', *Psychological Bulletin,* **108**: 499–514.

Phoenix, J. (2003) 'Re-thinking youth prostitution: national provision at the margins of child protection and youth justice', *Youth Justice,* **3**(3): 152–68.

Physicians for Human Rights and School of Public Health and Primary Health Care (2002) *Dual Loyalty and Human Rights in Health Professional Practice: Proposed Guidelines and Institutional Mechanisms,* Cape Town: University of Cape Town.

Picardie, R. (1998) *Before I Say Goodbye,* London: Penguin.

Pickford, J. (ed.) (2000) *Youth Justice: Theory and Practice,* London: Cavendish.

Pincus, A. and Minahan, A. (1973) *Social Work Practice: Model and Method,* Ithaca, IL: Peacock.

Pinkerton, J. (2000) 'Developing partnership practice', in P. Foley, J. Roche and S. Tucker (eds) *Children in Society: Contemporary Theory, Policy and Practice,* Basingstoke: Palgrave – now Palgrave Macmillan.

Pinkerton, J., Scott, B. and O'Kane, P. (1997) *Partnership Practice with Parents and Carers: An*

Approach to Practitioner Self Evaluation, Belfast: Centre for Child Care Research, Queen's University.

Pitts, J. (2000) 'The new youth justice and the politics of electoral anxiety', in B. Goldson (ed.) *The New Youth Justice*, Lyme Regis: Russell House Publishing.

Pitts, J. and Hope, T. (1998) 'The local politics of inclusion: the state and community safety', in C. Finer and M. Nellis (eds) *Crime and Social Exclusion*, Oxford: Blackwell.

Polack, P. (1993) 'Recovery from mental illness: the guiding vision of the mental health service system in the 1990s', *Psychosocial Rehabilitation Journal*, **16**(4): 11–24.

Popple, K. (1995) *Analysing Community Work: Its Theory and Practice*, Milton Keynes: Open University Press.

Powell, F. (2001) *The Politics of Social Work*, London: Sage.

Powell, J., Robinson, J., Roberts, H. and Thomas, G. (2007) 'The single assessment process in primary care: older people's accounts of the process', *British Journal of Social Work*, **37**(6): 1043–58.

Powers, A. (2007) *City Survivors: Bringing up Children in Disadvantaged Neighbourhoods*, Bristol: Policy Press.

Pozatek, E. (1994) 'The problem of certainty: clinical social work in the post modern era', *Social Work*, **39**(4): 396–403.

Pratchett, L. and Wingfield, M. (1994) *The Public Service Ethos in Local Government*, London: Commission for Local Democracy/Institute of Chartered Secretaries and Administrators.

Preston-Shoot, M. (1987) *Effective Groupwork*, London: Macmillan – now Palgrave Macmillan.

Preston-Shoot, M. (2007) *Effective Groupwork*, 2nd edn, Basingstoke: Palgrave Macmillan.

Price, V. and Simpson, G. (2007) *Transforming Society? Social Work and Sociology*, Bristol: Policy Press.

Priestley, P., McGuire, J., Flegg, D. et al. (1978) *Social Skills and Personal Problem Solving: A Handbook of Methods*, London: Tavistock.

Priestly, M. (2000) 'Dropping "Es": the missing link in quality assurance for disabled people', in A. Brechin, H. Brown and M. Eby (eds) *Critical Practice in Health and Social Care*, London: Sage/Open University.

Prilleltensky, I. and Prilleltensky, O. (2003) 'Towards a critical health psychology practice', *Journal of Health Psychology*, **8**(2): 197–210.

Prout, A. (2005) *The Future of Childhood*, London: Routledge Falmer.

Quinn, A. (1998) 'Learning from palliative care: concepts to underpin the transfer of knowl-edge from specialist palliative care to mainstream social work settings', *Social Work Education*, **17**(1): 9–19.

Quinn, M. (2003) 'Immigrants and refugees: towards anti-racist and culturally affirming practices', in J. Allan, B. Pease and L. Briskman (eds) *Critical Social Work: An Introduction to Theories and Practices*, Sydney: Allen & Unwin.

Quinsey, V.L. (1995) 'Predicting sexual offences', in J.C. Campbell (ed.) *Assessing Dangerousness: Violence by Sexual Offenders, Batterers, and Child Abusers*, London: Sage.

Quinton, D., Rushton, A., Dance, C. and Mayes, D. (1998) *Joining New Families: A Study of Adoption and Fostering in Middle Childhood*, Chichester: Wiley.

Quirk, A., Lelliott, P., Audini, B. and Buston, K. (1999) 'Performing the ct: a qualitative study of the process of mental health act assessments', National Research Register, www.dh.gov.uk.

Rabjee, P., Moran, N. and Glendinning, C. (2008) 'Individual budgets: lessons from early users' experiences', *British Journal of Social Work*, Advanced Access, 17 March, doi10.1093/bjsw/bcm152.

Ramon, S. (1997) 'Building resistance through training', *Breakthrough*, **1**(1): 57–64.

Ramon, S. and Williams, J.E. (2005) 'Towards a conceptual framework: the meanings attached to the psychosocial, the promise and the problems', in S. Ramon and J.E. Williams (eds) *Mental Health at the Crossroads: The Promise of the Psychosocial Approach*, Aldershot: Ashgate.

Ray, M. (2000) Continuity and Change: Sustaining Long-term Marriage Relationships in the Context of Emerging Chronic Illness and Disability, unpublished PhD thesis, University of Keele.

Raynor, P., Smith, D. and Vanstone, M. (1994) *Effective Probation Practice*, Basingstoke: Macmillan – now Palgrave Macmillan.

Read, P. (1981) *The Stolen Generations: The Removal of Aboriginal People in NSW 1883 to 1969*, Occasional paper no. 1, Sydney: NSW Ministry of Aboriginal Affairs.

Rees, S. (1991) *Achieving Power: Practice and Policy in Social Welfare*, London: Allen & Unwin.

Reid, T. ([1788]1977) *Essays on the Active Powers of Man*, New York: Garland.

Reid, W.J. (2000) *The Task Planner: An Intervention Resource for Human Service Planners*, New York: Columbia University Press.

Reid, W.J. and Epstein, L. (1972) *Task-centered Casework*, New York: Columbia University Press.

Reid, W.J. and Shyne, A.W. (1969) *Brief and Extended Casework*, New York: Columbia University Press.

Reisch, M. and Andrews, J. (2001) *The Road Not Taken: A History of Radical Social Work in the United States*, Philadelphia: Brunner-Routledge.

Reith, M. (1998) *Community Care Tragedies: A Practical Guide to Mental Health Inquiries*, Birmingham: Venture Press.

Rholes, W.S. and Simpson, J.A. (eds) (2004) *Adult Attachment: Theory, Research and Clinical Implications*, New York: Guilford Press.

Roberts, R. (1990) *Lessons from the Past: Issues for Social Work Theory*, London: Tavistock/ Routledge.

Robinson, L. (1995) *Psychology for Social Workers: Black Perspectives*, London: Routledge.

Robinson, L. (2000) 'Racial identity attitudes and self-esteem of black adolescents in residential care: an exploratory study', *British Journal of Social Work*, **30**: 3–24.

Robinson, L. (2007) *Cross-cultural Child Development for Social Workers: An Introduction*, Basingstoke: Palgrave Macmillan.

Robinson, L. (2008) *Psychology for Social Workers: Black Perspectives*, 2nd edn, London, Routledge.

Rochdale County Council (1986) *Report of Chief Executive to Social Services Committee, Study of Needs and Circumstances of Elderly Asians in Rochdale*, Rochdale: Rochdale Metropolitan Borough Council.

Rogalla, B. (2003) 'Modern-day torture: government-sponsored neglect of asylum seeker children under the Australian mandatory immigration detention regime', *Journal of South Pacific Law*, **7**(1), www.paclii.org/journals/fJSPL/vol07no1/11.shtml.

Rogers, A., Pilgrim, D. and Lacey, R. (1993) *Experiencing Psychiatry: Users Views of Services*, Basingstoke: Macmillan – now Palgrave Macmillan.

Rogers, C.R. (1942) *Counseling and Psychotherapy*, Boston: Houghton Mifflin.

Rojek, C., Peacock, C. and Collins, S. (1988) *Social Work and Received Ideas*, London: Routledge.

Rolfe, G., Freshwater, D. and Jasper, M. (2001) *Critical Reflection for Nursing and the Helping Professions: A User's Guide*, Basingstoke: Palgrave – now Palgrave Macmillan.

Rollnick, S. and Miller, W.R. (1995) 'What is motivational interviewing?', *Behavioural and Cognitive Psychotherapy*, **23**: 325–34.

Ronen, T. and Freeman, A. (2007) *Cognitive Behavior Therapy in Social Work Practice*, New York: Springer.

Rose, N. (1996) 'Authority and the genealogy of subjectivity', in Heelas, P., Lash, S. and Morris, P. (eds) *Detraditionalization: Critical Reflections on Authority and Identity*, Oxford: Blackwell.

Rose, S., Peabody, C. and Stratigeas, B. (1991) 'Undetected abuse amongst intensive case management clients', *Hospital and Community Psychiatry*, **42**(5): 499–503.

Rosenau, P.M. (1992) *Post-modernism and the Social Sciences: Insights, Inroads and Intrusions*, Princeton, NJ: Princeton University Press.

Rosenberg, M. (2007) 'Illegal foster homes in Guatemala', *The Vancouver Sun*: A7.

Rosenfield, S. (1992) 'Factors contributing to the subjective quality of life of the chronically mentally ill', *Journal of Health and Social Behaviour*, **33**: 299–315.

Rosenman, M., Holmes, A., Ackerman, R. et al. (2006) 'The Indiana chronic disease management program', *The Millbank Quarterly*, **84**(1): 135–63.

Ross, R.R., Fabiano, E. and Ross, R. (1989) *Reasoning and Rehabilitation: A Handbook for Teaching Cognitive Skills*, Ottawa: Cognitive Centre.

Rossiter, A. (2000) 'The professional is political: an interpretation of the problem of the past in solution-focused therapy', *American Journal of Orthopsychiatry*, **70**(2): 150–61.

Rossiter, A., Prilleltensky, I. and Walsh-Bowers, R. (2000) 'A postmodern perspective on professional ethics', in B. Fawcett, B. Featherstone, J. Fook and A. Rossiter (eds) *Postmodern Feminist*, London: Routledge.

Rowe, J. and Lambert, L. (1973) *Children Who Wait*, London: British Agencies for Adoption and Fostering.

Royal Courts of Justice (2008) *X and another v. London Borough of Hounslow*, [2008] EWHC 1168 (QB).

Russell, S. (1990) *Render Me My Song: African-American Women Writers from Slavery to the Present*, London: Pandora Press.

Rutman, D., Callahan, C., Lundquist, A. et al. (2000) *Substance Use and Pregnancy: Conceiving Women in the Policy-making Process*, Ottawa: Status of Women Canada.

Rutter, M. (2006) *Genes and Behavior: Nature–nurture Interplay Explained*, Oxford: Blackwell.

Sakamoto, I. and Pitner, R. (2005) 'Use of critical consciousness in anti-oppressive practice: disentangling power dynamics at personal and structural levels', *British Journal of Social Work*, **35**: 435–52.

Saleeby, D. (ed.) (1997) *The Strengths Perspective in Social Work Practice*, 2nd edn, New York: Longman.

Saleeby, D. (2002) 'The strengths approach to practice', in D. Saleeby (ed.) *The Strengths*

Perspective in Social Work Practice, 3rd edn, Boston: Allyn & Bacon.

Salzberger-Wittenberg, I. (1970) *Psycho-analytic Insight and Relationships: A Kleinian Approach*, London: Routledge & Kegan Paul.

Sanderson, H. (1997) *People, Plans and Possibilities: Exploring Person Centred Planning*, Edinburgh: Scottish Health Services.

Sands, R.G. and Nuccio, K. (1992) 'Postmodern feminist theory and social work', *Social Work*, **37**(6): 489–94.

Sanfacon, A. (2001) How Social Workers Address Ethical Dilemmas, unpublished PhD research paper, Leicester: De Montfort University.

Sarri, R. and Sarri, C. (1992) 'Organisation and community change through participatory action research, *Administration in Social Work*, **16**(3/4): 99–122.

Sayce, L. (2000) *From Psychiatric Patient to Citizen: Overcoming Discrimination and Social Exclusion*, Basingstoke: Palgrave – now Palgrave Macmillan.

Schofield, G. (1996) Inner and Outer Worlds in Child and Family Social Work, working paper, Norwich: Centre for Research on the Child and Family, University of East Anglia.

Schön, D. (1983) *The Reflective Practitioner: How Professionals Think in Action*, New York: Basic Books.

Schön, D. (1987) *Educating the Reflective Practitioner*, San Francisco, CA: Jossey-Bass.

Schön, D. (1991) *The Reflective Practitioner: How Professionals Think in Action*, Aldershot: Ashgate

Schore, A. (2001) 'Effects of a secure base attachment relationship on right brain development, affect regulation, and infant mental health', *Infant Mental Health Journal*, **22**(1/2): 7–99.

SCIE (Social Care Institute for Excellence) (2004) *Fostering Success: An Exploration of the Research Literature in Foster Care*, London: SCIE.

Scott, D. (1990) 'Practice wisdom: the disregarded source of practice research', *Social Work*, **35**(6): 564–68.

Scott, M. (1989) *A Cognitive-behavioural Approach to Clients' Problems*, London: Tavistock/ Routledge.

Scott, M. and Lyman, S. (1970) 'Accounts', in M. Lyman and M. Scott (eds) *A Sociology of the Absurd*, New York: Meredith.

Scott, M.J., Stradling, S.J. and Dryden, W. (1995) *Developing Cognitive-behavioural Counselling*, London: Sage.

Scourfield, J. (2002) *Gender and Child Protection*, Basingstoke: Palgrave Macmillan.

SCSI (Commission for Social Care Inspection) (2008) *The State of Social Care in England 2006/2007*, London: CSCI.

Seale, C. (1998) *Constructing Death: The Sociology of Dying and Bereavement*, Cambridge: Cambridge University Press.

Seale, C., Addington-Hall, J., and McCarthy, M. (1997) 'Awareness of dying: prevalence, causes and consequences', *Social Science and Medicine*, **45**(3): 477–84.

Secker, J. (1993) *From Theory to Practice in Social Work: The Development of Social Work Students' Practice*, Aldershot: Avebury.

Seden, J. (2005) *Counselling Skills in Social Work Practice*, 2nd edn, Maidenhead: Open University Press.

Seebohm Committee (1968) *Report of the Committee on Local Authority and Allied Personal Social Services*, Cmnd 3703, London: HMSO.

Segall, M.H., Dasen, P.R., Berry, J.W. and Poortinga, Y.H. (1990) *Human Behaviour in Global Perspective*, New York: Pergamon.

Segall, M.H., Lonner, W.J. and Berry, J.W. (1998) 'Cross-cultural psychology as a scholarly discipline: on the flowering of culture in behavioral research', *American Psychologist*, **53**(10): 1101–10.

Seligman, M.E.P. (1975) *Helplessness*, San Francisco, CA: Freeman.

Sellick, C. and Thoburn, J. and Philpot, T. (2004) *What Works in Adoption and Foster Care?* Barkingside: Barnardo's.

Senior, P. (1993) 'Groupwork in the probation service: care or control in the 1990s', in A. Brown and B. Caddick (eds) *Groupwork with Offenders*, London: Whiting & Birch.

SEU (Social Exclusion Unit) (1998) *Bringing Britain Together: A National Strategy for Neighbourhood Renewal*, London: TSO.

SEU (Social Exclusion Unit) (1999) *Teenage Pregnancy*, Cmnd 4342, London: TSO.

Sevenhuijsen, S. (1998) *Citizenship and the Ethics of Care: Feminist Considerations on Justice, Morality and Politics*, London: Routledge.

Sewpaul, V. (1998) The New Reproductive Technologies in South Africa, unpublished PhD thesis, Durban: University of Natal.

Shakespeare, T. (1999) 'When is a man not a man', in J. Wild (ed.) *Working with Men*, London: Routledge.

Shakespeare, T. (2006) *Disability Rights and Wrongs*, Abingdon: Routledge.

Shardlow, S. (1998) 'Values, ethics and social work', in R. Adams, L. Dominelli and M. Payne (eds) *Social Work: Issues, Themes and Dilemmas*, Basingstoke: Macmillan – now Palgrave Macmillan.

Shaw, M. (1996) 'Out of the quagmire: community care – problems and possibilities for radical practice', in I. Cooke and M. Shaw (eds)

Radical Community Work, Edinburgh: Moray House Publications.

Sheldon, B. (1994) 'Social work effectiveness research: implications for probation and juvenile justice', *Howard Journal of Criminal Justice*, **33**(3): 218–35.

Sheldon, B. (1995) *Cognitive-behavioural Therapy: Research, Practice and Philosophy*, London: Routledge.

Sheldon, B. and Chilvers, R. (2000) *Evidence-based Social Care: A Study of Prospects and Problems*, London: Russell House.

Sheldon, B. and Macdonald, G. (1999) *Research and Practice in Social Care: Mind the Gap*, University of Exeter: Centre for Evidence-based Social Services.

Sheldon, F. (1997) *Psychosocial Palliative Care*, Cheltenham: Stanley Thornes.

Sheppard, M. (1995) *Care Management and the New Social Work: A Critical Analysis*, London: Whiting & Birch.

Shotter, J. (1996) *Representing Reality: Discourse, Rhetoric and Social Construction*, London: Sage.

Showalter, E. (1987) *The Female Malady: Women, Madness and English Culture 1830–1980*, London: Virago.

Sibeon, R. (1991) 'Sociological reflections on welfare politics and social work', *Social Work and Social Sciences Review*, **3**(3): 184–203.

Siddell, M., Katz, J. and Komaromy, C. (1998) Death and Dying in Residential and Nursing Homes for Older People: Examining the Case for Palliative Care, unpublished research report, The Open University.

Silverman, P. (1996) 'Children's construction of their dead parents', in D. Klass, P. Silverman and S. Nickman (eds) *Continuing Bonds: New Understandings of Grief*, Philadelphia, PA: Taylor & Francis.

Simpkin, M. (1983) *Trapped within Welfare: Surviving Social Work*, London: Macmillan – now Palgrave Macmillan.

Sinclair, I. (2005) *Fostering Now: Messages from Research*, London: Jessica Kingsley.

Sinclair, I., Baker, C., Lee, J. and Gibbs, I. (2007) *The Pursuit of Permanence: A Study of the English Child Care System*, London: Jessica Kingsley.

Sinclair, R., Garnett, L. and Berridge, D. (1995) *Social Work Assessment with Adolescents*, London: National Children's Bureau.

Sinha, D. (1983) 'Cross-cultural psychology: a view from the third world', in J.B. Deregowski, S. Dziurawier and R.C. Annis (eds) *Explorations in Cross-cultural Psychology*, Lisse, Netherlands: Swets & Zeitlinger.

Skenridge, P. and Lennie, I. (1978) 'Social work: the wolf in sheep's clothing', *Arena*, **51**: 47–92.

Slade, J. (2006) *Pathways Through Fostering: Safer Caring*, London: The Fostering Network.

Smale, G. and Tuson, G. with Biehal, N. and Marsh, P. (1993) *Empowerment, Assessment, Care Management and the Skilled Worker*, London: NISW.

Smale, G., Tuson, G. and Statham, D. (2000) *Social Work and Social Problems*, Basingstoke: Macmillan – now Palgrave Macmillan.

Smart, B. (1999) *Facing Modernity: Ambivalence, Reflexivity and Morality*, London: Sage.

Smiles, S. (1875) *Thrift*, London: Harper and Bros.

Smiles, S. (1890) *Self-help: With Illustrations of Conduct and Perseverance*, London: John Murray.

Smith, C. and White, S. (1997) 'Parton, Howe and postmodernity: a critical comment on mistaken identity', *British Journal of Social Work*, **27**(2): 275–96.

Smith, C.R. (1976) 'Bereavement: the contribution of phenomenological and existential analysis to a greater understanding of the problem', *British Journal of Social Work*, **5**(1): 75–92.

Smith, S.C. and Pennells, M. (1995) *Interventions with Bereaved Children*, London: Jessica Kingsley.

Smith, S.R. (2007) 'Applying theory to policy and practice: methodological problems and issues', in S.R. Smith (ed.) *Applying Theory to Policy and Practice: Issues for Critical Reflection*, Aldershot: Ashgate.

Smith, T. (1995) 'Children and young people: disadvantage, community and the Children Act, 1989', in P. Henderson (ed.) *Children and Communities*, London: Pluto.

Snowdon, R. (1980) 'Working with incest offenders: excuses, excuses, excuses', in *AEGIS: Issues on Child Sexual Assault*, **29**.

Social Exclusion Task Force (2007) *Reaching Out: Think Family*, London: Cabinet Office.

Solomon, B.B. (1976) *Black Empowerment: Social Work in Oppressed Communities*, New York: Columbia University Press.

Southgate, J. (1990) 'Towards a dictionary of advocacy-based self analysis', *Journal of the Institute for Self Analysis*, **4**(1).

Spandler, H. (1996) *Who's Hurting Who? Young People, Self-harm and Suicide*, Manchester: 42nd Street.

Specht, H. (1972) 'The deprofessionalization of social work', *Social Work*, **28**(1): 3–15.

Specht, H. and Vickery, A. (eds) (1977) *Integrating Social Work Methods*, London: Allen & Unwin.

Spencer, M.B. (1988) 'Self-concept development', in D.T. Slaughter (ed.) *Black Children in Poverty: Developmental Perspectives*, San Francisco, CA: Jossey-Bass.

Spratt, T. and Houston, S. (1999) 'Developing critical social work in theory and practice: Child protection and communicative reason', *Child and Family Social Work*, 4(4): 315–24.

Stainton, T. (1994) *Autonomy and Social Policy: Rights, Mental Handicap and Community Care*, Aldershot: Avebury.

Stainton, T. (2007) 'Case management in a right-based environment: structure, context and roles', in C. Bigby, C. Fyffe and E. Ozanne (eds) *Planning and Support for People with Intellectual Disabilities: Issues for Case Managers and other Professionals*, London: Jessica Kingsley.

Stanworth, M. (ed.) (1987) *Reproductive Technologies: Gender, Motherhood and Medicine*, Cambridge: Polity Press.

Statham, D. (1978) *Radicals in Social Work*, London: Routledge & Kegan Paul.

Steinberg, D.L. (1997) *Bodies in Glass: Genetics, Eugenics, Embryo Ethics*, Manchester: Manchester University Press.

Stepney, P. (2006) 'Mission impossible? critical practice in social work', *British Journal of Social Work*, 36: 1289–307.

Stevens, I. and Hassett, P. (2007) 'Applying complexity theory to risk in child protection practice', *Childhood*, 14(1): 128–44.

Stevenson, H. and Davis, G.Y. (2004) 'Racial socialization', in R.L. Jones (ed.) *Black Psychology*, 4th edn, Berkeley, CA: Cobb & Henry.

Stephenson, M., Giller, H. and Brown, S. (2007) *Effective Practice in Youth Justice*, Cullompton, Willan.

Stickley, T. (2006) 'Should service user involvement be consigned to history? A critical realist perspective', *Journal of Psychiatric and Mental Health Nursing*, 13(5): 570–7.

Strier, R. (2007) 'Anti-oppressive research in social work: a preliminary definition', *British Journal of Social Work*, 37: 857–71.

Stroebe, M. (1998) 'New directions in bereavement research: exploration of gender differences', *Palliative Medicine*, 12: 5–12.

Stroebe, M. and Schut, H. (1995) *The Dual Process Model of Coping with Loss*, paper presented at the International Work Group on Death, Dying and Bereavement, St Catherine's College, Oxford.

Stroebe, M. and Schut, H. (1998) 'Culture and grief', *Bereavement Care*, 17(1): 7–11.

Stroebe, M. and Schut, H. (1999) 'The dual process model of coping with bereavement: rationale and description', *Death Studies*, 23: 197–224.

Stubbs, P. (1988) The Reproduction of Racism in State Social Work, unpublished PhD thesis, University of Bath.

Sue, D.W. and Sue, D. (1990) *Counselling the Culturally Different*, New York: Wiley.

Sullivan, M. (2008) 'Social workers in community care practice: ideologies and interactions with older people', *British Journal of Social Work*, Advance Access, 2 May, doi:10.1093/bjsw/bcn059.

Sullivan, W. and Poertner, J. (1989) 'Social support and life stress: a mental health consumer's perspective', *Community Mental Health Journal*, 25(1): 21–32.

Survivors Speak Out (1988) *Self-advocacy Action Pack: Empowering Mental Health Service Users*, London: Survivors Speak Out.

Sutton, C. (1994) *Social Work, Community Work and Psychology*, Leicester: British Psychological Society.

Sutton, C. (1999) *Helping Families with Troubled Children: A Preventive Approach*, Chichester: Wiley.

Sutton, C. (2000a) 'Cognitive-behavioural theory: relevance for social work', *Cognitive Behavioural Social Work Review*, 21: 22–46.

Sutton, C. (2000b) *Child and Adolescent Behaviour Problems: A Multidisciplinary Approach to Assessment and Intervention*, Leicester: British Psychological Society.

Sweeting, H. and Gilhooly, M. (1997) 'Dementia and the phenomenon of social death', *Sociology of Health and Illness*, 19(1): 93–117.

Tadd, W. (1994) 'Accountability and nursing', in R. Chadwick (ed.) *Ethics and the Professions*, Aldershot: Avebury.

Tam, H. (1998) *Communitarianism: A New Agenda for Politics and Citizenship*, Basingstoke: Macmillan – now Palgrave Macmillan.

Tanner, D. (2005) 'Promoting the well-being of older people: messages for social workers', *Practice*, 17(3): 191–205.

Taylor, C. and White, S. (2000) *Practising Reflexivity in Health and Welfare: Making Knowledge*, Buckingham: Open University Press.

Taylor, G. (1996) 'Ethical issues in practice: participatory social research and groups', *Groupwork*, 9(2): 110–27.

Taylor, I. (1996) 'Reflective learning, social work education and practice in the 21st century', in N. Gould and I. Taylor (eds) *Reflective Learning for Social Work*, Aldershot: Arena.

Taylor-Gooby, P. (1994) 'Postmodernism and social policy: a great leap backwards?', *Journal of Social Policy*, 23(3): 385–405.

Tebbutt, C. (1994) 'After suicide', *CRUSE Chronicle*, 3/4 July/August, CRUSE Bereavement Care, CRUSE House, 126 Sheen Road, Richmond, Surrey, TW9 1UR.

Therborn, G. (1983) *The Power of Ideology and the Ideology of Power*, London: Verso.

Thoburn J. (ed.) (1992) *Participation in Practice: Involving Families in Child Protection*, Norwich: University of East Anglia.

Thoburn, J. (1994) *Child Placement: Principles and Practice*, 2nd edn, Aldershot: Arena.

Thomas, E.J. (ed.) (1974) *Behaviour Modification Procedure: A Sourcebook*, Chicago, IL: Aldine.

Thompson, A. (2000) 'The body politic', *Community Care*, 2–8 November: 20–1.

Thompson, N. (1993) *Anti-discriminatory Practice*, Basingstoke: Macmillan – now Palgrave Macmillan.

Thompson, N. (1995) 'Men and anti-sexism', *British Journal of Social Work*, **25**: 459–75.

Thompson, N. (1996) *People Skills: A Guide to Effective Practice in the Human Services*, Basingstoke: Macmillan – now Palgrave Macmillan.

Thompson, N. (2003) *Promoting Equality: Challenging Discrimination and Oppression in the Human Services*, Basingstoke: Palgrave Macmillan.

Thompson, N. (2006) *Anti-discriminatory Practice*, 3rd edn, Basingstoke: Palgrave Macmillan.

Thompson, N., Murphy, M. and Stradling, S. (1996) *Meeting the Stress Challenge: A Training and Staff Development Manual*, Lyme Regis: Russell House Publishing.

Thorpe, D., Smith, D., Green, C. and Paley, J. (1980) *Out of Care: The Community Support of Juvenile Offenders*, London: Allen & Unwin.

Thorpe, M. (1986) Child Abuse and Neglect from an Aboriginal Perspective, paper presented at the Sixth International Congress on Child Abuse and Neglect, Sydney.

Throssell, R. (1975) *Wild Weeds and Wind Flowers*, Sydney: Angus & Robertson.

Tober, G. (1998) 'Learning theory, addiction and counselling', in K. Cigno and D. Bourn (eds) *Cognitive-behavioural Social Work in Practice*, Aldershot: Ashgate.

Tolson, E.R., Reid, W.J. and Garvin, C.D. (1994) *Generalist Practice: A Task-centred Approach*, New York: Columbia University Press.

Townsend, P. (2007) 'Using human rights to defeat ageism: dealing with policy-induced "structured dependency"', in M. Bernard and T. Scharf (eds) *Critical Perspectives on Ageing Societies*, Bristol: Policy Press.

Trevithick, P. (2005) *Social Work Skills: A Practical Handbook*, 2nd edn, Maidenhead: Open University Press.

Trieman, N., Leff, J. and Glover, G. (1999) 'Outcome of long stay psychiatric patients resettled in the community: prospective cohort study', *British Medical Journal*, **319**(7201): 13–16.

Trinder, L. (2000) 'A critical appraisal of evidence-based practice', in L. Trinder and S. Reynolds (eds) *Evidence-based Practice: A Critical Appraisal*, Oxford: Blackwell Science.

Triseliotis, J., Borland, M. and Hill, M. (2000) *Delivering Foster Care*, London: British Agencies for Adoption and Fostering.

Triseliotis, J., Shireman, J. and Hundleby, M. (1997) *Adoption: Theory, Policy and Practice*, London: Cassell.

Tronick, E.Z., Morelli, G.A. and Ivey, P.K. (1992) 'The Efe forager infant and toddlers pattern of social relationships: multiple and simultaneous', *Developmental Psychology*, **28**: 568–77.

Turner, B.S. (1990) 'Periodisation and politics in the postmodern', in B.S. Turner (ed.) *Theories of Modernity and Post Modernity*, London: Sage.

Twelvetrees, A. (2008) *Community Work*, 4th edn, London: Macmillan – now Palgrave Macmillan.

UN (United Nations) (1989) *Convention on the Rights of the Child*, Geneva: UN.

Underdown, A. (1998) *Strategies for Effective Offender Supervision: Report of the HMIP What Works Project*, London: Home Office.

Ungerson, C. (1987) *Policy is Personal: Sex, Gender and Informal Care Work*, London: Tavistock.

Ussher, J. (1991) *Women's Madness: Misogyny or Mental Illness*, Hemel Hempstead: Harvester Wheatsheaf.

Vanstone, M. (1995) 'Managerialism and the ethics of management', in R. Hugman and D. Smith (eds) *Ethical Issues in Social Work*, London: Routledge.

Vernelle, B. (1994) *Understanding and Using Groups*, London: Whiting and Birch.

Walter, T. (1994) *The Revival of Death*, London: Routledge.

Walter, T. (1996) 'A new model of grief: bereavement and biography', *Mortality*, **1**(1): 7–25.

Walter, T. (1997) 'Book review', *Mortality*, **2**(2): 73–4.

Walter, T. (1999) *On Bereavement*, Buckingham: Open University Press.

Ward, A. (1993) 'The large group: the heart of the system in group care', *Groupwork*, **6**(1): 64–77.

Ward, D. (ed.) (1996) Groups and Research, special edition of *Groupwork*, **9**(2).

Ware, T, Matovesic, T., Hardy, B. et al. (2003) 'Commissioning care services for older people in England: the view from care managers, users and carers', *Ageing and Society*, **23**: 411–28.

Warner, J. and Gabe, J. (2008) 'Mental disorder and social work practice: a gendered landscape', *British Journal of Social Work*, **38**(1): 117–34.

Washington, S. (2003) 'Ruddock's secret report', *Business Review Weekly*, (9–15 October): 18.

Watkins, T.R. (1997) 'Mental health services to substance abusers', in T.R. Watkins and J.W. Callicutt (eds) *Mental Health Policy and Practice Today*, Thousand Oaks, CA: Sage.

Wattam, C. (1999) 'Confidentiality', in N. Parton and C. Wattam (eds) *Child Sexual Abuse:*

Responding to the Experiences of Children, Chichester: Wiley.

Wearing, B. (1986) 'Feminist theory and social work', in H. Marchant and B. Wearing (eds) *Gender Reclaimed: Women in Social Work*, Sydney: Hale & Iremonger.

Webster-Stratton, C. and Herbert, M. (1994) *Troubled Families – Problem Children*, Chichester: Wiley.

Weiner, K., Hughes, J., Challis, D. and Pederson, I. (2003) 'Integrating health and social care at the micro level: health care professionals as care managers for older people', *Social Policy and Administration*, **37**(5): 498–515.

Weiner, K., Stewart, K., Hughes, J. et al. (2002) 'Care management arrangements for older people in England: key areas of variation in a national study', *Ageing and Society*, **22**: 419–39.

Welch, B. (1998) 'Care management and community care: current issues', in D. Challis, R. Darton and K. Stewart (eds) *Community Care, Secondary Health Care and Care Management*, Aldershot: Ashgate.

Welshman, J. (2007) *From Transmitted Deprivation to Social Exclusion*, Bristol: Policy Press.

Wendell, S. (1996) *The Rejected Body: Feminist Philosophical Reflections on Disability*, London: Routledge.

Westwood, S. and Bhachu, P. (1988) 'Images and realities', *New Society*, 6 May.

Wheal, A. (ed.) (2005) *The RHP Companion to Foster Care*, Lyme Regis: Russell House Publishing.

Whitaker, D.S. (1985) *Using Groups to Help People*, London: Tavistock/Routledge.

White, J.L. (2004) 'Toward a black psychology', in R.L. Jones (ed.) *Black Psychology*, 4th edn, Berkeley, CA: Cobb & Henry.

White, M. (1993) 'Deconstruction and therapy', in S. Gilligan and R. Price (eds) *Therapeutic Conversations*, New York: Norton.

White, M. and Epston, D. (1990) *Narrative Means to Therapeutic Ends*, New York: W.W. Norton.

White, S., Fook, J., and Gardner, F. (eds) (2006) *Critical Reflection in Health and Social Care*, Maidenhead: Open University Press.

White, V. (1995) 'Commonality and diversity in feminist social work', *British Journal of Social Work*, **25**(2): 143–56.

White, V. (2006) *The State of Feminist Social Work*, London: Routledge.

Whiteford, J. (2005) 'Let's face it! Young people tell us how it is', in D. Crimmens and I. Milligan (eds) *Facing Forward: Residential Child Care in the 21st Century*, Lyme Regis: Russell House Publishing.

Whyte, G. (1998) 'Recasting Janis's groupthink model: the key role of collective efficacy in decision fiascoes', *Organisational Behaviour and Human Decision Processes*, **73**(2/3): 185–209.

Williams, F. (1989) *Social Policy*, Oxford: Polity Press.

Williams, F. (2004) *Rethinking Families*, London: Calouste Gulbenkian Foundation.

Wilson, A. and Beresford, P. (2000) '"Anti-oppressive practice": emancipation or appropriation?', *British Journal of Social Work*, **30**: 553–73.

Wilson, E. (1980) 'Feminism and social work', in R. Bailey and M. Brake (eds) *Radical Social Work and Practice*, 2nd edn, London: Edward Arnold.

Wilson, M. (1993) *Crossing the Boundaries: Black Women Survive Incest*, London: Virago.

Winnicott, C. (1964) *Child Care and Social Work: A Collection of Papers*, Oxford: Codicote Press.

Winston, R. (1987) *Infertility: A Sympathetic Approach*, London: Optima.

Winter, K. (2006) 'Widening our knowledge concerning young looked after children: the case for research using sociological models of childhood', *Child and Family Social Work*, **11**: 55–64.

Wise, S. (1985) 'Becoming a feminist social worker', in L. Stanley and S. Wise (eds) *Feminist Praxis*, London: Routledge.

Women in MIND (1986) *Finding our Own Solutions: Women's Experiences of Mental Health Care*, London: MIND.

Wood, G. and Tully, C. (2006) *The Structural Approach to Direct Practice in Social Work: A Social Constructionist Perspective*, 3rd edn, New York: Columbia University Press.

Worden, W. (1991) *Grief Counselling and Grief Therapy: A Handbook for the Mental Health Practitioner*, 2nd edn, London: Routledge.

Worden, W. (1996) *Children and Grief*, London and New York: Guilford Press.

Wortman, C.B. and Silver, R.C. (1989) 'The myths of coping with loss', *Journal of Consulting and Clinical Psychology*, **57**: 349–57.

Yalom, I. (1970) *The Theory and Practice of Group Psychotherapy*, New York: Basic Books.

Yeh, C.J. and Huang, K. (1996) 'The collectivistic nature of ethnic identity development among Asian-American college students', *Adolescence*, **31**: 645–66.

Yelloly, M. (1980) *Social Work Theory and Psychanalysis*, London: Van Nostrand Reinhold.

Yelloly, M. and Henkel, M. (1995) *Learning and Teaching in Social Work: Towards Reflective Practice*, London: Jessica Kingsley.

Youll, P. (1996) 'Organisational or professional leadership? Managerialism and social work education', in M. Preston-Shoot and S. Jackson (eds) *Educating Social Workers in a Changing Policy Context*, London: Whiting & Birch.

Young, M. and Cullen, L. (1996) *A Good Death*, London: Routledge.

Younghusband, E. (1951) *Social Work in Britain*, London: Carnegie UK Trust.

Author index

Subject index